Jim & Pam —

May this book
help you in your life
fitness as much as
it has helped Carol
and me.

My best regards,

Pat

THE
La Costa
BOOK OF
NUTRITION

Other books by Patrick Quillin:

The La Costa Prescription for Longer Life
Healing Nutrients

THE
La Costa
BOOK OF
NUTRITION

PATRICK QUILLIN, Ph.D., R.D.
A. GORDON REYNOLDS, M.D.

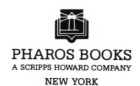

PHAROS BOOKS
A SCRIPPS HOWARD COMPANY

NEW YORK

Pharos Books are available at special discounts on bulk purchases for sales promotions, premiums, fundraising or educational use. For details, contact the Special Sales Department, Pharos Books, 200 Park Avenue, New York, NY 10166

Cover and text design: Nancy Eato

First published in 1988.
Library of Congress Cataloging-in-Publication Data:
Quillin, Patrick.
    The La Costa book of nutrition/Patrick Quillin, A. Gordon Reynolds.
    p.   cm.
    Bibliography: p.
    Includes index.
    ISBN 0-88687-343-6 : $24.95
    1. Nutrition. I. Reynolds, A. Gordon, 1926-   . II. Title.
RA784.Q55 1988
613.2—dc19   87-37380
                                                     CIP

Printed in the United States of America.

Pharos Books
A Scripps Howard Company
200 Park Avenue
New York, NY 10166

10   9   8   7   6   5   4   3   2   1

CONTENTS

Acknowledgments   viii
Foreword   ix

Part One: Your Life Is at Stake   1

1. Why Nutrition Is Important to Everyone   5
2. Malnutrition in the Land of Plenty   10
3. Why All the Confusion?   20
4. Assessing Your Nutritional Status   27
5. The Seven General Rules of Nutrition   33

Part Two: Essential Dietary Components   35

6. Carbohydrates   37
7. Fiber   47
8. Protein   55
9. Fats   62
10. Water   74
11. Vitamins   81
12. Minerals   102
13. Quasi-Vitamins   126

Part Three: Nonessential Dietary Components   143

14. Alcohol   145
15. Caffeine   153
16. Food Additives   159
17. Naturally Occurring Toxins in Food   168

Part Four: Nutrition Throughout the Life Cycle   179

18. Pregnancy   181
19. Infancy   190
20. Childhood   199
21. Adolescence   206
22. Older Adulthood   212

Part Five: Nutrition and Disease   219

23. Obesity   221
24. Heart Disease   232
25. Cancer   237
26. Diabetes   241
27. Osteoporosis   246
28. Arthritis   249
29. Food Allergies and Sensitivities   252
30. Smokers   258
31. Mental Functions   262
32. Sex   267
33. The Athlete   274

Part Six: Nutrition and the Government   281

34. United States Recommended Daily Allowances   283
35. Senate Dietary Goals   286
36. Regulation of the Vitamin Industry   288
37. Food Labeling   291

Part Seven: Practical Applications of Nutrition   295

38. The Exchange System   297
39. Making It Nutritious and Delicious   304
40. Super Foods   314

Afterword   325
Notes   327
Index   351

For Noreen,
Without your emotional, spiritual, and physical support of this project, we would still be working on the outline. Carino y besos.

PATRICK QUILLIN

This book is dedicated to all my loyal patients who have taught me so much over the years and to my family who have oft served as guinea pigs in my search for optimal nutrition.

A. GORDON REYNOLDS

ACKNOWLEDGMENTS

"NO MAN IS AN ISLAND," WROTE JOHN DONNE. THAT STATE-ment certainly applies to book writing. This Herculean task required a talented and energetic support of compassionate editor Shari Jee and the incredibly versatile Noreen Quillin.

We extend a special thanks to the thousands of dedicated researchers throughout the world who daily bring forth stunning revelations, to the applause of almost no one. Without you, this book would not have been possible.

FOREWORD

WE ARE ENTERING A NEW ERA OF MEDICINE BY RETURN-
ing to and taking seriously one of its oldest frontiers: nutrition. I foresee
some of the most important breakthroughs in the medical sciences emerg-
ing from this direction. Not only will nutrition become the centerpiece for
new preventive medicine, but nutrients themselves will become important
treatment modalities. Out of this will evolve a more gentle medicine in
which the human organism will be treated with substances that are not so
foreign and will have fewer side effects. There are many who believe the
future of medicine to be bleak. On the contrary, I foresee an optimistic future if, and only if, mainstream medicine assumes responsibility in this vital
area.

The scientific data base has progressed more in the last thirty years than
the previous three thousand years combined. I have had a unique vantage
point from which to view these changes, first as a researcher in biochemistry, then as a physician. Today, the healing arts are perched on the very edge
of a major transition. Medicine, chemistry, and nutrition are merging into
one. I was quite fortunate to have been a student, friend, and cohort of the
father of modern biochemistry, Dr. Sol Spiegelman of Columbia University. His vision was to use substances found in nature, such as the nutrition
information found in this book, for the betterment of mankind.

Science is like a giant and complicated jigsaw puzzle. All the answers to
science and all the pieces to the puzzle are somewhere on earth, yet it requires great diligence and brilliance to put them together. Every so often,
someone finds a key missing piece in the puzzle, and immediately after-
wards scientists are able to proceed at a much more rapid pace than before.
Dr. Spiegelman found several major pieces of this great biochemical puzzle
of life. In this book, Professor Quillin and Dr. Reynolds have gathered the
entire puzzle for a comprehensive macro view of how optimal nutrition fits
into the healing arts.

I am enthralled with the completeness, the readability, and the documentation of this book. The chapter on quasi-vitamins is particularly relevant to
the message of Dr. Spiegelman and his protégés. The chapter on malnutrition in the land of plenty thoroughly documents the myth of the well-nourished average American.

The healing arts are merging, like Great Northern geese joining to fly in
formation. One goose flying alone must continually fight headwinds and

therefore proceeds at a slower pace with more wasted effort. In the classic "V" formation, geese take turns in the lead as the wind break, then fall back to rest. They work much more efficiently that way and for the betterment of all. The "geese" are merging in health care. The aerodynamic and symbiotic "V" is being formed. You are very lucky people. You hold in this book one of the key ingredients to a long and vigorous life. The only ingredient missing now is the knowledge and motivation to use these nutrition principles. May you be educated, motivated, and live into your second century.

SHELDON SAUL HENDLER, M.D., PH.D.
Author of The Complete Guide To Anti-Aging Nutrients; *instructor of medicine at the University of California at San Diego; specialist in internal medicine; researcher in biochemistry and medicine.*

PART ONE

YOUR LIFE
IS AT STAKE

"LADIES AND GENTLEMEN, THIS IS YOUR CAPTAIN SPEAKING. I have good news and bad news. First the bad news: we're lost. Now the good news: we're making excellent time."

This book is an answer to a problem. The problem is the health of Americans and the dinosaurlike health care system we use. In 1950, health care costs totaled 5 percent of the gross national product. Today, health care costs total almost 12 percent of the gross national product, or $450 billion annually, compared with about 3 percent in Britain and Japan.[1] From 1974 through 1982, hospital costs in the U.S. rose over 300 percent.[2] In 1980, more than a third of all health insurance policies had no deductible (i.e., patient pays nothing), but today only 6 percent of the policies written can afford such a luxury. If all that money was curing people and bringing longer and more energetic lives, it would be easier to swallow. But the billions of dollars spent have been to little avail. It becomes more obvious each year that money cannot buy health. Only continued lifestyle efforts, including optimal nutrition, can bring us the health and vitality we are seeking.

The U.S. produces more Nobel laureates and spends more money on scientific research and applied health care than any other nation on earth. Yet twenty-six countries have a better record of healthy hearts; twenty-three countries have a better infant survival rate. (Curiously enough, the nations with the lowest rates of infant mortality are the ones with the highest rates of home deliveries.[3])

American workers are far from fit: 70 percent have poor nutrition habits; 50 percent are overweight; 50 percent are physically inactive; 33 percent smoke an average of one pack of cigarettes daily; 25 percent have hypertension; 15 percent have mental or drug abuse problems; 8 percent abuse alcohol. This collection of unhealthy workers costs industry $25 billion each year and causes 132 million lost workdays each year.[4]

You have a fifty-fifty chance of dying of cardiovascular disease.[5] You have a one in four chance of dying of cancer. You have a one in five chance of developing diabetes and falling prey to its many insidious effects throughout the body. You have a one in three chance of developing osteoporosis, a hollowing of the bones. Thirty-seven million Americans have high blood pressure.[6] Twenty million have arthritis that limits their lives. The average American wears glasses, is overweight, has six colds per year, will have dentures by age fifty lacks energy and vitality enough for even the mildest recreational pursuits, and will spend about ten years in a state of semiambulatory retirement before dying in his or her seventies. There is indeed a health problem in America.

Yet there is good news. There is a very good chance that you can prevent the above mentioned diseases. You can increase the chances of living an exuberant, healthy, long life if you want to. But don't count on others to provide that health and long life for you. A study done at Mt. Sinai Hospital in Chicago revealed some rather amazing attitudes among the public.[7] The people in the study were aware of the seriousness of the major killing diseases in America and could even identify some of the symptoms. Sixty-one percent knew that lifestyle factors, including nutrition, were related to the incidence of these diseases and that these factors were under voluntary control. Yet these people did not feel vulnerable to these diseases. Their reasoning for continuing their semisuicidal lifestyle: their confidence in medical science was so great that they believed science could cure them of any condition they might contract from poor health practices. Don't believe it! Many of the killing conditions today are only marginally treatable. If you want a vibrant body and mind, you are going to have to earn it, through lifestyle. And one of the most important factors in lifestyle is nutrition.

Today's science is much more fascinating than yesterday's science fiction. Forty years ago only the wildest imaginations dreamed of landing on the moon. We have saddled the energy of the atom, stared into the bottom recesses of the oceans, and sent messages to other galaxies. Medical science has been equally productive. Microsurgery techniques allow the surgeon's deft hands to suture vessels as tiny as a hair. CAT scan devices allow scientists to see more within a live body than yesterday's autopsies could reveal. Pacemakers can stimulate a tired heart. Drugs can induce or block many chemical processes within the body. Life support systems give the premature infant and the heart transplant patient an opportunity to recover.

Because of all this, people are living well into their eighties. But that is less exciting when you realize that, 200 years ago, Benjamin Franklin and Thomas Jefferson also lived into their eighties. And our progress dims even further when you consider that, 400 years ago, Michelangelo reached his eighties. And Hippocrates, father of modern medicine, lived into his eighties, about 2,500 years ago.

Science, through vaccination and hygiene programs, has been able to markedly improve the general health and welfare of the people. Yet people place an inordinate amount of faith in science to cure whatever comes along. The fact is that the keys to health and long life still lie in prevention. In getting inoculations before a disease strikes, because polio still cannot be cured. In cleaning water and food before consuming it to prevent typhoid or hepatitis, because these don't have a cure either. In avoiding heart disease before the need for triple bypass surgery develops, because this often-used procedure may not increase lifespan. In avoiding cancer before the need arises for the oncologist, because many cancer patients will die from the disease, in spite of the physician's efforts.

You can eat your way into an early grave after much illness and undo suffering throughout life. Or you can use this book as a guide to help you stay healthy and perhaps live considerably longer than the seventy some years that the statistics promise us. The choice is yours: to live a "normal" life and accept your fate with the Grim Reapers of today, or to pack your own parachute and take charge of your life. Optimal nutrition, as thoroughly explained in this book, can help you to suck the marrow out of life.

Note: Throughout this book, we have abbreviated the nutritionists' term "kilocalorie" to the better-known term, "calorie." A kilocalorie is actually equal to 1,000 calories.

1
WHY NUTRITION IS IMPORTANT TO EVERYONE

"If medical science has made so much progress, why do I feel so much worse than I did twenty years ago?"

—ROBERT ORBEN

We all want more out of life: more love, more money, more sex, more travel, more friends, more years, and so on. But none of this is worth last week's newspaper unless we are healthy and feeling good. Experts now estimate that up to 90 percent of our diseases today are preventable. There are six crucial factors that decide your health, performance and longevity:

- genetics
- exercise
- nutrition
- physical environment
- body maintenance
- attitude

Each of these relates directly to your ultimate enjoyment of life. And, since they all interrelate, they form a complex web in which they magnify one another.

Genetics

In the center of all the cells in your body is a spiral strand of DNA, which contains all the "blueprints" necessary to make another identical you. This genetic material was passed on from your parents. At the time of conception, when sperm met egg, many parameters of your life were locked in, such as color of hair, eyes, and skin, as well as certain genetic diseases. Other parameters were more flexible, such as intellect, emotions, and physical stature. Given optimal nutrition, emotional support, and exercise, you could develop to the peak capacity of the genes given to you.

You cannot choose your parents. But by being aware of family characteristics, you can make the most of the genetic cards that were dealt you at conception. If obesity, food allergies, heart disease, or other maladies run in your family, then be particularly aware of these conditions and make a specific point to avoid the lifestyle factors that encourage these diseases.

Exercise

No better panacea exists today than regular and vigorous exercise. Scientists have documented a list of benefits of consistent exercise:[1]

1. Proper weight maintenance, by burning calories, lowering the "set point" (weight at which the body wants to stay), and helping to control appetite.[2]

2. Improving fat levels in the blood and lowering the risk for heart disease.

3. Lowering blood pressure. Sedentary people with normal blood pressure are at greater risk for developing high blood pressure.[3]

4. Improving the heart and lung capacity and ability of the body to deliver oxygen and nutrients to the cells.

5. Reducing risk of heart disease.

6. Improving emotional and intellectual functions, making people happier, more confident, and more stable.

7. Stabilizing blood sugar for more predictable energy levels.[4]

8. Improving digestion and efficiency of absorption. You end up getting more nutrients from your food when you stay active.

9. Improving sex life by aiding general fitness, circulation, and attitude.

10. Lowering the percentage of body fat for a lean, healthy, and attractive body.[5]

11. Enhancing disease resistance, wound healing, and recovery time.

12. Enhancing the effectiveness of insulin, to improve the diabetic's condition.[6]

13. Increasing the quantity and quality of life.

You could follow all the principles in this book and still not feel as well as you should if you are sedentary. Your program should be fun, vigorous, and regular (at least three times per week). You should strive for strength, flexibility, and endurance (cardiovascular fitness). Consult your fitness-oriented physician if you are in the least bit concerned about your health, and especially if you are more than forty years old. Unfortunately, less than 7 percent of all medical doctors recommend exercise programs for their patients.[7]

Nutrition

Your body is a complex coordination of 60 trillion cells. In order to perform the processes of life, these cells manufacture thousands of chemicals. Your diet provides all of the raw materials to perform all of these life processes. You are, in the most literal sense, a product of your diet. The rest of this book will provide specifics on how to optimize your nutrient intake.

Physical Environment

Many things outside your body—bacteria, virus, light, noise, smog, tobacco smoke, pollution, radiation, ultraviolet light—can influence your health and lifespan.

In the earlier part of this century, the primary causes of death came from the environment. Infectious diseases such as tuberculosis and influenza, plagues of typhoid, polio, diptheria, cholera, and others used to kill thousands and maim thousands more. Thanks to proper hygiene and modern vaccinations, we no longer have to dread outbreaks like the Black Death, which killed 75 million people, or half the known world, in 1347. Nevertheless, though the physical environment in the developed nations has been tamed of its devastating plagues, there is a new threat from the environment: pollution. Lead, formaldehyde, soot, carbon monoxide, and other deadly substances fill our air. PCB (polychlorinated biphenyl), mercury, crude oil, dioxin (the active ingredient of Agent Orange), chlorine (bleach), and other chemicals fill our water. Foods contain unacceptable levels of pesticides, dangerous additives, and hormones. Our modern technological society has brought us many fabulously productive tools and chemicals. Yet with them has come a need to dispose of these toxic substances in a responsible manner. In 1979 as conservative an agency as the United States Department of Health, Education, and Welfare, through the Surgeon General's office, issued a book, *Healthy People*, which estimated that 20 percent of the death and disability in the United States is due to wallowing in our own effluvia.

If your water is laden with deadly chemicals and your air is full of lead, then even optimal nutrition can only slightly lower these risks. Avoid the hazards that you can while supporting measures to clean up our environment.

Body Maintenance

Your body is the most amazing servomechanism ever designed. It deserves better maintenance than it usually gets. Feet often hurt and become a hindrance, not because of poor nutrition, but from ill-fitting shoes. Backs become a source of pain when furniture, posture, and exercise are at their worst. Deafness can be a result of excessive exposure to noise. Poor sight can result from abuse and neglect to the 70-millimeter stereo cameras called your eyes. Although obesity may seem to fit into this category, it is regulated by other forces of diet and exercise. Obesity will be discussed in its own chapter later. Maintain your body and be good to it. It will reward you in years to come. Optimal nutrition can do little to overcome decades of abuse of your body.

Attitude

We are only beginning to understand the capacity of the brain. It can create, think, remember, love, forgive, and perform other tasks unique to the human brain. There now exists a scientifically documented area called "psychogenic diseases," in which the mind (psycho) begins ("genic" as in genesis) a disease. Studies have shown that the mind can raise or lower immune bodies, depending on your mood.[8] Emotions can dictate how well food will be digested, since a direct connection exists between the brain and the gastrointestinal tract. The mind can release potent euphoric pain killers, literally writing your own prescription, if we can learn how to control these endorphins. Attitude has been found to be relevant to the incidence of heart disease, cancer, arthritis, and even premature death. Researchers have found a strong correlation between the number of social connections people have and the length of life.[9] Guided imagery has been used to treat some rather tenacious diseases. The recommendations given in this book will not be as effective if you hate your job, your companions, and yourself. Nutrition cannot totally compensate for an ailing mind and soul.

The mind influence four of the other factors: nutrition, exercise, body maintenance, physical environment. While nutrition can influence your emotions and intellect, emotions can affect your digestion, absorption, and turnover rate. Exercise improves mental function, yet only the proper attitude will make exercise enjoyable.

Beyond the physical connection between brain and body lies another crucial relationship: the attitude you have toward change. No doubt you will need to make some changes in your lifestyle if you heed the message in this book. Your attitude will dictate whether you will make those changes and whether you will enjoy it. We guarantee that the foods recommended in this book are extremely tasty, once you give yourself a chance to adapt to something new.

2

MALNUTRITION IN THE LAND OF PLENTY

"O beautiful for spacious skies, for amber waves of grain, for purple mountains majesty, above the fruited plain."

—AMERICA THE BEAUTIFUL

We produce enough food within our borders to feed our people, to have about half of them get overfat, to waste enough in trash cans to feed another 50 million people per day, and to ship enough overseas to help our foreign trade deficit. America is unquestionably the most agriculturally productive nation in the history of mankind. How can there be malnutrition in such a land of plenty?

There is. Put simply, we make the wrong choices. Ten percent of Americans are starving, and although the rest have ample food available, many Americans make poor decisions at the dinner table. The ideal strata of population for being properly nourished should be those who are wealthy, young, healthy, and intelligent. Yet in a study of Yale students, 18 percent were found to be iron anemic.[1] It is ironic that poor people in America have two to three times the incidence of obesity that the wealthy do. At the turn of the century, the few overfat individuals probably had no vitamin or mineral deficiencies. Today, many overfat people eat so much nutrient-robbed food that they are undernourished in addition to being overfat. ("Overfat" refers to an excessive amount of bodyfat stores, while "obesity" is based upon height/weight tables and can be misleading.)

Until this century, very few people had enough to eat. Most cultures ate as much as they could whenever they could find it, and it was not enough. The few cultures that had food abundance had no refined "junk food" to select from. In other words, we are one of the first societies to have not only enough food but many depleted foods to tempt the palate and ruin the body.

Recently in a supermarket we saw one corpulent man in his forties unloading his cart onto the checkout stand. His purchases typified the American attitude on nutrition. Hot dogs, buns, chips, candy, beer, vodka, and canned olives were followed by a bottle of generic vitamins. This rather unhealthy-looking fellow had some vague notion that nutrition was related to health, so he was willing to make the ineffective concession of buying the cheapest vitamins available to somewhat compensate for his cornucopia of nonfoods.

Each of the following factors contributes to the malnutrition that is so abundant in this nation of plenty:

1. We are deficient in numerous nutrients.

2. Our rapidly changing modern lifestyle has spawned many poor dietary habits.

3. We have deviated substantially from our evolutionary heritage of what our ancestors ate.

4. The plethora of drugs, alcohol, and tobacco being consumed create serious malnutrition.

5. Our polluted environment creates higher-than-normal nutrient demands.

6. Food refining removes many valuable nutrients. Modern agricultural techniques often do not properly nourish the soil.

Even if all other factors were ignored, we are the first nation in history to have the potential for optimal health rather than just survival. So why settle for anything but the best?

Dietary Surveys

The Ten State Survey, conducted by the Department of Health, Education, and Welfare, thoroughly examined over 60,000 low-income people with respect to their diet and many medical parameters. Many people were found to be low in iron, calcium, vitamin A, thiamin, riboflavin, and ascorbic acid. Height and bone growth was considerably retarded in many people. One-third of the children were low in serum vitamin A, while 4 percent of the people had scorbutic gums from serious vitamin C deficiency.[2] One out of six were low in protein levels in their blood. Five percent showed blatant protein malnutrition.

From 1971 to 1974 the Health and Nutrition Examination Survey (HANES I) found low levels of vitamin A, iron, and calcium throughout the land. Thiamin was clinically low in 14 percent of whites and 29 percent of blacks.

The Nationwide Food Consumption Survey, which measured all strata of the population, added the nutrients B_6 and magnesium to its list. For most nutrients surveyed, roughly one-third to one-half of the population was at risk for being deficient. Other studies have found that many other nutrients are low in the American food supply, including folacin, chromium, copper, zinc, pantothenic acid, and selenium. The vast majority of people in this country are probably low in one if not more nutrients.

In 1977, the Senate Select Subcommittee on Nutrition and Human Needs gathered a blue-ribbon panel to review the nutritional problems in this country. These scientists found that our diet contributes substantially to our health dilemma.

We consume twice the cholesterol that we should.

Our fat levels are 50 percent higher than they should be, and we are eating the wrong types of fat.

Our sodium intake is about three times what it should be.

We eat too little naturally occurring complex carbohydrates but consume twice the refined sugar that is recommended.

Our fiber intake is ridiculously low.

We consume far too much animal protein and not enough plant protein.

In 1983, the National Research Council published a significant collection of the best scientific research, which proved that diet in America is a substantial contributor to the incidence of cancer.[3]

Ironically, these surveys have all found that, although we have a serious problem with overfatness in America, we actually eat fewer calories than past generations. Our sedentary lifestyle is at fault here. Experts have calculated that few sedentary people, even when following an ideal nutrition program, could consume their RDA for all nutrients without causing overfatness. Because we exercise so little that we need less food, it is difficult to get the nutrients we need from food. Enter the subject of nutrient density and quantity of food. Not only do we eat less, but the food that we do eat is refined into a depleted state. Nutrient density refers to the amount of vitamins, minerals, fiber, and protein per 100 calories of food. The higher the nutrient density, the more nourishing the food.

Since these major dietary surveys, others turned up equally impressive deficiencies among Americans. Excellent studies show that areas of America that have low selenium levels in their soil, and hence in their diet, also have significantly higher cancer rates.[4] Low chromium in the American diet is a major factor in the incidence of heart disease, diabetes, and probably other ailments, such as cataracts. The average daily intake of chromium for men is 33 micrograms and women 25.[5] The RDA board recommends 50 to 200 micrograms as a safe range, while other scientists have called 500 micrograms a more ideal intake.[6] Older adults are experiencing an epidemic of osteoporotic broken bones. Hollowed bones are caused by, among other things, too little calcium and vitamin D. Though the RDA for calcium is 800 milligrams for older adults and may be raised to 1,500 with good reason, most adults get about 500 to 600 milligrams per day. Our vitamin D intake is equally atrocious.

Reports in prestigious scientific journals show that one-third to one-half of the population is low in folacin.[7] This deficiency is probably a factor in birth defects,[8] anemia, mental disturbances, and uterine functional abnormalities (which often lead to hysterectomy).[9]

The term pantothenic acid is derived from a Greek word meaning "everywhere." Everywhere but in the refined American diet, one might add. One study found that nursing home residents were consuming only one-third of their RDA for this often ignored nutrient.[10] Another study found that adolescents consumed about half of their RDA for this "everywhere" nutrient.[11] Pantothenic acid is lost in wheat milling and other food processing.

The American diet has excessive levels of fat. Most nutrition textbooks consider that the requirement for the essential fatty acid is easily satisfied since we eat so much fat. Yet 60 percent of the fats consumed in this country are hydrogenated,[12] meaning saturated and forced into an unnatural configuration through refining techniques. Hydrogenated fats do not satisfy the body's need for the essential fatty acid. They also surreptitiously fill the crucial roles of the essential fatty acid yet do not perform as they should.

Alcohol, though not nutritious, is a nutrient by virtue of its seven calories per gram. Americans consume 10 to 20 percent of their total calories from alcohol, which is two to four times the recommended upper limit.

The so-called balanced mixed diet has been proved to be insufficient. Many health care professionals say the four food groups make up a balanced diet. Studies have shown that a person might meet all the criteria of the four food groups and still be blatantly deficient in vitamins E, B_6, folacin, magnesium, zinc, and iron.[13] Goiter, long thought to be extinct in America, was found in more than one out of three schoolchildren in rural Kentucky, even though their iodine intake seemed adequate.[14]

Drug-Nutrient Interactions

The sales of legal prescription drugs have long since passed the $20-billion-per-year mark. Ninety-eight percent of older adults in America take some form of medication.[15] This does not take into consideration those consuming over-the-counter drugs like aspirin, diuretics, and dangerous diet aids like phenylpropanolamine (PPO). Nor could it possibly allow for the "recreational drugs" that are plaguing our nation. Nor does it account for the most abused drug of all: alcohol. Two-thirds of all adults drink, with one-third of those consuming five or more drinks at any given session.[16] Medicine for high blood pressure often ends up lowering body potassium, which further elevates blood pressure.[17] This is a typical drug-nutrient interaction.

Table 1 shows just some of the drug-nutrient interactions, as well as their effects on appetite.[18] Check with your physician or pharmacist to fully understand your medication.

TABLE 1: Appetite and Nutrients Affected by Drugs

Alcohol (ethanol)	Thiamin, folacin, B_6, B_{12}, magnesium
Amphetamines	Decreased appetite
Antacids	Phosphorus, calcium, D, magnesium
Antibiotics neomycin, penicillin, chloramphenicol	Fat, protein, cholesterol, sugars, carotene, iron, K, B_6, B_{12}, potassium, folacin; decreased appetite
Anticonvulsants (for epilepsy)	D, K, B_6, B_{12}, folic acid
Antihistamines (some)	Increased appetite
Antihyperlipidemics (for lowering cholesterol and fats in the blood) clofibrate, cholestyramine	Fat-soluble vitamins, calcium, iron, B_{12}, K, fat, folic acid; constipation
Antihypertensives hydralazine	B_6; decreased appetite, nausea
Biguanides (for diabetes) metformin	B_{12}
Cancer drugs	Decreased appetite
Colchicine (for gout)	Fat, protein, sugars, B_{12}
Corticosteroids (for severe allergies and inflammations such as rheumatic arthritis) cortisone, cortisol, prednisone	Protein, B_6, C, D, calcium, zinc, potassium; increased appetite
Digitalis (for heart disease)	B_1, Zinc; decreased appetite
Diuretics (for congestive heart failure) spironolactone	Potassium, calcium, magnesium, A; decreased appetite

INH (anti-TB drug)	B_6, niacin
Insulin	Increased appetite

Laxatives
    mineral oil, Epsom salts,
    methyl cellulose, guar gum,
    phenolphthalein
	Fat-soluble vitamins, potassium,
	calcium; decreased appetite

L-Dopa (for Parkinson's disease)	B_6
Methotrexate (antileukemia drug)	B_{12}, calcium, folic acid; nausea, decreased appetite
Nitrites	C
Oral contraceptive agents	Folic acid, B_6, phosphorus, magnesium, calcium, A, thiamin, riboflavin, C, B_{12}, E
Pesticides	Niacin, A
Potassium chloride (nutrient supplement)	B_{12}
Psychotropic drugs	Increased appetite
Pyrimethamine (antimalaria drug)	Folic acid
Salicylates aspirin	Iron, A, B, C, folic acid
Sedatives barbituates, chloral hydrate	Folic acid, D, C
Tobacco	C

Effects of Pollution

Vitamin E supplements help to protect against lung damage due to air pollution.[19] E and selenium together are potent antioxidants against radiation.[20] Selenium helps prevent heavy-metal toxicity[21] and harm from certain dangerous chemicals.[22] Selenium supplements lower the cancer-causing ability of various toxins.[23] Vitamin C protects against harm from radiation and sun exposure.[24] The abundance of lead in our air from leaded-gasoline exhaust can be somewhat offset by higher selenium in the diet.[25] C also protects the gastrointestinal tract from the cancerous effects of nitrates and burned meats.[26] Vitamin A helps protect nonsmokers from their often smoke-ridden office environments.[27] Zinc helps to offset the possible toxic levels of cadmium in water pipes and canned foods. In other words, because of our polluted environment, the need for many nutrients is much higher.

Our Evolutionary Design

If an automobile manufacturer designed a car to be driven at sixty miles per hour in a forward direction, and you constantly drove it sixty miles per hour backward, one could say that you were not using the machine the way it was designed to be used. The manufacturer's warranty would be null and void. Humans, too, have a way in which we were designed. Based upon several million years of evolution, our cells have certain nutrient requirements for maintaining a healthy body. We are not following these "factory specifications."

A study of diabetic Australian aborigines hints at how badly we are deviating from the "owner's manual" in using our bodies. Ten adult male aborigines were living in the cities and eating like other city dwellers. They returned to their bushland and their former life as hunters and gatherers and lost an average of 16 pounds each in spite of making no effort to reduce. Though animal foods were 64 percent of their calorie intake, their diet was low in fat (only 13 percent) due to the low fat content of wild game. All blood indices improved markedly. Within seven weeks, their type II diabetes was under control.[28] We are not encouraging everyone to go out to the bush country and hunt and gather. Yet this does illustrate how far the human species has drifted from the lifestyle from which we evolved.

Look at the following contrasts between our evolutionary heritage and our modern conditions:

We evolved	We now
as active creatures	are sedentary
as self-reliant and independent creatures	are very dependent
eating fresh vegetables and wild meat	eat highly refined foods with fat, sugar, salt, and little fiber
in clean atmosphere	have polluted air, water, food, and soil
under occasional stress	are under regular daily stress
without drug use	have much drug use

We need not return to the Stone Age. We have no intentions of turning in our microwave ovens, efficient cars, and the computer we wrote this book on. Yet while enjoying the bliss of technology, we need to keep in mind our heritage. If you deviate far from your evolutionary diet, your "warranty" for a healthy body will likely be null and void.

Nutrient Losses in Food Refining

The food technologist has not been sleeping for the past twenty years. Techniques have been developed to modify the color, taste, texture, and shelf life of nearly every food. But problems can hide in excess technology. There are additives, flavorings, and other cosmetic touch-ups to make not-so-fresh food seem appealing. We make excessive use of pesticides, herbicides, and incomplete fertilizers to grow plants. Animals are raised amidst the use and abuse of hormones, drugs, and antibiotics.

Foods are continually robbed of their inherent nutritive value in the food factory.[29] White flour has only 14 percent of the vitamin E, 50 percent of the pantothenic acid, about 1 percent of the chromium, and 28 percent of the B_6 once found in the whole wheat kernel.[30] Only 2 percent of the flour sold in the United States is whole wheat.[31] Doughnuts can be made with nonfortified white flour and so are even more useless than normal white flour. Potato chips have almost none of the fiber and vitamin C found in potatoes.

The food need not be refined in order for grand theft of nutrients to occur. Long-term storage, canning, transportation, and freezing can seriously lower vitamin and mineral levels.[32] Canned salmon loses more than half of its B_6. Canned spinach loses 80 percent of its pantothenic acid and 82 percent of its manganese. Canned beans lose 60 percent of their zinc. Frozen vegetables lose 44 percent of their B_6. Orange drinks match fresh oranges only in their vitamin C content, certainly not in rutin, bioflavonoids, fiber, fructose, and the hundreds of other substances in oranges that may have nutritive value in the body. Without the pectin the apple skin is so rich in, processed apple juice is little more than sugar water. Fresh cheese, with an ideal calcium-to-phosphorus ratio of 2 to 1, is refined into an aerosol can cheese spread that has had a fourfold deterioration in this important ratio.

Even assuming that the consumer selected the fresh orange instead of the orange drink, there may be little vitamin C left, considering the time and heat that these oranges were exposed to. Much of our fresh produce, like oranges, is picked green. This significantly reduces the flavor, texture, and nutrients. Fresh oranges from the grocery store have been found to have zero vitamin C content.[33] Transportation and storage time, being picked unripe, and exposure to the sun and fluorescent lighting can all combine to deplete otherwise healthy foods.

The table of nutrient composition, gathered by the United States Department of Agriculture decades ago and long held as being inscribed in stone, has now been found to be inaccurate.[34]

Vitamin and mineral content varies considerably within the same species of plant. For example, 100 grams of fresh, raw carrots can contain anywhere from 70 to 18,500 international units of beta-carotene (vitamin A).[35]

Humans require about 50 nutrients in their diet to maintain health. Most plants require only 15 nutrients. Thus a plant can appear to be perfectly healthy while growing on soil depleted of fluoride and selenium. Commercially fertilized soil is probably low in other trace elements as well. Nitrogen, phosphorus, and potassium are the primary constituents used in conventional fertilizers. All other nutrients essential to plant growth are rarely if ever used. Soil that is calcium- or zinc-depleted will still grow plants, although not as prolifically. The consumer ends up with food having subpar nutrient levels. Big-business farming in America does not usually replace these trace elements in the soil. Yet the fields would be more prosperous and the consumers more healthy if the soil were properly fertilized.

Malnutrition in Hospitals

Since there are highly trained dieticians and physicians on hospital staffs and a cost of about $1,000 per day, one would think that ideal nutrition would exist in hospitals. It doesn't. Although many patients arrive at the hospital already malnourished—which is not surprising, since their diet might have precipitated their ill health—once there, these people might well experience an even further decline in health through poor diet. Dietetic staffs are given low-priority support and funding by hospital administrators. There is a grim lack of nutrition knowledge among physicians. And, ironically, the sickest patients are put on tube feedings, which are often devoid of certain minerals and other known essential nutrients.[36] Just when optimal nutrition could assist their recovery, these patients are literally starved by unknowing health care specialists. The sick often get sicker.

Surviving Versus Thriving

The recommended daily allowances were determined by finding the level at which blatant deficiency symptoms would occur, then adding 50 to 100 percent to that intake level for safety. Arguments abound today that the RDA provides only for a lack of deficiency symptoms in *most* people. Even by its own standards, the RDA board admits that 2.5 percent of the population is not covered by their recommendations, which means that for each nutrient about 6 million people will suffer a deficiency even at RDA levels of intake.

There is a great deal wrong with the state of nutrition in America. There is also much right about it. First and most important, we have the agricultural abundance to eat whatever we want. Also, Americans are willing to change their dietary habits if they are convinced a change will be beneficial. Scientists in the 1970s erroneously indicted eggs as a primary cause of heart disease. The poultry business nearly died as a result. Scientists told the people that plant oils were better than animal fats. Margarine sales skyrocketed.

The real question is not, "Why is there so much sickness and premature death in America?" Given the nutritional deficiencies, the abundant excesses, the abuses of drugs, alcohol, and tobacco, the continual exposure to pollutants and psychological stress, and the normal semi-suicidal lifestyle that people have in this country, the question is, "Why are so many people alive today?" The answer is the incredible tenacity of the human body. Once you have studied this book, think of the many people who live on coffee and doughnuts, cigarettes, alcohol, stress, sedentary lifestyles, drugs, and empty nonfoods, and you too will shake your head in amazement at the resilience of the human body.

People do survive anyway. And get sick too often. And live most of their lives in a state of low productivity and listlessness. And die too young. Consider how much more mental, physical, and sexual vigor we could have. How intelligent could a human being become if provided with ideal emotional and nutritional nourishment? No one really knows. But few people would consider today's brightest students to be at the maximum level of accomplishment.

Why settle for just existing, when we could perhaps thrive in a longer and fuller life? Most Americans are just surviving. The most common complaints that physicians deal with are depression, fatigue, constipation, lethargy, and other such ailments. With optimal nutrition and an ideal lifestyle, these lackluster health problems might become nearly extinct.

Even if Americans ate the right foods in the right proportions, and avoided drugs, tobacco, and alcohol, and lived in pristine environments and avoided excess stress, and did not indulge in bizarre diets or fasting, they still might be considered malnourished if one were measuring health based on the ideal rather than the normal. Normal people live a lethargic and disease-riddled existence until they finally lose their health in their fifties and sixties. That is "normal." Shouldn't we strive for something better?

3

WHY ALL
THE CONFUSION?

"You say yes, I say no . . . You say stop and I say go, go, go!"
—THE BEATLES FROM "HELLO, GOODBYE"

Outside of politics and religion, nutrition may be one of the most controversial subjects of the day. One expert tells you to eat this. Another expert says that that food is bad for you. It is this storm of controversy that is holding back the nutrition field from seriously improving the lives of Americans. Some examples of the contradictory statements:

While even the most conservative scientists agree that calcium supplements could prevent and even reverse the course of osteoporosis,[1] a small band of influential scientists at the University of Wisconsin recently stated in the prestigious *American Journal of Clinical Nutrition:* "Until definitive studies conclusively show efficacy and demonstrate safety, calcium must be viewed as an experimental drug."[2]

Helen Guthrie, Ph.D., D.Sc., R.D., professor of nutrition at Pennsylvania State University, adamantly states: "Supplements at anything but minimum levels should be taken only when evidence of a deficiency has been established and then only under medical supervision."[3] While Sheldon Saul Hendler, M.D., Ph.D., professor of medicine at the University of California at San Diego, has compiled a rather convincing argument in favor of supplements both for the general population and therapeutic use.[4] Victor Herbert, M.D., J.D., says vitamin B_{12} supplements are "used by megahustlers to make megabucks selling oral tablets containing megaquantities . . . for . . . nonexistent effects."[5] Roger Williams, D.Sc., discoverer of the B vitamin pantothenic acid and professor of nutrition at the University of Texas has written several books on the subject of supplement usage to achieve optimal health and cure diseases.[6]

Frederick Stare, M.D., formerly of Harvard University, has repeatedly defended sugar and sugared "junk food" as being an acceptable part of the diet. Meanwhile, a legion of other scientists have documented the potential harm of a high-sugar diet.

What is the lay person to do? Not all of these "experts" can be right at the same time. Such confusion often drives a well-meaning person back into old harmful dietary habits.

Waiting for unequivocal and reproducible evidence takes decades. On the other side, there are the impressionable few who leap at the latest preliminary evidence as being sound fact. Neither extreme approach is valid.

The purpose of this chapter is to give you an understanding of scientific research principles and levels of credibility in evidence. Some "experts" draw premature conclusions from poorly designed studies while other "experts" ignore the evidence or fear censorship from peers if they believe something different from mainstream thought.

It is usually years before a scientific fact filters down to the public. This chapter should help you separate the scientists' facts from the charlatans' promises.

Levels of Credibility

This sequence, the actual way in which vitamin B_6's value against autism became known to the scientific community, demonstrates the three levels of credibility or data.

Anecdotal Evidence

These are case studies of individuals who found that something worked for them. Mrs. J. has a child with autism, an incurable condition in which an infant withdraws from the outside world. In her desperation, Mrs. J. tries various medications, herbs, vitamins, and other therapies to help her autistic child. She finds that vitamin B_6, although no cure, helps her child's behavior noticeably. This is weak evidence, but research has to begin somewhere. Many popular health magazines thrive on anecdotal evidence for "proving" their point. Yet some very prestigious scientific journals also use anecdotal evidence (case studies) in letters to the editor to keep their colleagues informed. Half of all articles in the *New England Journal of Medicine* are reports of anecdotal studies.[7] Nearly all useful ideas began as anecdotal evidence.

Clinical Observations

This is a gathering of case studies compiled by a research scientist or licensed health care professional. Mrs. J. writes to a reknowned expert on autism, Dr. Bernard Rimland, about her discovery that vitamin B_6 helped her autistic child. Dr. Rimland finds that many other mothers of autistic children have written in with the same information. These clinical observations make the evidence much stronger.

Controlled Scientific Study

This is a study done by unbiased scientists that attempts to create one variable and assess the effect this has on research subjects. Dr. Rimland, being both personally and professionally involved in autism, is curious about this B_6 treatment. He gathers prestigious cohorts to work with, designs a valid experiment, finds the funding, and performs a controlled scientific experiment. The results once again find that B_6 helps a significant number of autistic children.[8] The evidence is now very strong.

Even within the realm of controlled scientific studies there are varying levels of credibility.

Animal versus human studies. Since most creatures make their own vitamin C, a study using rats to test vitamin C deprivation would provide data useless for humans. Cows can digest fiber, while people cannot, so studies on fiber comparing the two would be useless. Other differences between humans and laboratory animals make animal studies questionable for human application, unless an animal's particular function is very similar to a human's.

Vitro (test tube) versus vivo (life) studies. When money and time are limited, some experiments are done in test tubes. These studies may have little validity when applied to humans. They do not take into consideration what the body's other chemicals and pH might do to the tested substance, nor is anything known about its safety. But these studies can be useful and are at least a start.

Blind versus double blind studies. If a physician could convince a group of ten people that a certain pill would help them, it is likely that up to five of them would improve even if the pill had nothing in it.[9] This placebo effect must be taken into consideration. Belief in something can be a very strong medicine. Thus, the blind experiment was designed to remove belief and the placebo effect. Ten people (the experimental group) would be given a pill, and nothing would be said about what is in it or what it should do. Another ten (the control group) would be given an identical pill (a placebo sugar pill) and, again, no promises would be made.

Yet, if the experimental group showed some improvement, the results would be questioned by some scientists because the person passing out the pills could have projected something inaudible to the subjects being studied. To take away this possibility, the double blind experiment was designed. In this procedure, none of the subjects being tested, nor any of the researchers handing out the pills, know what is being given to whom. This completely eliminates the placebo effect and satisfies most scientists.

Statistically significant results. Statisticians apply all evidence from an experiment to an equation and come up with statistical significance. This is a number that expresses the likelihood that the experimental results could occur as a result of random chance. The lower the number, the more convincing the results are. Thus an experiment with a probability of less than 0.05 means that 5 out of 100 times, or one out of 20, these results could have been obtained through random chance. However, with the great external diversity of the human race, is there any reason to believe that we are identical inside? When only a few people respond to a treatment, the statistician tells us to disregard the results. But should we listen to numbers or people?

Time span. The longer a study is carried on, the more credible the results. In the Framingham study, a group of Harvard researchers examined the diet, smoking, and exercise habits of thousands of Americans for over a decade. It is considered a classic in understanding the role that lifestyle plays in heart disease.

Vested interests. Food is the number one industry in the United States. When a multibillion-dollar food company finds that scientific evidence might indict its products, the facts can be shelved or hidden. Powerful food lobbies stifle the efforts of government to make some nutritional guidelines in the school cafeterias.

Reproducible results. Scientists are trained skeptics. In some ways this is good. Skepticism prevents one poorly designed experiment from swinging the entire community toward a new idea. Yet in other ways this can be dreadful. Vitamin E was shown twenty years ago to prevent the rampant blindness that occurs in premature infants exposed to the high-oxygen environments of intensive care units. Scientists wanted better data. So another study confirmed this again in a controlled experiment.[10] Retinal damage was much worse in the control group of infants than in the group treated with vitamin E. None of the infants receiving vitamin E went blind. Vitamin E has no side effects in the amounts being used, so the risk/benefit ratio strongly favors using vitamin E to prevent blindness in premature infants. How many times must results be reproduced and at what expense to the human subjects?

Another tragedy of skepticism is occurring with respect to folic acid's (a B vitamin) preventing neural tube defects in infants. Large and well-controlled studies have proved that folic acid given to pregnant women prevented this birth defect. Without the folic acid supplement, many women gave birth to infants with neural tube defects,[11] which are permanent and disastrous. Yet many researchers called for another study to reproduce the same results.[12] With an abundance of evidence favoring folate supplementation and no risks whatsoever, why sacrifice other infants to create "unequivocal and reproducible results"?

Time Lags

Until the twentieth century, Americans thought that tomatoes were poisonous, in spite of their widespread use in Europe. In the late nineteenth century, aspirin was an effective treatment for arthritis until the medical community decided that arthritis was an infectious ailment and ceased using aspirin. It wasn't until 1950 that aspirin was revived as a treatment.[13] A Scottish physician, Dr. James Lind, proved that limes could both cure and prevent scurvy, but it wasn't until forty-eight years later that the British navy mandated lime juice aboard all ships. In 1915, Dr. Goldberger found that foods rich in niacin (meat, milk, eggs) prevented and cured pellagra, the scourge of the southeastern United States. There were 10,000 deaths annually and over 10 percent of all mental patients suffering from this condition, but the public and scientific community did not welcome Dr. Goldberger's discovery until 1937, twenty-two years later.[14]

Time lags have not faded, even in our computer-assisted modern science, because of poor communication, a public that is resistant to change, and scornful and skeptical scientists. The radicals of today may be proved correct tomorrow.

The Quick Fix

If you went to your physician with severe pain, he or she could give you an injection of demerol or morphine that would give instant pain relief. Nitroglycerine placed under the tongue of a patient with angina (pain from constriction of vessels near the heart) gives immediate relief as it dilates the blood vessels. Other medications work quickly on high blood pressure, water retention, and many other health problems.

Nutritional supplements (vitamins, minerals, amino acids, etc.) and foods don't have such swift effect. Most healthy people could probably drink soda pop for years before any serious health problems developed. No one drops dead after smoking one cigarette. Supplements, though valuable, usually take weeks before subtle changes occur in a person's health. A group of nutrients designed to bolster low blood count would likely take weeks or months to really help the patient, since red blood cells take time to be built.

While drugs are unnatural agents that work at blocking or exciting a certain process in the body, nutrients are natural substances that slowly become part of the body's tissues. Nearly all drugs have a toxicity level and side effects, there are few dramatic medicine shows with nutrients. Although in extreme cases nutrients can have ill effects, usually there are few to no side effects with most nutrients.

Why All the Confusion?

Look around at a room full of people. There are as many different noses in size, shape, and color as there are people there. If people are so different outside, who says they are identical inside? They aren't.

You have a unique fingerprint and voiceprint. You also have a unique internal biochemistry. This biochemical individuality is what makes nutrition research even more confusing to some people. It has been found that most humans make their own carnitine (required in fat burning) out of various components in the diet. But some people do not make carnitine fast enough to prevent fatty buildup in arteries and tissues.[15] Blacks have a significantly higher "normal" serum B_{12} level than whites.[16] Thus, a black person could be diagnosed normal yet actually be deficient in B_{12}. All humans use GTF (a chromium complex) to help get sugar into the cells. Yet some people cannot efficiently make enough of their own GTF to stay healthy even if given adequate dietary chromium.[17] Careful scientific studies have found a sixfold variance in blood levels of vitamin C in lactating women, with a twofold variance in the levels of vitamin C in their milk.[18] In another study there was a fourfold difference in the absorption of C once the subjects were saturated.[19]

This lack of rigid formal rules bothers some scientists, but such is the great diversity of life. The bottom line in health care should be whatever works, without harmful side effects.

Nutrition is also a uniquely controversial field because it is relatively new. It is a science of the twentieth century, with essential nutrients still being uncovered. Controversy abounds in a new area of study until the dust settles.

Nutrition is not currently supported by the medical community. Medical doctors, the backbone of the healing professions, do not study, practice, or necessarily believe in nutrition as part of health care. Until doctors study nutrition, it is likely to be embroiled in controversy by sincere but uneducated physicians.

There is no accepted and state-licensed "nutritionists." Anyone can take on the name, from the teenager who is part-time help at a vitamin store to the self-proclaimed nutritionist with a regular flow of patients into an office. Since nutrition is so crucial to health, we need state certification of this healing modality. State certification would provide better quality control of nutritionists, a disciplinary panel, and the cartel that comes from exclusive rights to a field.

Much of the public is looking for a quick fix. People do not want to change lifestyle but would rather take a few vitamins with their cigarettes, coffee, and doughnuts. And there are plenty of hucksters willing to tell the public what it wants to hear.

Few scientists are willing to make the unconventional statement. Scientists, like other people, fear rejection and ostracism. Animals in the wild attack others that exhibit unusual behavior. Educated humans often attack others with unusual ideas, in spite of documentation to support the new ideas. This predatory approach to the introduction of new facts seriously slows down the process of change and improvement.

What This Book Offers

As you can see, nutritional science is not as cut and dried as we all would like it to be. We are in the rudimentary stages of understanding what the body needs and how it processes these nutrients. Some evidence is stronger than other evidence. Some is irrefutable yet still not incorporated into the healing arts. Some "experts" just refuse to keep up with the new scientific literature or refuse to change their minds.

Many scientists avoid giving answers. They skirt the issues with such elusive comments as "we really don't know for sure" or "the evidence is not conclusive yet." They want to avoid recommendations until all possibility of error has been removed.[20] By then you may be dead or irremediably ill.

You are a concerned citizen with an interest in your health and longevity. That is why you are reading this book. You want answers and guidance. Nutrition may be controversial and sometimes confusing, but it is also a science with much data available. There is enough evidence to make numerous recommendations regarding ways to improve your health through optimal nutrition. On the basis of our extensive educational and professional background, we will assess the evidence of scientific data and make specific recommendations for you to follow. No more lag time. No more confusion. No more a vague avoidance of answers.

4

ASSESSING YOUR NUTRITIONAL STATUS

"It is what we think we know already that often prevents us from learning."
—CLAUDE BERNARD

So far we have proved that nutrition is critical to your health and that many Americans are malnourished. The next question is, how does this apply to you specifically? There are five primary tools that help assess an individual's nutritional status and then tell the nutritionist what needs to be done to improve matters.

Dietary analysis. What you have been eating is an excellent barometer of your nutritional status. This tool will tell you what nutrients are likely to be in excessive or deficient levels in your diet. You will have a chance to take a dietary questionnaire at the end of this chapter.

Physical examination. There are tell-tale signs of deficiencies of various vitamins, minerals, and protein. The skin, nails, eyes, muscle tissue, and other physical attributes can tell the physician or nutritionist a great deal about the nutritional status of your body. Cracked skin or gray skin pallor can be warning signs of malnutrition. Percent body fat can be measured with skin-fold calipers or an electrical resistance device.

Blood chemistry. When the physician or nurse sends the patient's blood sample to the lab, the lab then sends back a computer printout indicating levels of fats, sugars, amino acids, certain enzymes, red blood cells, and certain vitamins and minerals found in the blood. Blood potassium can be misleading, since most of the body's potassium is found within, not outside, the cells. Blood calcium can also be misleading. The bones can be robbed of their calcium stores to maintain adequate blood calcium levels to keep the heart pumping. Only a few vitamins and minerals can be accurately assessed through blood samples. So blood is a good but not totally accurate indicator of nutrient status. Lymphocytes (disease resistance cells in the blood) have recently been found to be very accurate indicators of nutrient status.

Excreta analysis. Urine, feces, spit, nails, and mucous can give further details about your body's nutrient status. What comes out of your body is a very good indicator of what's going on inside.

Hair analysis. Hair analysis involves clipping a section of hair from near the base of the skull and sending it to a lab that specializes in this work. This tool has been much abused and has gained a huckster reputation.[1] Some hair salons, nutrition supplement shops, and grifter nutritionists have used this technique extensively to sell their products. An expensive computer print-out of the hair analysis impresses many clients.

Still, hair analysis is not without some value. Hair is readily available, stores and ships easily, provides information on the long-term status of certain minerals, and the procedure is noninvasive. Hair analysis cannot tell anyone about vitamin or protein status, nor does it necessarily find the levels of all minerals in the blood. There is great discrepancy in the preparation of the hair sample for analysis, the quality of equipment used to determine mineral levels, population norms with which to compare the results, and interpretation of the results.[2] But hair analysis is particularly suited to telling the health care professional about long-term exposure to toxic minerals, like lead and cadmium.[3] It also can accurately indicate the body pools of some essential trace elements, like chromium and zinc.[4] Though not yet widely used, toenails have been found to be even more valid records of mineral metabolism than hair.[5]

Of these methods of assessment, dietary analysis is the most important. The longer the record is kept (a record of six to seventeen days is usually necessary), the more accurate the results will be. Unfortunately, this is usually followed only in research studies. The diet history is more accurate if the person writes foods down as they are consumed, thus avoiding inaccuracies due to poor memory. Some people may want to impress the nutritionist with their good eating habits and so may not tell the truth about what or how much they ate. A study of dietary surveys found that male patients underestimated their food intake by an average of 500 calories per day while women underestimated by an average of 900 calories per day.[6] Some patients may change their eating habits temporarily while recording the foods, in order to look good. As you can see, the diet history, even when analyzed by computer, is still not a totally accurate measurement of nutritional status.

In order to evaluate your own diet, take the following test. Answer the questions truthfully, since you don't have to tell anyone. You can interpret your results from the scores at the end of the test. For more specifics in assessing your diet, look under each vitamin and mineral for those at risk. For even more specific information on your nutrient status, have a computer diet analysis performed by a qualified nutritionist/dietician.

Diet Analysis Questionnaire

Circle the answer that most closely applies to your situation

*1. The amount of weight I have gained since age 20 is about
   1) 30 or more lbs.   2) 20-29 lbs.   3) 10-19 lbs.   4) less than 10 lbs.

2. My weight now is about _____ pounds from ideal.
   1) 30 or higher   2) 15-29   3) 14 or less   4) My weight is now ideal.

3. I have tried
   1) many diets.   2) a few diets.   3) no diets.   4) I do not need to lose weight.

4. The largest skin-fold thickness I have on either the back of my arm or just above my hip bone measures
   1) 3 or more inches.   2) 2-3 inches.   3) 1-2 inches.   4) less than an inch of "earned thinness."

*5. I eat a good breakfast (coffee and doughnuts do not count)
   1) rarely.   2) sometimes.   3) usually.   4) almost always.

*6. My meal pattern is
   1) skip many meals but eat a few large ones.   2) skip some meals and eat a few large ones.   3) eat a lot of food and often.   4) eat small frequent meals.

7. Before swallowing, I chew my food
   1) less than 5 times.   2) 5-10 times.   3) 10-20 times.   4) 20 or more times.

*8. I spend _____ minutes eating each meal
   1) 5-10   2) 11-15   3) 16-20   4) more than 20

*9. Most of my meals are eaten at
   1) office, restaurants, planes, out.   2) home or sometimes restaurants.   3) home or sack lunch.   4) home.

10. I usually eat the following types of foods:
   1) fried, deep fried, boiled, canned, prepared.   2) baked, canned, frozen.   3) broiled, steamed, microwaved.   4) mostly fresh or unprocessed, baked or steamed.

*11. In my budget, the buying of wholesome foods rates
   1) low priority, can't afford it.   2) only when guests are coming.   3) relatively high priority.   4) very high priority.

*12. I salt my food
   1) always at the table and often while cooking.   2) always, but lightly.   3) sometimes.   4) rarely.

13. Snack and dessert foods such as soft drinks, candy, pastry, sweetened breakfast cereal, and potato chips are in my diet
    1) at least once each day.   2) sometimes once each day.   3) only a few times each week.   4) rarely.

14. My daily consumption of alcoholic beverages is (one drink equals one ounce of distilled spirits, 4 ounces of wine, or 12 ounces of beer)
    1) 4 or more drinks.   2) 2-3.   3) 1-2.   4) none.

*15. The following identifies my consumption of dairy products:
    1) I don't eat many.   2) I eat cheese, whole milk, butter, and ice cream.   3) I eat some butter, cheese, and ice cream, but mostly low- and nonfat milk.   4) I eat three or more servings each day of low- and nonfat milk, yogurt, or cottage cheese, with rare samplings of butter, cheese, and ice cream.

16. The following identifies my consumption of fruit:
    1) canned fruit, jams and jellies, pies.   2) dried fruit, canned fruit.   3) some fresh fruit, mostly canned, dried, prepared.   4) mostly fresh fruit, abundantly and daily.

17. My consumption of vegetables would best be described as
    1) rare.   2) canned, creamed, in TV dinners.   3) some fresh, mostly canned and prepared.   4) mostly fresh or steamed, abundantly and daily.

*18. The following identifies my consumption of fat (nuts, oils, bacon, salad dressings, margarine, butter, fried foods, etc.):
    1) I like these foods, eat them often, and am overweight.   2) I like fried foods and use dressings, gravies and margarine regularly, but I'm not overweight.   3) I try to restrict my intake.   4) My low intake is primarily from cold-pressed vegetable oils and nuts. I am not overweight.

*19. Of the protein group, I eat
    1) red meat and eggs often.   2) a little of every kind of meat, often fried.   3) occasionally red meat and eggs, primarily from fish and poultry.   4) much vegetable protein with proper matching, some fish and poultry, and occasional meat and eggs.

20. My intake of breads and grains would best be described as
    1) usually white bread, instant potatoes, crackers etc. 2) sporadic; these "carbs" make me fat.   3) some whole grain, much white bread and pastas.   4) mostly whole grain, regularly and abundantly.

*21. I take vitamin and mineral supplements
    1) never. 2) daily, in large quantities. 3) sometimes. 4) in the form of a high quality, broad spectrum supplement daily.

*22. My eating environment is usually

1) away from home and hectic.   2) equally divided between home and away.   3) mostly at home.   4) usually at home in a relaxed surrounding.

*23. Of the following symptoms, constipation, nausea, heartburn, diarrhea, gas, food allergies, food intolerance, I experience
   1) most of these regularly.   2) some of these often.   3) some of them, but rarely.   4) rarely any.

*24. The following foods are in my diet: fresh fruits, fresh and steamed vegetables, whole grains, legumes (beans)
   1) rarely.   2) sometimes.   3) several times each week.   4) each of them daily.

Evaluating Your Results

To get your total number of points, add the number of each answer you circled. For example, if you circled number three for question one, you count three points for that question.
   If you scored:

24-41   Very poor. Your diet may be your own demise. Get a complete dietary analysis. Have a physician examine you. Take some supplements. Read on; this book could save your life.

42-60   Poor. You need major improvements in your diet. You should seek proper nutritional counseling. You will find this book most informative.

61-78   Good. Try to improve in your areas of weakness (those questions for which you did not answer with a number 4). Congratulations for your efforts.

79-96   Excellent. Keep up the good work.

---

*Explanation

Questions 1-4 identify a problem with overfatness.

   5. Breakfast eaters are usually more alert, energetic, healthier, and better nourished.

   6. "Grazers" are healthier and longer-lived than "gorgers."

   8. "Speed eaters" have weight and digestive problems, while slow eaters can better enjoy, digest, and absorb their nutrients with less likelihood of overfatness problems.

   9. When others prepare your food, you lose control of what goes into it and how much you will eat. Oftentimes, healthy foods are not even available when dining out.

   11. Many people consider food a secondary expense, with clothes, cars, records, and other items rating a higher priority. Good food is not expensive. People who buy only cheap prepared foods are increasing their food bill and doing so at their health's expense, which is definitely not cheap.

12. High sodium intake can lead to high blood pressure.

13. These foods are high in salt, fat, and sugar, while being almost totally devoid of vitamins, minerals, fiber, and protein.

15. Dairy products are high in many nutrients, yet high-fat dairy products can create health problems. Low-fat and nonfat dairy selections are preferable.

18. A high-fat diet is a major health risk, especially if the individual is overfat.

19. Red meat is a primary contributor of fat and cholesterol to the American diet. Fish and poultry are lower in fat and cholesterol. Plant protein options are low in fat and higher in fiber and other valuable nutrients.

21. Supplements can improve nutrient intake, but random supplements or megadoses can be harmful.

22. A friendly and conducive environment aids digestion and absorption.

23. These symptoms can indicate not only a health problem but poor digestion and absorption of nutrients.

24. These foods should be the backbone of a healthy diet, since they are high in naturally occurring complex carbohydrates, fiber, protein, vitamins, minerals, and water.

5

THE SEVEN
GENERAL RULES
OF NUTRITION

"Keep it simple." —BUSINESS PROVERB

We live in an information age. Many of you may be deluged with the amount of data that you must read to keep up with your profession. Many people do not have the time or inclination to fully understand every field. They want to know what to do rather than always be concerned with why they should do it. If you have a competent mechanic, you do not need to understand transmissions to have your car fixed. This chapter is dedicated to those individuals who are interested in nutrition for their health's sake but are too busy to become fully involved in all the whys behind nutrition principles. We condensed thousands of pages of complex biochemical studies into this ultimate digest of nutrition.

1. Eat foods in as close to their natural state as possible. Refining food often does one or more of the following:

a) Removes valuable nutrients like fiber, vitamins, minerals, and protein. Grains, which are normally low in the amino acid lysine, have much lysine destroyed when they are overcooked.[1] The milling of whole wheat flour removes twenty-four nutrients and adds back only four. Only recently has vanadium been considered an essential mineral; refining eliminates most of the vanadium.[2] Since no one even knew it was necessary, vanadium was not added to any food or vitamin supplement. Only those eating natural foods got their share of this essential trace mineral.

b) Adds agents of questionable value like fat, salt, sugar, and additives. Potato chips, compared with fresh baked potatoes, have 800 percent more calories, nearly 40,000 percent more fat, 34,000 percent more sodium, not to mention other additives used by various potato chip manufacturers.

c) Increases cost. Potato chips are ten times the cost of the same weight of regular potatoes.

2. Eat a wide variety of foods. Studies have shown that people who consume a widely varied diet also have a higher nutrient intake.[3] This will help you to:

a) Include all essential nutrients, especially those not currently recognized as essential. Remember that the science of nutrition is in its infancy and we do not know all there is to know about optimally nourishing a human being.

b) Avoid excess toxins, both naturally occurring and synthetic.

c) Minimize risks of food allergies, since it is the most frequently consumed foods that often cause allergies and sensitivities.

3. Eat small and frequent meals (four to six per day), beginning with a substantial breakfast and tapering down to a smaller supper. Snackers following this program have a lower incidence of obesity,[4] heart disease, diabetes, hypoglycemia, and gastrointestinal problems.[5] "Grazers" live longer than "gorgers."

4. Minimize your intake of fat, salt, sugar, cholesterol, alcohol, and caffeine. These nutrients and substances are probably not harmful in small quantities but can be deadly in the high quantities that Americans normally consume. Avoid processed meats and additives. Luncheon, smoked, and salted meats, monosodium glutamates, nitrates, and food colorings are risky even in small quantities.

5. Maximize your intake of fresh vegetables, fruit, whole grains, legumes, low-fat dairy products, fish, poultry, and clean water. These should be the backbone of your diet.

6. Get your nutrients with a fork and spoon whenever possible. Foods provide all essential nutrients while vitamin pills contain only a select few. Yet, because of modern lifestyles (i.e., stress, dieting, smoking, alcohol, drug use, poor eating habits), nutritional supplements can be quite valuable to many people. Take a broad-spectrum vitamin and mineral insurance product with meals and in divided dosages.

7. Balance calorie intake with expenditure. Maintain ideal body fat composition (less than one inch of skin-fold thickness just above the hip bone). For a rough estimate of daily calorie needs, multiply weight in pounds times 10 for sedentary people, 12 for low-activity people, 14 for moderately active people, and 17 for very active people. Thus, a 150-pound moderately active person would maintain weight on 2,100 calories per day. For a rough estimate of average daily protein needs in grams (not including pregnancy, lactation, illness, or rapid growth), divide weight in pounds by 2.2. Thus, a 150-pound normal healthy adult would require 68 grams of protein per day.

PART TWO

ESSENTIAL DIETARY COMPONENTS

FOOD CONTAINS MANY THOUSANDS OF CHEMICALS. ABOUT fifty are essential for proper health. This section discusses only those substances recognized as being essential in the diet of humans in order to maintain health. There are also substances not currently considered essential but that may be useful. We call them "quasi-vitamins," and they are what may make the difference between surviving and thriving.

6

CARBOHYDRATES

"Breakfast foods grow odder and odder; It's a wise child that knows its fodder."

—OGDEN NASH

It all starts 90 million miles away on a thermonuclear fireball called the sun. In seconds, energy reaches our small planet and is used by green plants to combine carbon dioxide and water to form a simple six-carbon sugar. This process is called photosynthesis. This is the essence of carbohydrates and even life itself. From this process many sugars may be bound together to form a starch. Or the sugars may be altered with a nitrogen group attached to form an amino acid, the beginning of a protein. Of the 16 billion tons of carbon bound each year in this incredible act of energy conversion, about half is available to humans in the form of dietary carbohydrate; the remainder is unavailable for human absorption and is called fiber.[1]

The primary macronutrient need of the human body is energy. The human body has evolved a very adaptable fuel capability. We humans can "burn" carbohydrates, fats, protein, and even alcohol. Yet the preferred fuel source for most cells of the body is carbohydrates. Given a high-carbohydrate diet, most people have more energy, especially for athletic events. Carbohydrate foods provide the brain fuel glucose, which helps to keep mood, behavior, and intellect on an even keel. Yet, in spite of their health value, carbohydrates have earned a dubious reputation because most carbohydrates in America are highly refined starches or simple sugars.

There are two types of carbohydrates: simple and complex. Simple carbohydrates are the sugars that are sweet to the taste buds. Complex carbohydrates are the starches. Within these two categories there are both refined and naturally occurring versions.

Until the 1960s, many nutritionists were teaching that refined carbohydrates were equal to the nutritive value of natural carbohydrates. That idea has since been proved wrong. When whole wheat is refined to enriched white flour, about twenty-four nutrients are lost with only four being added back. This staple of Western civilization thus is robbed of many valuable nutrients including magnesium, vitamin E, and chromium. A lifetime of consuming these nutritionally depleted refined carbohydrates may be responsible for considerable disease in Western society.

Under the auspices of the Senate Select Subcommittee on Nutrition and Human Needs, a gathering of prestigious scientists recommended that we lower our intake of refined carbohydrates and increase our intake of complex and naturally occurring carbohydrates. The health benefits of these foods are amazing. A person consuming a diet high in these naturally occurring carbohydrate foods will be much less likely to suffer from heart disease, obesity, diabetes, hypertension, gastrointestinal problems (like hemorrhoids, constipation, and cancer), hypoglycemia, dental caries, and radical swings in emotional and physical energy levels.

TABLE 2: Types of Carbohydrates

	Simple	*Complex*
Naturally Occurring	fruits, honey, milk sugar, some vegetables, molasses	whole grains, legumes, nuts, vegetables
Refined	white sugar, brown sugar, sugar, confectioner's sugar	white bread, white flour, crackers, white pasta, potato chips

TABLE 3: Sources of Naturally Occurring Carbohydrates

Whole Grains	*Fruit*	*Vegetables*	*Legumes*
rice	berries	squash	soybeans
barley	cherries	broccoli	navy beans
quinoa	melons	potatoes	split peas
wheat	bananas	tomatoes	garbanzo beans
amaranth	apples	onions	lima beans
millet	citrus	cauliflower	lentils
rye	papaya	parsley	pinto beans
oats	apricots	carrots	kidney beans

In addition to these extensive health benefits, naturally occurring carbohydrate foods are less expensive than high-fat, high-protein foods like meat and cheese; have a longer shelf life, especially dried legumes and whole grains; and offer considerable fiber and fluid, essential nutrients we will discuss in their own sections.

The basic unit of all carbohydrate food is one six-carbon molecule. This unit is usually glucose, fructose, or galactose, which are called monosaccharides (meaning one sweet unit). When combined, these units form one of the following disaccharides (two sweet units):

glucose + glucose = maltose (in cereals and beer)
glucose + fructose = sucrose (table sugar, fruits, some vegetables)
glucose + galactose = lactose (milk sugar)

Fiber is a polysaccharide whose glucose units are joined in such a way that human digestive enzymes will not break it down.

Functions of Carbohydrates in the Diet

Carbohydrates are an essential part of the diet for the following reasons:

1. To provide energy, thus sparing the body the need to create its own carbohydrates by scavenging protein from lean tissue. A high-carbohydrate diet will increase one's exercise capacity.[2]

2. To maintain water and sodium levels. The kidneys rely almost entirely on carbohydrates for energy. Once the diet becomes low in carbohydrates, the inefficient kidneys begin losing water and sodium. Water is the essence of the quick weight loss in a low carbohydrate diet.[3] This is both a risky and fleeting method of losing weight, since the water weight returns within a few days.

3. To become part of the body's tissues. Functional components like the anticlotting compound heparin and structural parts like the connective tissue hyaluronic acid are derived primarily from carbohydrates in the diet.

4. To stimulate the growth of helpful intestinal bacteria. Some bacteria produce vitamins like K and biotin, while others help stave off other disease-causing bacteria. Lactose in foods such as milk is particularly efficient at encouraging beneficial bacteria in the intestines (although lactose causes intestinal problems in people who are unable to digest it).

5. To aid in the absorption of nutrients. Glucose provides energy for the active transport mechanisms in the intestinal wall, aiding in the uptake of various nutrients.

6. To provide bulk in the form of indigestible fiber. See the chapter on fiber for the numerous health benefits of this carbohydrate.

7. To provide satiety to the diet. Carbohydrate foods have much color, taste, texture, and aroma to offer. They make eating more enjoyable.

What Happens to Carbohydrates in the Body

Once carbohydrates are absorbed into the blood, the body has a number of metabolic routes on which to send them. The carbohydrates could be:

1. Burned immediately for energy (glycolysis).
2. Stored as fat for future energy needs (lipogenesis).

3. Converted to glycogen for future quick energy needs (glycogenesis).

4. Used to create a structural bodily component, such as the connective tissue hyaluronic acid.

5. Used to create a functional bodily component, such as the anticlotting compound heparin or a liver detoxifying agent.

6. Broken down in the hexose monophosphate shunt (HMPS) to provide energy for various anabolic building processes within the body.

The human body stores about 340 grams, or roughly three-fourths of a pound, of carbohydrates. Of these 340 grams, one-third is in the liver and two-thirds in the muscles. The liver slowly releases glycogen into the blood in order to maintain a certain level of the preferred energy substrate glucose. Most of the body's energy is stored as fat, since fat weighs less, takes up much less space than protein and carbohydrates, and produces considerable water as it is being burned. Most tissues favor blood glucose for fuel and some are almost entirely restricted to it, including the lens of the eye, kidneys, and brain.

Blood Glucose and Diabetes

Problems in carbohydrate metabolism often result in marginal functioning of the glucose-dependent body sites, such as the eyes, kidneys, and brain. Diabetes, also called hyperglycemia (above-normal sugar in the blood) and hypoglycemia (below-normal sugar in the blood) is a form of erratic blood sugar regulation that can cause health problems.

Hypoglycemics experience many problems as their nervous and muscular systems suffer from fuel shortages: weakness, malaise, trembling muscles, headache, blurred vision, depression, nausea, radical mood and energy swings, sweating, and light-headedness.

The Andes mountains in Peru are home to the Qolla Indians, who are proud of their reputation as being "the meanest and most unlikeable people on earth." An anthropologist was curious to see if there might be an explanation for their truculent nature and found a significant relationship between the level of meanness and low blood sugar.[4]

Diabetics suffer a myriad of subtle changes within the body that increase their risk for heart disease, renal failure, gangrene, and blindness. Initial symptoms of diabetes might be thirst, frequent urination, and poor wound healing.

There are two questions to answer in order to understand the importance of blood glucose regulation: (1) How does the glucose get into the cells of the body? (2) What causes the fluctuations in blood glucose levels?

Glucose into the Cells

Glucose does not pass easily through the cell membrane and into the cell. Glucose must have several other substances available for it to enter into the cells and thus be burned, including cyclic AMP (a hormone), insulin (a hormone produced by the beta cells of the pancreas), and glucose tolerance factor (GTF), a chromium-containing complex.

All three of these must be present at the right time, in the right ratio, in order for the glucose molecule to slip through the membrane and into the cell. Someone with emphysema is suffocating to death, even though he or she lives in a "sea" of air. The diabetic has a similar problem: plenty of glucose in the blood, yet the glucose molecule is unable to enter the cell. Thus, many cells begin to starve and deteriorate.

Blood Glucose Curves

In a glucose tolerance test, the subject is asked to fast from the evening supper until the test the next morning. Then the subject drinks a measured amount of glucose solution. A blood sample is drawn from a vein at the start of the test and every thirty to sixty minutes for the next three to six hours. The glucose consumed is absorbed into the blood and then into the cells. The amount of glucose in the blood tells the clinician how well that person responds to a carbohydrate load. These blood glucose levels can be plotted on a graph. The closer one stays to within 70 to 100 milligrams percent (a measurement of how much sugar is in the blood) for the first and last measurement, and the more gradual the curve, the better the subject's glucose tolerance is, according to normal Western values. When blood glucose falls below normal, the person will begin to experience symptoms of hypoglycemia mentioned above.

Program to Stabilize Blood Glucose Levels

If you experience any or all of the symptoms of hypoglycemia, it would be wise to follow a program to stabilize blood glucose. Many clinicians have found great success with patients having various nerve disorders by placing the patients on the hypoglycemic program. If this program helps the symptoms, then continue with it. If it doesn't, see your doctor about a glucose tolerance test and/or advice on other possible remedies.

Minimize simple refined carbohydrates. Cut them in half or less. Some people may even need to avoid certain high-sugar fruits like dates and raisins.

Minimize caffeine intake. Caffeine influences insulin output, which then drives blood glucose down. One cup of weak tea (15 mg. caffeine) might bother some people, while others can consume 200 mg. of caffeine per day (four cups of coffee) without any immediate untoward effects. Millions of people in the civilized world begin their day with pastries and a cup of strong coffee. The caffeine from the coffee helps produce insulin to drive the sugar from the pastry into the cells, thus leaving the person with a fleeting sense of energy and well-being. This is followed shortly by a fall in blood glucose level and a subsequent nadir in mental and physical energy. Sound familiar?

Maximize complex naturally occurring carbohydrate foods. These foods, especially legumes, have been proved to provide the most stable blood glucose curve of all.[5] Complex and naturally occurring carbohydrates with high fiber, such as whole grain instead of white bread, must be slowly broken down in the digestive tract, thus providing a more gradual influx of glucose into the blood. This avoids the peaks and valleys in energy levels.

Eat small, frequent meals. This routine has been shown to provide more continuous and higher levels of energy, resulting in a more stable blood glucose curve.[6]

Regular exercise is nearly miraculous at helping to bring about more stable blood glucose curves. Diabetics, hypoglycemics, and everyone else can benefit from exercise for a more dependable energy level throughout the day and improved glucose tolerance.

Lactose Intolerance

Lactose (milk sugar) is a disaccharide that must be digested by the enzyme lactase into its component sugars of galactose and glucose. People who don't make enough lactase in their intestines experience discomfort when they drink milk because bacteria use the lactose and create bloating, flatulence and diarrhea. Hard cheeses do not usually affect these people because the lactose there has been converted to lactic acid by bacteria or by the enzyme rennin. Yogurt, with live bacteria cultures of lactobacillus, is usually well tolerated by these people because the bacteria aids in lactose digestion. About 75 percent of blacks, at least 5 to 10 percent of whites, nearly all Asians, and 70 percent of the Jewish population experience at least some degree of lactose intolerance.[7] Sixteen percent of healthy American adolescents from various ethnic backgrounds were found to be lactose intolerant.[8] For these people, the consumption of either yogurt or lactose-reduced milk will allow them to obtain the many nutritional benefits of dairy products without intestinal discomfort. Lactose also aids in calcium absorption by stimulating bacterial growth and increasing acidity in the gut.

Sugar

It was cultivated as early as 325 B.C. in India, yet it remained a scarce luxury until Columbus brought sugar cane to the Caribbean in 1493. Sugar quickly became one of the most valued products in the New World; pirates plundered ships for their gold, silver, and sugar.[9]

Sugar presents a health hazard in what it is: a concentrated calorie source that is quickly absorbed into the blood; an irresistible temptation to some people's taste buds; the favorite "food" of bacteria in the mouth that cause cavities.

Sugar also presents a hazard in what it isn't: no protein, fiber, vitamins, minerals, or other redeeming nutritive quality.

It offers the body a fuel, but none of the critical nutrients needed to burn it, including thiamin, niacin, riboflavin, pantothenic acid, biotin, and chromium. Heavy sugar users run the risk of creating a deficiency of these nutrients, and some diseases are more prevalent in areas that have a high consumption of refined sugar. Americans consume 132 pounds of sugar per year per person.

Sugar contributes to a number of health problems.

Dental caries. There is an undisputable relationship between the amount of sucrose (white sugar) consumed and the incidence of cavities.[10] Factors that encourage cavity-causing bacteria are adhesive simple sugars, time, moisture, and darkness. Your mouth provides all but one of these: sticky sugar. Sticky dried fruits and honey can be even more cavity-causing than some white sugar products. Certain detergent foods like carrots, apples, celery, and other crisp fresh produce can help cleanse the sticky sugar from the tooth surface. The toothbrush and dental floss are more lethal weapons against caries. Dental caries are the most prevalent disease in Western society, affecting over 90 percent of the population. Since a recent study found 80 percent of all dentists' children to be cavity-free, this is obviously a quite preventable disease.[11]

Obesity. Sugar products (candy, pastries, soda pop) and sugar-fortified products are more concentrated in calories than their natural counterparts. The sweet tooth of many people is their girth downfall.

Heart disease. Obesity doubles the risk of heart disease.[12] Constant high levels of insulin, such as would occur on a high-sugar diet, are associated with heart disease risk.[13] Sugar itself is a heart disease risk factor.[14]

Nutrient deficiencies. A high sugar intake provides a fuel to burn, but not the metabolites to burn it. A key problem now seen by many scientists is the chromium lost in sugar and wheat refining. Molasses (the residue from the sugar refining process) and whole wheat have considerable chromium, while their refined counterparts have none. The chromium deficiency created by a high intake of refined carbohydrates may be one of the key links in the rampant problems of heart disease and diabetes in America.[15,16]

Hyperactivity and affected mental functions. Good studies have shown that the more sugar a child eats, the lower his or her intellectual abilities become.[17] Sugar has an effect on the brain of sensitive individuals and may cause edema or erratic blood glucose. A high-sugar diet has been linked to hyperactivity in children and mood swings in adults. It was even used as a plausible defense for murder. A San Francisco man was acquitted of murdering the mayor and an assistant because of temporary insanity provoked by a high-sugar diet, a.k.a. the "Twinkies" defense. Ask a teacher what the elementary classroom is like on the day after Halloween. There is definitely a difference in the behavior and attention span of many sugar-laden children.

Radical energy and mood swings. Glucose from the sucrose molecule is literally pumped into the blood from the intestinal area, thus causing a radical rise in blood glucose levels. Contrast this with fructose from honey, fruits, corn syrup, and molasses, which is absorbed only at 30 percent the rate of glucose from white table sugar. This rapid influx of glucose into the blood can cause the body to produce an excessive amount of insulin, thus overcompensating and producing a subsequent drop in blood glucose levels and hypoglycemic symptoms. Sucrose worsens diabetic symptoms,[18] while fructose is better tolerated by diabetics.

Beta cell burnout. Through excessive and continual demands of insulin supply (from the beta cells of the pancreas), sugar may literally exhaust the pancreas. Obesity (i.e., excess calories) can cause beta cell burnout, especially if the diet is high in sugar. Nonobese individuals with high sugar intake also may suffer beta cell burnout. This effect could be compared to continually drag racing with a small economy car. Neither the engine nor the pancreas is built for that type of continuous, stressful demand.

TABLE 4: Types of Sweeteners

Nutritive (Provides Calories)		Nonnutritive (No Calories)
corn syrup	levulose	cyclamates (now banned)
dextrose	maltose	saccharin (possibly harmful)
fructose	mannitol*	aspartame, Equal (breaks down in long
glucose	sorbitol*	storage and under high heat)
honey	sucrose	
lactose	xylitol*	

*Will not cause cavities; other nutritive sweeteners will.

People consuming ridiculous amounts (four quarts of diet soda and a gallon of lemonade per day) of aspartame may bring on epileptic seizures.[19] The consumption of soft drinks has increased so dramatically in the past five decades that it is nearly impossible to watch television without seeing a soft drink commercial. Better than half the United States consumes soft drinks regularly (two to three per week) with one out of eight people consuming three or more per day.[20] Most soft drinks are composed of sugar (nine teaspoons per can), caffeine, artificial flavoring, synthetic food dye, and phosphoric acid; it is staggering to compute the health cost of each person's drinking the equivalent of a bathtub full of this nonfood each year.

Much of our sugar intake is hidden. Ketchup has a higher percentage of sugar (29 percent) than ice cream (21 percent). Russian dressing is 30 percent sugar. Nondairy creamer is 65 percent sugar compared with 51 percent sugar in a chocolate bar. Americans get about one-fourth of their calories from sugar, of which 3 percent is from fruits and vegetables, 3 percent is from milk sugar lactose, and the remaining 18 percent is added to our foods. Three-fourths of all sugar used is in commercial food preparation— the hidden sugar load.[21]

Recommendations

If it takes a little sweetness to help make very nutritious foods become tasty, then the sweet substance has some value. Small amounts of sweeteners on otherwise nourishing foods like oats or soybeans is an acceptable nutritional compromise. Sugar foods like soda pop and pastries are without any redeeming value. Some experts consider saccharin to be safe in normal amounts.[22]

Use one third (or less) the amount of sugar a recipe calls for. It has been estimated that if the average consumption of sugar in the United States were cut to 33 pounds per year from the current 132 pounds, cavity incidence would fall sharply and quickly.[23] Molasses, honey, dried fruit, and corn syrup are higher in fructose, which has nearly twice the sweetness of sucrose, so these are preferable sweeteners, since less fructose needs to be used to provide the same level of sweetness. Fructose has been shown to be a more efficient fuel for athletic endurance.[24]

Check labels and avoid foods high in added sugar. Some food manufacturers will separate the various types of sugar on the label just to avoid having to put sugar as the leading ingredient in the package. Levulose, dextrose, sucrose, glucose and others are all simple refined sugars. Note that "sugar-free" gum probably contains one of the alcohol sugars, which, though it won't cause cavities, does have calories and can contribute to weight problems.

TABLE 5: Food Sources of Carbohydrates

Food Group	% Calories from Carbohydrates
muscle glycogen (the small amounts found in beef, poultry, and fish), lactose, fruits	nearly 100%
whole grains	about 90%
vegetables	about 66%
legumes	most are about 60%-70%; soybeans are 33%
nuts	5% (Brazil nuts) to 20% (cashews)
seeds	about 10%-15%

Daily Carbohydrate Intake

RDA: None stated.

Senate dietary goals: 58 percent of total calories.

Average U.S. intake: 46 percent of total calories, of which about 40 percent (18 percent of total calories) is sugar. Daily intake of carbohydrates in the Orient and Africa is about 80 to 85 percent of total calories.

Minimum intake: Less than 60 grams a day will produce ketosis and other undesirable effects. Experts recommend no less than 100 grams a day, although it is known that the brain itself uses about 140 grams a day.

Energy value: 4 calories per gram; thus the 340 grams stored in the body will provide about 1,360 calories, enough for one sedentary day or ninety minutes of intense exercise.

Optimal intake: Carbohydrates should be 60 to 75 percent of total calories in the form of those foods listed in table 3. The greater your activity level, the higher the percentage should be. Less than 10 percent of total calories should come from refined simple sugars.

7

FIBER

"Men who call salads 'rabbit food' should remember what such food does for rabbits. The male rabbit is light on his feet, has no paunch and maintains lively romantic interests."
—DR. W.W. BAUER

Fiber has no nutrient value whatsoever. It cannot be digested or absorbed into the blood stream. Yet it is because of its indigestibility that fiber is so essential to human health. For many centuries, the common country physician has known the value of roughage in the diet. In the twentieth century, much of this was forgotten, ignored, or rebuked as being primitive medicine. Since 1900, the consumption of refined low-fiber foods has been increasing. So too has the incidence of the many degenerative diseases of civilization.

In the early 1970s Drs. Dennis Burkitt and H.C. Trowell, two English physicians, returned from a lifetime of medical service in Uganda with a novel and sensible explanation for many of the diseases in Western society. While the Western world consumed five to twenty grams of fiber daily, its counterparts in underdeveloped Africa and Asia were getting 50 to 60 grams per day. Dr. Burkitt found a near zero incidence of overweight, heart disease, diabetes, and gastrointestinal problems among these people.

In 1980, Dr. James Anderson of the University of Kentucky found a high-fiber version of the Exchange System (see chapter 39) to be extremely effective in the treatment of adult diabetes. As data are gathered, it appears that fiber, through its "useless" and indigestible nature, is a dietary essential and a formidable weapon in clinical nutrition.[1]

Functions of Fiber

1. To provide bulk to the fecal matter, making it nature's "soft broom" to clean the intestinal tract. This soft fecal matter is less likely to irritate the delicate sphincter muscle, or anus; such irritation can lead to hemorrhoids and other problems.

2. To absorb fat, cholesterol, and bile salts and carry them out in the feces. The net effect is to lower the levels of all fats in the blood.[2] The soluble fibers of pectin, mucilage, and gum are the most effective at lowering fat levels in the blood and stabilizing blood glucose.

3. To absorb toxic elements and metals in the intestines and make them unavailable for absorption.

4. To reduce the amount of time that various toxins are exposed to the intestinal wall. Cholesterol is degraded by bacteria in the intestines to deoxycholic acid, a known cancer-causing agent. With fiber to hurry the food along, carcinogens have less time to attack the intestines.

5. To interfere with digestion and absorption of food, thus slowing the entrance of calories into the blood stream. This more gradual infusion of glucose makes it easier for the body to maintain a more constant blood glucose level.

6. To maintain a smooth and constant flow of water-binding fecal matter in the intestines, thus avoiding the intestinal "nuggets" from low-fiber diets and the diverticulae (weakened spots in the intestines) that are caused by the pressure from these nuggets.

Hazards of Excess Fiber

1. Fiber binds such toxic metals as lead, which is good. Fiber also binds such essential metals as calcium, iron, magnesium, and zinc, which is not so good, since these minerals are already in low supply in Western diets. Too much fiber may cause deficiencies of these and other minerals.[3]

2. Fiber binds water and carries it out of the intestinal tract. Too much fiber and not enough fluids to compensate for it can cause diarrhea and dangerous dehydration if this situation continues too long. Since fiber binds water, it is essential for people on a high fiber diet (especially the older adult) to consume more water than normal.

3. Fiber provides bulk and speeds food through the intestines. With the food having less time available for exposure to the intestinal walls, the efficiency of absorption of all nutrients is reduced somewhat. This can create malnutrition with some people, especially rapidly growing children, who need more calories and nutrients than they need fiber bulk.

4. Excess flatulence brought on by excess fiber, though certainly not dangerous, may cause undue social discomfort.

Optimal nutrition is a quest for balance; too much or too little of any nutrient can create problems. Fiber is no exception. Those accustomed to the typical Western diet should slowly increase their fiber intake until it reaches fifty grams or so per day. (The average American consumes twenty grams.) Consume enough fiber in your diet to maintain one or more floating soft stools daily. The buoyancy occurs from the gas bubbles produced by bacteria acting on the high carbohydrate and fiber foods.

Types of Fiber

Scientists initially had a difficult time calculating the amount of fiber in food. They would expose a food substance to a hot acid bath, then a hot alkali bath, then consider whatever survived that ordeal to be fiber—a form called crude fiber. This is far too harsh to compare to the human digestive tract. Current estimates of fiber—dietary fiber—are based upon a much more reasonable approach to simulating the body's digestive processes. Yet most books, in listing fiber content, still refer to crude fiber because the technique for finding true dietary fiber is so new. Crude fiber can be as little as 8 percent of actual dietary fiber.

The plant kingdom has numerous versions of fiber, including:

Insoluble	*Soluble*
lignin	pectin
cellulose	gums and mucilages
hemicellulose	

All of these, except lignin, are carbohydratelike substances. Cellulose forms the cell wall of plants but is slowly converted to lignin as the plant ages. Thus, the soft flowerets of broccoli contain cellulose while the chewy bottom part contains more lignin. Cellulose is nearly identical to amylose (digestible starch).

Cows and other ruminants are able to digest cellulose. Helpful bacteria, which thrive in the multichambered stomach of the ruminant, have the enzyme to break down cellulose to its elemental glucose: a perfect symbiotic (both host and guest win) relationship. Cotton and paper are nearly 100 percent cellulose. Moths can digest cotton down to its glucose units, as some people find after storing clothes for a time. Experiments are being conducted on using microorganisms that consume newspaper to provide an eventual food source for people.[4]

Pectin is a formless substance that joins like a spiderweb and binds water molecules within its structure to give jellies and jams their gelatinlike texture. All fiber is valuable and better than no fiber at all.

Sources of Fiber

There is virtually no fiber in animal foods. Plant foods vary considerably in their fiber content. Whole grains (wheat, barley, oats, rice, corn, etc.) are

TABLE 6: Fiber Values of Various Foods
(Percent per 100 Grams Dry Matter)

	Insoluble*	Soluble+	Dietary Fiber	Crude Fiber
Fruits and Vegetables				
Apples‡	12	17	29	9
Cabbage	14	5	19	8
Carrots	9	19	28	6
Lettuce	17	4	21	12
Oranges‡	4	12	16	3
Potatoes‡	5	7	12	1
Squash	15	3	18	6
Grains				
Whole barley	27	tr	27	7
Whole corn	13	tr	13	3
Whole oats	31	tr	31	3
Whole wheat	14	tr	14	3
Corn bran	60	tr	60	14
Wheat bran	45	tr	45	11
Rice bran	24	tr	24	13

tr: trace amount
* hemicellulose, cellulose, lignin
+pectin
‡ peeled
Source: G.A. Spiller and S.G. Sorenson, "Dietary Fiber and Human Intestinal Microflora." In *Dietary Fiber: Proceedings of the Miles Symposium* (Nova Scotia, 1976).

high in fiber primarily from their outer bran coating. In the refining of grains, this outer coating is removed and leaves a food product with one-fourth or less the amount of dietary fiber. The same is true of fresh produce. The peels of apples and potatoes provide a significant amount of those foods' total fiber. By removing the peels, much fiber, vitamins, minerals, and time is wasted. Most armed forces groups have a predilection toward serving refined starchy foods. Imagine the time and health benefits if the mountains of wasted potato peels were left on.

The best sources of fiber are also the best sources of naturally occurring carbohydrates: fruits, vegetables, whole grains, and legumes. Nuts and seeds contain some fiber but are too high in fat to be considered valuable fiber sources.

TABLE 7: **Dietary Fiber in Selected Foods**
(Total Percent per 100 Grams)

Bran	48.0
Whole-wheat flour	11.7
Brown flour (90% extraction)	8.7
Peas	7.7
Carrots	3.7
White flour (72% extraction)	3.4
Cabbage	2.9
Pears	2.4
Strawberries	2.1
Bananas	1.8
Plums	1.5
Apples	1.4
Tomatoes	1.4

Source: Southgate, D.A.T., "The Definition and Analysis of Dietary Fiber," *Nutrition Reviews*, 35:31, 1977.

Flatulence

Here is another topic that is avoided by most nutrition books. Everyone produces some intestinal gas, with some people emitting up to three dozen flatus (farts) per day. Since food causes flatulence and dietary modification has proved to be the most effective treatment for excess flatulence,[5] the subject is worthy of discussion under the topic of nutrition.

Some families (about 30 percent of the population) have an inherited trait that encourages methane-producing bacteria in the intestines. In most other people, gas is produced either by swallowing air, through hasty eating and drinking, or by bacteria working on fiber and partially digestible foods in the intestines (especially the colon).

At high altitudes and changes in pressure, carbon dioxide leaves the blood, enters the intestines, and exits the body as flatulence. These have been some of the more unusual discoveries of mountain expeditions and space travel.

Partially digestible polysaccharides make up about 2 percent of diets on the average. These substances include raffinose, stachyose, inulin, galactogens, mannosans. They are found in beans, certain grains, nuts, and vegetables. People who have not been used to eating high-fiber foods, especially beans, will experience some flatulence. In a study that overloaded the hu-

man subjects with beans (56 percent of their calories), flatulence production rose elevenfold.[6] The partially digestible carbohydrates found in these
foods are consumed by bacteria in the gastrointestinal tract, yielding various
gases as by-products. This effect can be somewhat defused by soaking legumes in water overnight, then dumping out the water and cooking them as
usual. Or bring beans to a boil, let stand for one hour, then dump out water
and cook as usual. Also, when sprouted, beans and lentils become less flatu-
lence-producing.

The cruciferous vegetable family (broccoli, cabbage, cauliflower, Brussels sprouts) and dried apricots are high in sulfur. These can cause intestinal
discomfort along with a hydrogen sulfide rotten-egg smell in some people.
Lactose-intolerant individuals produce inordinate amounts of flatulence
when drinking milk. Yogurt prevents this problem. Flatulence has been
shown to be very individualized, and dietary records are extremely valuable
in locating the troublesome foods. If one slowly builds up a tolerance to
these various high-fiber foods, flatulence will be a minimal problem.

Studies have shown drug therapy to be of little value here.[7] Stress can increase flatulence by hurrying foods toward the colon, where the bacteria
thrive and produce gas. Fasting is an effective treatment for flatulence. It is
also very important to defecate when the urge strikes. Allowing feces to sit
in the colon creates the ideal conditions for flatulence-causing bacteria. Yogurt, kefir, and other live bacteria dairy products are usually very effective
in reducing flatulence.

After dietary modification, the next most effective treatment for flatulence is drinking a blended beverage containing activated charcoal (twenty
to fifty grams daily).[8]

Health Benefits of a High-Fiber Diet

A high-fiber diet will lower your risk for certain health problems.

1. Obesity is nearly nonexistent in societies with high-fiber intake. Fiber
foods slow the emptying rate of the stomach, which delays hunger pangs.[9]
Fiber has the capacity to fill you up, not out, which reduces the tendency to
overeat.[10] Certain fiber foods (guar gums and mucilage) reduce the appetite.[11] Seaweed, high in gum-type fibers, is a favorite of the rarely overweight Asians. High-fiber diets are extremely effective in maintaining an
ideal weight throughout life.

2. Heart disease would decrease merely by the reduction in obesity alone.
Add to that major benefit the value of lowering the amount of fat and cholesterol absorbed,[12] and the risk of cardiovascular ailments drops markedly.[13] Blood pressure is reduced when fiber intake is increased.[14]

3. Diabetes would be less severe in some people and nonexistent in others.[15] Dietary fiber helps to create a more gradual blood glucose curve. Most people feel better and are less likely to be labeled diabetic or hypoglycemic. Whole grains also contain significant amounts of chromium, while refined grain products contain almost none. Chromium is intimately related to the body's ability to metabolize glucose properly.

4. Cancer of the gastrointestinal tract would drop off markedly, since fiber absorbs various toxins and provides a daily soft brush to cleanse the intestines.[16] Cruciferous and green vegetables in general are particularly effective at this anticancer protection.[17] Beans and whole grains, with their phytate fiber, are also proven anticancer substances.[18]

Cancer elsewhere in the body would be much less likely because of the reduced absorption of fat, cholesterol, and toxins. Rats on a low-fiber diet were exposed to a variety of drugs and food additives that were acutely toxic; some died, many became ill. Similar rats fed a high-fiber diet and exposed to the same levels of toxins were unaffected.[19]

5. General nutritional deficiencies would diminish because high-fiber foods are also richer in vitamins and minerals.

6. Energy levels would be more stable and predictable. Pectin in fruits and vegetables slows the emptying rate of the stomach and helps stabilize blood sugar levels.[20] The incidence of hyperactivity in children, if related to hypoglycemia, and depression and temper tantrums would be reduced through a high-fiber diet. Many people would find a noticeable improvement in their mental and physical energy levels.

7. Gallstones would nearly disappear from physicians' worries if people ate adequate fiber.[21] Fiber binds cholesterol and carries it out of the digestive tract, thus forcing the body to convert more of its own cholesterol to bile salts. The gallbladder is charged with concentrating and storing these bile salts. A "constipation" of this cholesterol conversion to bile salts probably is one main cause of gallstones.

8. Gastrointestinal ailments would diminish throughout the population. Hemorrhoids are enlarged vessels in the anus caused by straining to defecate. The abrasion of hard feces against the delicate sphincter muscle then exacerbates the condition. These problems would almost disappear.[22] Cramps from constipation (a major nuisance in Western nations) would all but cease to exist on a high-fiber diet.[23] Children with high-fiber diets have half the risk of developing appendicitis.[24]

The average American has a 600 percent greater chance of developing cancer of the colon than his African counterpart. A low-fiber diet triples the risk for many types of diseases.[25] Many people take for granted that the "diseases of civilization" are here to stay, along with our satellite weather forecasts and microwave cookery. Not true. Humans evolved over millions of years as consumers of whole foods. Our systems are adjusted to this high-fiber intake. Given a few million years of living on refined low-fiber food, humans might evolve an intestinal tract more suited to our current low-fiber diet. But we don't think too many people will want to wait that long.

8

PROTEIN

—DUTCH CHEMIST MULDER UPON DISCOVERING PROTEIN IN 1838

About four and a half billion years ago the primordial soup of life was being stirred by winds, sun, and volcanic activity. It wasn't until carbon combined with nitrogen to form a primitive protein that life on earth began. Mulder's statement was not far off because protein is the essence of all forms of life. Millions of humans suffer and die from insufficient protein, while millions in affluent nations have proved that it is possible to consume excess protein. After water, protein is the most prevalent substance in the human body.

Functions of Protein

Structural. Tough, fibrous proteins become part of the body's support system of bones, muscles, teeth, tendons, cartilage, collagen and elastin connective tissue, hair, and nails. Protein is critical to wound healing.

Functional. Essential tasks in the chemical factory of the human body are performed by protein substances such as red blood cells to carry oxygen; hormones to do everything from providing sexual characteristics to regulating blood glucose; immunoglobins and antibodies to fight off disease-causing organisms; building blocks for DNA and RNA; lining of the intestinal tract so that the body does not digest itself; raw materials for vital brain chemicals; cysteine, which participates in DNA repair and slows aging.[1] Protein is also essential to enzyme production, fluid balance, maintaining proper pH balance, and energy (protein provides four carlories per gram).

Enzymes are essential to the human body. The body has substance A and wants to convert it to substance B. The laws of chemistry state that the only way to speed up the rate of a reaction is to either change the temperature, pressure, concentration of reactants, concentration of enzymes, alter the pH, or expose more surface area. Since the body depends on a steady state of most of these factors, it is enzymes that accelerate the rate of most reactions. Enzymes are primarily protein in nature, with some carrying a vitamin and/or mineral to enhance their effectiveness.

Fluid balance is a very important job for proteins. There is a tendency for nature to try to equalize the concentration of substances on each side of a membrane, a process called osmosis, which in the body is greatly dictated by the concentration of amino acid (protein) molecules in the blood. In osmosis, one of two things can occur: (1) the particles can move across the membrane and equalize; or (2) the fluid can move across the membrane until it dilutes the side with the heavier concentration of particles. Usually, the second option is the easiest, since not all particles can move with ease across membranes.

There is a slight gap, called the synapse, between all nerve cells, which is bridged by chemicals known as neurochemical transmitters. Tyrosine, an amino acid, is converted to dopamine or norepinephrine in the brain. Tryptophan, an essential amino acid is converted to serotonin in the brain. Serotonin, dopamine, and norepinephrine are vital "bridges" that allow nerve impulses to get from one nerve cell to another. They are derived from protein in the diet and are vital to normal thought, intellect, and emotions.

Protein Deficiency Symptoms

Since protein is found throughout the body and in most life processes, the results of protein deficiency are devastating. Infections become more common and sustained. Fatigue is likely. A shortage of red blood cells will create anemia. All structural proteins of hair, skin, nails, bones, muscles, and so on begin to deteriorate, since they are not being adequately repaired. The amino acid tyrosine provides material for the body to manufacture the pigment melanin. Lacking enough dietary protein, dark-skinned people can lose some skin pigmentation and even develop a red or orange tint to the hair. Confusion and irritability is the result of the brain's not receiving enough precursors for neurochemical transmitters. If the lining of the intestinal tract is not properly repaired, the protein-deficient victim is left with poor digestion and absorption. The role of hormones and enzymes in the body is so important that a protein deficiency here will surface more as general chaos within the body than as an easily identified set of symptoms. Some victims of the concentration camps of World War II reverted to a neutral gender—reduced breasts and hips in women and no sex drive—since their diet did not allow enough protein to maintain normal sex hormone production.

Without enough protein in the diet, fluid balance goes awry. Edema, or water retention, is common, resulting in the bloated belly of starving young children. In pregnancy, the bloating from protein deficiency may occur throughout the body.

The Building Blocks

Proteins are composed of smaller units called amino acids. There are approximately twenty-one amino acids found in nature. We say approximately because some amino acids have one or more slight variations, such as proline and hydroxyproline.

TABLE 8: Naturally Occurring Amino Acids

alanine	glutamine	phenylalnine+
arginine	glycine	proline
asparagine	histidine*	serine
aspartic acid	isoleucine+	threonine+
cysteine	leucine+	tryptophan+
cystine	lysine+	tyrosine
glumatic acid	methionine+	valine+

* Histidine is essential for infants and possibly for adults during illness.
+ Essential for all humans.

Table 8 shows that, of the twenty-one naturally-occurring amino acids, some are considered nonessential. This is somewhat misleading. Nonessential means that they are needed in the body but can be produced from the other essential amino acids found in the diet. Thus, all amino acids are essential in the body, yet some do not have to be in the diet.

The great diversity of life on earth is due to the limitless possible combinations of these twenty-one amino acids, known as the "alphabet of life." With at least five hundred amino acids found in any protein, nature can create an unending variety of proteins by varying the sequence of amino acids and changing the length of the protein. Thus, the same fundamental building blocks make up a gnat, a newt, a redwood tree, or a human being.

Quantity Versus Quality of Protein

Consider the body's needs for protein to be like a major construction site. Wood, nails, concrete, steel beams, and other supplies are shipped to the building site. If the building has been completed and there are few leftover parts, then the suppliers met the needs of the contractor. If there were not enough steel beams to finish the last two stories of a skyscraper, then the supply was not adequate for the needs and the project is in big trouble. Let us say that the body is trying to build a gathering of enzymes and it requires a certain collection of amino acids to finish the job. If a person's diet was not adequate in protein quantity or quality then there would not be enough of a given amino acid to complete the construction. There may not be enough nails or lumber available. The result would be a scrapped project, with the incomplete enzyme's being broken down and probably used for fuel.

Protein quality is based upon how well the amino acids in the food match the needs of the human body. Generally speaking, animal proteins are higher in quality than plant proteins because they provide the right amino acids in the right ratio. There are exceptions, and there are ways vegetarians can create their own high-quality proteins by properly combining lower quality proteins.

Vegetarians

For financial, religious, philosophical, and health reasons, the ranks of vegetarians are swelling rapidly. There are various types of vegetarians: the *vegan* consumes no animal tissue at all; the *lacto-vegetarian* consumes plant food plus milk and other dairy products; the *lacto-ovo-vegetarian* consumes plant food plus milk and egg products; those who have given up red meat.

There are some nutrients the vegetarian does not consume as readily as the nonvegetarian.

Vitamin B_{12}, even for the strict vegan, is available from tempeh, miso (both fermented soy products), B_{12}-fortified brewer's yeast, spirulina, and certain seaweeds.

Vitamin D deficiency (rickets) is more common among strict vegetarians,[2] especially children who do not consume vitamin-D-fortified milk. Fifteen to thirty minutes of daily exposure to sunshine can provide the body with adequate vitamin D if sun conditions are right. Fish liver oil tablets are highly recommended as vitamin D insurance for strict vegans.

Iron is more concentrated and more available from animal sources, yet the vegetarian can get iron from seaweed, cream of wheat, spinach, prunes, raisins, and asparagus. Researchers were startled to find no anemia among a group of lacto-ovo-vegetarians, even though their dietary iron intake was low.[3] Using cast iron cookware can easily double the iron intake.

Zinc, though normally associated with animal foods, is also found in wheat germ, bran, oatmeal, nuts, peas, and carrots.

Vitamin B_6 is found in higher levels in animal foods, yet one of its richest sources is soybeans, with bananas, lima and other beans, avocados, and nuts also containing some B_6.

There is no carnitine in a vegetarian diet. Though the body makes some from lysine, carnitine is essential for fat burning. See the chapter on quasivitamins for more on carnitine.

There is less eicosapentanoic acid (EPA, from fish oil) in a vegetarian diet. Notable exceptions to this role include spirulina (ocean algae) and purslane (a salad vegetable common in Mediterranean countries). Some scientists consider EPA to be essential to the human body.

There are numerous advantages to the vegetarian diet. High protein plant foods include grains, legumes, nuts, and seeds, which are:

1. Cheaper. Steak is twenty-four times the cost of soybeans.
2. Lower in fat; contains no cholesterol.
3. Higher in polyunsaturated fats and the essential fatty acid.
4. Higher in fiber and complex carbohydrates.
5. Lower in phosphorus.
6. Higher in potassium.
7. More efficient. Easier to digest. Foods are less bulky, easier to store, have longer shelf life, and are tasty when properly prepared.
8. Significant health and longevity benefits. As the intake of plant protein increases, heart disease risk goes down.[4] The vegetarian is less likely to have high blood pressure,[5] and has a lower risk of cancer.[6] Vegetarians have a lower percent body fat.[7] Meat eaters suffer a higher rate of colon cancer.[8] Vegetarianism actually helps to promote bone density.[9] Vegetarian women were found to have a much lower incidence of gallstones than meat eaters.[10] Vegetarian men were found to have a lower risk for prostate cancer.[11] Vegetarians are at half the normal risk for becoming diabetics.[12] Almost as impressive was the fact that diabetic vegetarians were at a much lower risk for dying from a diabetes-related ailment.

Basically, vegetarians need not worry about malnutrition if they are nutrition-wise. While meat-eating consumers can often haphazardly stumble across most of the nutrients they need, the vegetarian must actively plan a balanced diet to avoid potential health pitfalls.

Protein can easily be obtained even in the strict vegan diet as long as the vegetarian is intelligent in matching complementary proteins to insure adequate quality of protein. This is especially critical for the pregnant woman and growing child.

Complementary Proteins

By matching the right combination of proteins, the deficit of one is compensated for by the excess of the other. In other words, there is a synergistic relationship in which one plus one equals three. Grains are inherently low in lysine yet have a surplus of methionine. Legumes are usually low in methionine yet have a surplus of lysine. Matching the two results in a protein of similar quality to that of steak.

Protein enhancement is most commonly achieved by combining:

1. Grains (corn, wheat, amaranth, rye, millet, quinoa, rice, oats, barley) with legumes (soybeans, lentils, split peas, garbanzo beans, navy beans, pinto beans, peanuts).

2. Grains with nuts or seeds (walnuts, pecans, cashews, sesame seeds).

3. High-quality (meat, fish, poultry, eggs, or dairy foods) with medium-quality proteins (grains, nuts, seeds, legumes). Milk or eggs will complement virtually any protein.

Various societies around the world have developed some rather creative means of combining complementary proteins. Small amounts of meat on large amounts of grains and vegetables are common in the Orient and satisfy method three. Tortillas and beans from Mexico are a classic example of method one. Tahini (sesame seed spread) on rice cakes satisfies method two. Milk on cereal, cheese on wheat (pizza), and chili beans on cornbread are more of the unending array of high-quality proteins with little to no animal protein.

Protein Requirements

Protein needs are based on growth and repair requirements. Therefore, pregnant and lactating women, growing infants and children, and recuperating burn and surgery patients have very high needs. People under stress have high needs, due to poor absorption and higher protein loss. There is also growing evidence that protein requirements for the older adult should be higher.[13] In order to calculate daily protein needs in grams for an average healthy person, multiply body weight (in pounds) by:

newborns (0-½ year)	1.0
infants (½-1 year)	0.9
young children (1-3 years)	0.8
children (4-10 years)	0.5
early teens (11-14 years)	0.45
later teens (15-18 years)	0.4
adults (19 and up)	0.36
for pregnancy	add 30 grams/day
for lactation	add 20 grams/day

There is a great diversity in the efficiency of protein use. Some people could get along with half of these amounts, while a few may not be adequately nourished at this level. These numbers are designed to cover almost all healthy individuals.

Protein Excess

Excess protein will stress the liver and kidneys, since these are the organs that must process any extra protein. The body has a minimal capacity to store protein, so any extra can be converted to fat or excreted. Too much protein in the diet can be stored as fat, thus creating weight problems and the many complications of being overfat. Excess protein also causes calcium to be lost from the bones. Protein excess is common in the U.S. and may be partly responsible for the abudance of osteoporosis victims. High-protein diets cause zinc to be lost in the urine.[14]

Daily Protein Intake

Recommended: Depending on age, sex, weight, and other physiological factors, most normal healthy adults require 45 to 76 grams per day.

Senate dietary goals: Protein (at 4 calories per gram) should constitute about 12 percent of your total daily calories. About half of this protein should be from animal sources and the other half from plant sources.

Supplemental: For the older adult, pregnant and lactating woman, surgery or burn patient, and occasionally for the serious athlete, another 20 to 60 grams per day of protein could be essential.

Toxicity: More than 100 grams per day may induce calcium loss from the bones. Even for the special cases listed above, no more than 150 grams per day of protein should be consumed.

Recommendations

Since there are advantages in vegetarianism yet certain unique contributions made by animal products, we recommend a quasi-vegetarian diet. Make plant products the bulk of your diet, with animal products used in smaller quantities. Some cheese on your bean burrito, some meat on your spaghetti, some fish on your rice and vegetables, some chicken in your soup. Mankind has evolved as an omnivorous creature (eating a little of everything) and there seem to be good reasons for eating this way. Yet if you choose vegetarianism, do so with an intelligent plan in mind.

9
FATS

"I saw few die of hunger; of eating, a hundred thousand."
—BENJAMIN FRANKLIN, 1736

Fat is an amazing substance. It is such a lightweight and concentrated energy source that the average adult would weigh 130 pounds more if all their calories were stored as carbohydrates (glycogen) rather than fat. Without fat as a flotation device, muscular people sink in the water. Fat makes living in cold climates tolerable. Eskimos even have fat pads over their eyelids. Fat padding in the chest and stomach region allows delicate organs to be protected against minor bumps. Without fat, your food would taste bland and your fat-soluble vitamins would be poorly absorbed. You also would not have the raw materials to make some very important substances in your body called prostaglandins. There is a definite need for fat.

Yet, if you consume too much fat, or the wrong kind of fat, or not enough nutrients that allow your body to properly deal with the fat, then fat could be your health downfall. More Americans die each year from cardiovascular disease than all Americans lost in all of our wars combined. High-fat diets are also major contributors to corpulence in the United States.[1] Cancer, arthritis, and osteoporosis may be at least partly induced by high-fat diets. It is important to realize that fat in the diet does not necessarily have to end up as fat in the body.

TABLE 9: Functions of Fat

In the Body	In the Diet
energy storage	concentrated energy source; fat has
buoyancy; fat floats	more than twice the calorie value
organ padding, protects delicate	of carbohydrates or protein
internal parts	absorption of fat-soluble vitamins
insulation, prevents heat	(A, D, E, K)
loss	essential fatty acid
	satiety: flavor; slows digestion to
	delay hunger pangs

What Is Fat?

Fats are a group of substances containing carbon, hydrogen, and oxygen that can be dissolved in solvents like ether and alcohol. Of all the fatty substances, 93 percent are triglycerides (normal dietary fats), 6 percent are phospholipids (including lecithin), and the remainder are composed of cholesterol, sphingomyelins, glycolipids, and others. Of these, we will spend some time elaborating on triglycerides, cholesterol, and lecithin. Lecithin is also discussed in the chapter on quasi-vitamins.

Triglycerides

Triglycerides (normal fat found in the diet) are composed of saturated and unsaturated fats. The greater the unsaturation the more liquid (low viscosity) the fat becomes. Corn and linseed oil are highly unsaturated, and thus do not harden even when placed in the refrigerator. But olive oil, which is low in unsaturated bonds, will become very thick when cooled.

Polyunsaturated fats (which has more unsaturated areas on its atoms) have a tendency to grab onto destructive substances. Vitamin E and selenium can prevent this "lipid rancidity" or "bad fat" situation from occurring, therefore the higher your intake of polyunsaturated fats, the higher your intake of vitamin E and selenium should be. Fortunately, the richest sources of vitamin E are also some of the richest sources of polyunsaturated fats, like safflower, cottonseed, and wheat germ oil. Unfortunately, many of these oils are heat processed. Steam heats up oils and allows the food manufacturer to extract more fat from corn, soy, safflower, and the like. This heat also destroys some of the vitamin E. Cold pressed oils, though more expensive, are higher in vitamin E than commercial oils.

Polyunsaturated fats can lower heart disease risk. Yet, once again, more is not always better. Studies have found a higher incidence of cancer in areas where overall fat intake is low but intake of polyunsaturated fats is high.[2] At high intake levels or if unprotected by various antioxidants, they are more vulnerable to lipid peroxidation, which can be the beginning of a cancerous growth.

Polyunsaturated fats are found in higher levels in plant oils (except coconut and palm oil). Saturated fats are higher in animal fats, with poultry and fish oils having decent levels of unsaturated fats. All fats are mixed, with some polyunsaturated fatty acids, some monounsaturated, and some saturated; it is the percentage of each that is critical. A ratio of 1 to 1 to 1 is considered ideal according to the Senate Diet Goals. We currently have a fatty intake ratio of 1 to 3 to 2.

TABLE 10: Relative Content of Fatty Acids in Selected Foods

More saturated fatty acids ↑	beef tallow lard poultry fat egg yolk fat butterfat fish fat and oil peanut oil soybean oil cottonseed oil corn oil safflower oil	↓ More unsaturated fatty acids

TABLE 11: Fatty Acid Composition of Selected Foods

		Fatty Acid Percentage		
	Total Fat	Sat.	Monounsat.	PUFA
Salad and cooking oils				
Safflower	100%	10%	13%	74%
Sunflower	100	11	14	70
Corn	100	13	26	55
Cottonseed	100	23	17	54
Soybean	100	14	25	50
Sesame	100	14	38	42
Peanut	100	18	47	29
Olive	100	11	76	7
Coconut	100	80	5	1
Vegetable fats				
Shortening	100	23	23	6-23
Margarine				
Safflower	80	11	18	48
Corn oil (tub)	80	14	26	38
Corn oil (stick)	80	15	33	29
Partially hardened or				
hydrogenated fat	80	17	44	14
Butter	81	46	27	2
Animal fats				
Poultry	100	30	40	20
Beef, lamb, pork	100	45	44	2-6

Fish, raw				
Salmon	9	2	2	4
Tuna	5	2	1	2
Mackerel	13	5	3	4
Herring, Pacific	13	4	2	3
Nuts				
Walnuts, English	64	4	10	40
Walnuts, black	60	4	21	28
Brazil	67	13	32	17
Peanuts or Peanut butter	51	9	25	14
Pecan	65	4-6	33-48	9-24
Egg yolk	31	10	13	2
Avocado	16	3	7	2

Note: Total is not expected to equal "total fat."
sat. = saturated; monounsat. = monounsaturated; PUFA = polyunsaturated fatty acids.
Source: *Fats in Food and Diet*. Agriculture Information Bulletin no. 362. Washington, D.C.: U.S. Department of Agriculture, 1974.

The Essential Fatty Acid

Most fats consumed by the body are stored as fuel reserves or burned immediately for energy requirements. Some fats are incorporated into the cell membranes or become specialized fats in the brain, reproductive organs, or lens of the eye. Your body uses the raw materials of linoleic acid to build prostaglandins and other essential substances, which is why linoleic acid is called the essential fatty acid. Most authorities now agree that linolenic acid is also an essential dietary fat. Current recommendations state that 1 to 2 percent of total calories from linoleic acid are enough to satisfy the body's requirements. Since these are based on the absence of disease symptoms, it could be that this mere three to six grams per day of linoleic acid is a low estimate. People with high blood pressure have been successfully treated with gamma linolenic acid.[3] This indicates that the requirements for linoleic acid may be understated for some people or that the true effect of this fatty acid is only beginning to be felt. Fish oil (EPA, or eiosapentanoic acid, a special omega-3 fat), docosahexanoic acid (DHA), and gamma linolenic acid (GLA, or evening primrose oil) are fascinating and new subjects in the field of nutrition. They are all more thoroughly discussed in the chapter on quasi-vitamins.

Hydrogenated Fats

Plant oils are usually liquid at room temperature. This liquid state, plus their vulnerability to rancidity, plagued food manufacturers. Food technologists solved the problems with a process known as hydrogenation, in which hydrogen atoms are catalytically added to a fat to make it more saturated. The food technologist can even carefully control the degree of saturation, thus shaping the viscosity and shelf life of the fat. It was a technological achievement for food merchants that offered an inexpensive alternative to the more costly butter fats. Then, when scientific studies found that there were health benefits to eating plants oils as well, the margarine market grew.

But evidence is gathering that these fats may be more harmful than the saturated animal fats they were intended to replace. The newly created fats pose a unique dilemma for the body. Hydrogenated fats impair the liver's ability to create other essential fats.[4] The essential fatty acid is used to make important fat substances including cell membranes and prostaglandins. The trans fatty acids from hydrogenation are similar enough to be incorporated into the body like a normal fat but do not have the exact chemical properties.[5] The body has been fooled.

Hydrogenated fats raise the levels of serum lipids.[6] Indeed, the hydrogenated fats in these margarines and many other foods are probably a greater risk for heart disease.[7] Since the type of fat in the diet will dictate the fat to be found in mother's milk, lactating women should minimize intake of hydrogenated fats.

Sixty percent of the fats consumed in this country have been either partially or totally hydrogenated.[8] This is worthy of concern. We suggest that you seriously limit your intake of hydrogenated fats and choose your margarine/butter in the following order of preference:

BEST: tub margarine—minimal hydrogenation, high polyunsaturation.

OKAY: butter—higher in saturated fats but has no questionable trans fatty acids.

WORST: stick margarine—usually highly hydrogenated or uses coconut oil (more saturated than beef lard, yet still considered a vegetable oil).

Cholesterol

Cholesterol is truly one of the more versatile and important substances in the human body. It is also a lethal weapon when deposited along the blood vessel walls. The average diet in the West contains about 600 milligrams of cholesterol per day, with most of it coming from red meat. Recommendations are to reduce cholesterol intake to 300 milligrams per day. Dietary cholesterol relates to blood levels of cholesterol. Yet the human body manufactures far more cholesterol than most people consume—up to 2,000 milligrams each day, the same amount found in eight egg yolks. So the problem of cholesterol-clogged arteries is more involved than just avoiding cholesterol in the diet.

Functions of Cholesterol in the Body

1. It provides the raw materials to build bile salts for fat digestion.
2. When exposed to sunshine on the skin, cholesterol is converted into vitamin D, which is involved in calcium and magnesium use.
3. The fatty wrapping around the 10 billion nerve cells in the body is primarily made up of cholesterol. It makes sense that egg yolks (soon to become the central nervous system of the chicken) and brains (a dietary delicacy in some cultures) are rich in this electrical insulator.
4. It is a precursor to build the sex hormones estrogen (female) and testosterone (male).
5. It is involved throughout the body in all cell membranes.

TABLE 12: Dietary Sources of Cholesterol

1 egg or egg yolk	274 mg
cream	20 mg per fluid ounce
milk, whole	33 mg per cup
cheese	30 mg per ounce
beef, pork, poultry, lobster	75 mg per 3 ounces
shrimp	130 mg per 3 ounces
heart	230 mg per 3 ounces
liver	370 mg per 3 ounces
kidney	680 mg per 3 ounces
brains	1,700 mg per 3 ounces

Note: These are all animal foods; there is no cholesterol in plant foods.

Cholesterol and Disease

A high-cholesterol diet increases the risk for various types of cancer, especially of the colon.[9] Fiber in the diet significantly lowers these risks. The more cholesterol there is in the diet, the higher the cholesterol levels are in the blood.[10]

Cholesterol, as do all other nonwater soluble substances in the body, requires an escort to be carried in the blood. Lipoproteins (composed of part fat and part protein) serve this purpose. Apparently, the more cholesterol that is carried by high-density lipoproteins (HDL), the less likely one is to develop heart disease. The HDLs seem to prevent the cholesterol from creating fatty roadblocks. Several factors have been shown to improve one's HDL levels: exercise, meditation and other relaxation forms, small amounts of alcohol daily, daily garlic intake, one or more of the vitamins and minerals.

Lecithin

Lecithin is somewhat like a soap because it can dissolve in both fat- and water-soluble agents at the same time. For this reason, it is used to keep the fat from separating out of solution in many food products on your grocer's shelves. Lecithin is a natural emulsifier in egg yolk. The fatty acids in lecithin can be as diverse as the other fatty acids in your diet, and of varying degrees of saturation. Basically, lecithin in egg yolk has saturated fatty acids, while lecithin from soybean contains primarily polyunsaturated fatty acids. This difference is significant. Lecithin from soy has been shown to lower serum cholesterol levels,[11] while the lecithin from egg yolk will not.

Lecithin contains choline, which is discussed later as a quasi-vitamin.

Like any other fat, lecithin contains calories and therefore should not be consumed excessively. It is the primary ingredient in the low-calorie frying fats found in aerosol cans.

Lecithin is sold as small yellow granules, a translucent thick liquid, or in gelatin capsules of the liquid. One capsule or one tablespoon of granules contains about 1,200 milligrams of lecithin. One or two tablespoons of granular lecithin mixed with yogurt, apple sauce, pudding, or bread may be of some health value to many individuals.

Sources of Dietary Fat

Table 13 helps illustrate where we get our fat. Food groups that are high in fat include:

fats and oils, margarine, butter, mayonnaise;
nuts and seeds;
beef, especially hamburger, franks, bologna, prime rib;
dairy products, particularly cream, ice cream, whole milk;
added fat, such as fried foods, pastries, and fat in recipes.

TABLE 13: Percentage of Fat Calories in Food

75% or More

Avocado
Bacon
Beef—choice chuck, rib, sirloin, loin
   untrimmed, hamburger (regular)
Coconut
Cold cuts—bologna, salami
Coleslaw
Cream—heavy, light, half-and-half,
   sour
Cream cheese

Frankfurters
Headcheese
Nuts
Olives
Peanut butter
Pork—sausage, spareribs, butt,
   loin, ham (untrimmed)
Salt pork
Seeds—pumpkin, sesame
sunflower

50% to 75%

Beef—rump, corned
Cake, pound
Canadian bacon
Cheese—blue, cheddar, American,
   Swiss, etc.
Chicken, roasted with skin
Chocolate candy
Cream soups
Eggs
Ice cream (rich)

Lake trout
Lamb chops, rib
Oysters, fried
Perch, fried
Pork—ham, loin, shoulder
   (trimmed lean cuts)
Tuna with oil
Tuna salad
Veal salad

40% to 50%

Beef—T-bone (lean), hamburger (lean)
Cake, devil's food with chocolate icing
Chicken, fried
Ice cream (regular)
Mackerel
Milk, whole

Pumpkin pie
Rabbit, stewed
Salmon, canned
Sardines (drained)
Turkey pot pie
Yogurt (whole milk)

30% to 40%

Beef—flank steak, chuck, pot roast
   (lean)
Cake—yellow, white (without icing)
Chicken, roasted without skin
Cottage cheese, creamed
Fish—flounder, haddock (fried),
   halibut (broiled)
Granola

Milk, 2% fat
Pizza
Seafood—scallops and shrimp
   (breaded and fried)
Soups—bean with pork
Tuna in oil (drained)
Turkey, roasted dark meat
Yogurt (low fat)
Ice milk

20% to 30%

Beef—sirloin (lean only)
Corn muffin
Fish—cod (broiled)
Liver
Oysters, raw

Pancakes
Shake, thick
Soups—chicken noodle,
tomato, vegetable
Wheat germ

Less than 20%

Beans—peas, lentils
Bread
Buttermilk
Cabbage, boiled
Cake—angel food, sponge
Cereals—breakfast (except granola)
Cottage cheese, uncreamed
Fish—ocean perch (broiled)
Frozen yogurt
Fruits

Grains
Milk, skim
Seafood—scallops and shrimp
(steamed or boiled)
Soups—split pea, bouillon,
consommé
Tuna in water
Turkey, roasted white meat
Vegetables

Digestion and Absorption of Fats

Fats do not dissolve in water. Were it not for a complex series of enzymes and bile salts, fat would sit in your intestines like an oil slick on a lake. Among protein, fat, and carbohydrates, fats are the most complicated to digest. Most of the digestion occurs in the small intestine, where the fatty acids are emulsified (broken up into smaller globules) with bile salts so that more of their surface area is exposed. They then move toward the walls of the intestines to be absorbed into the lymph system. Once they have passed through the intestinal mucosa, these fatty acids are coated with a thin layer of protein to make them slightly water soluble and carried through the lymph to the thoracic duct (near the left shoulder), where they are dumped into the blood, then used by the body in a number of ways.

Fat lingers the longest of all macronutrients in the stomach, staying perhaps three and a half hours before being emptied into the intestines. This delayed stomach emptying is valuable in preventing frequent hunger pangs. Total fat digestion time could be a day or more, varying considerably with the health of an individual's digestive tract and the quantity of fiber ingested. A healthy person will absorb about 95 percent of the fat consumed.

Once fat is absorbed, it performs a number of functions in the body. It is (1) used immediately for energy by muscle and other cells (beta oxidation);

(2) stored in fat cells for later use (lipogenesis); (3) made part of the structure of cells, like the cell membrane (structural anabolism); (4) used in the making of vital compounds, such as prostaglandins (functional anabolism), which help regulate maternal labor contractions, nerve transmissions, blood pressure, and smooth muscle contraction.

Fat Deficiency Symptoms

The absence of the essential fatty acid will produce symptoms of poor growth, skin problems (dermatitis), and failure of the reproductive glands. As often happens in nutrition, these deficiency symptoms were discovered in patients on long-term parenteral (other than by mouth) feedings. Tube feedings are often grossly inadequate nourishment for someone too sick to eat.

Fats for Fuel

Beyond the small amount of essential fatty acid required by the body, the primary need for fat is in its incredible energy value: 9 calories per gram. This is more than twice the calorie density of carbohydrates or proteins. Thus, fat becomes essential for active people and growing children to obtain enough calories to sustain life processes. There are individuals who are so active in their athletic training that their 10,000-calorie-per-day needs must be met by occasionally dipping a spoon into the peanut butter jar. Growing children present a similar problem. With their high-calorie demands, small stomachs and whimsical appetites, fat in the diet becomes a vital energy need.

It is in the sedentary individual that fat becomes a problem. It is not necessarily the fat consumed that does people so much harm but the fat that is left over in the body and blood vessels that can be the saboteur from within. If you eat fat, you had best burn it in exercise. Also, as we age, naturally elevated blood fat means that fat consumption should be reduced. The heart is a unique organ since it prefers to burn fats rather than carbohydrates like the rest of the body. With this constant flow of fats to the vessels of the heart, a high-fat diet becomes a tightrope walk for many sedentary and stress-prone people.

Carnitine is a substance critical for the burning of fats anywhere in the body. It can be consumed in the diet or made internally with the raw materials of lysine, methionine (both amino acids), vitamins C, B_6, niacin, and iron. Carnitine is a shuttle system to allow fats to get into the "furnace" of the cell to be burned. Without it, fat oxidation can be very inefficient. There is more on carnitine in the chapter on quasi-vitamins.

Inefficient burning of fats could lead to a buildup of ketone bodies. Ketosis is common in diabetics and fasting individuals.

It has been well established that calories from fat are more likely than carbohydrates and proteins to end up being stored as fat.[12]

Fat and Disease

A thrombus is a gathering of blood elements, including platelets and fibrin (a clotting agent), which often causes obstruction in a blood vessel. If your blood cells clump together, they may form a clot. The clot will start gathering fat, which will block off blood flow to some area of the body. There are two different and somewhat antagonistic substances your body can make that help determine whether your blood forms clots or not. Table 14 shows some of the factors that encourage either thromboxane (the villain) or prostacyclin (the hero). These are but a few of the known players in this extremely complex game of heart disease.

TABLE 14: Nutrient Factors That Affect Heart Disease Risk

Thromboxane—aggregatory, clotting tendency; vascular problems	Prostacyclin—antithrombotic, prevents vascular problems
high-fat diet	eicosapentanoic acid
saturated fats	gamma linolenic acid
smoking	polyunsaturated fats
	selenium
	vitamins C and E

Fat is also involved in the incidence of cancer, especially of the breast and colon.[13] Women with the highest intake of eggs (cholesterol) or fried foods (fat) had three times the risk for cancer of the ovaries.[14] Fat also may be an irritant in arthritis.

Recommendations

As you can see, the subject of fats in the diet is one of great complexity. Fats are essential in the diet. Yet consuming too much or the wrong kind can lead to serious health problems, especially in sedentary and overweight individuals. These people should take adequate fish and vegetable oils and enough vitamin E and selenium for protection. On the basis of abundant data, we can make several valuable recommendations to improve your health:

1. Eat less fat from all sources. Cut your intake in half if possible.

2. Of the fat that you do consume, eat more polyunsaturated fats and less saturated animal fats.

3. Avoid hydrogenated fats. The more solid in texture the fat is, the more it has been hydrogenated.

4. Add vitamin E (100 to 400 IU per day) and selenium (200 micrograms daily) to your diet in food or supplement form to help prevent these polyunsaturated fats from free radical destruction.

5. Select fats in the following order of preference:
   Best—sunflower, safflower, corn, soy, cottonseed, olive, and fish oils.
   Acceptable—peanut oil, fat from poultry and nuts.
   Worst—coconut and hydrogenated oils; lard, bacon, beef, lamb, or pork drippings.

6. Avoid fatty parts of meat and poultry (marbling, skin, etc.). Since most pesticides, hormones, drugs, and other toxic substances are fat soluble, these end up in the fatty tissue of the animal.

7. Once again nutrition is a quest for balance. While excess saturated fats may provoke heart disease, excess polyunsaturated fats may provoke cancer. Do not overconsume either type of fat.

10

WATER

"We've got to do something about water pollution. My kid has a water pistol that jams!"

—ROBERT ORBEN

Two-thirds of your body weight is water. It is the essence of life, and yet few people think of water as an essential nutrient. And there is overwhelming evidence that our water supply is not only dwindling but suspiciously tainted. With the average adult body containing forty to fifty quarts of water, there is indeed much to discuss here.

Functions of Water in the Human Body

1. Provides structure. Seventy-five percent of the muscles and 22 percent of the bones are water.

2. Cushioning. Much of the padding for delicate internal organs is provided by water. Your brain and spinal cord are bathed in a water medium to protect them from shock.

3. Medium for bodily fluids. Eighty-three percent of blood is water. Blood is the "river of life," carrying nutrients to the cells and bringing waste products from them. Nearly all substances in the human body that are not water soluble must have an "escort" in the blood. Lipoproteins escort cholesterol and fats, retinol binding protein (RBP) escorts vitamin A, and transcobalamin carries vitamin B_{12}. Much of the cellular fluid inside and outside the cells is water.

4. Solvent. Most substances in the body dissolve readily in water.

5. Reactant. The digestion of foods inserts molecules of water to split large complex substances into smaller, more usable parts for absorption.

6. Product of energy metabolism. When protein, alcohol, fats or carbohydrates are metabolized in the body, water is the final product. Upon being burned, fats produce more than their own weight in water. This is how the camel's fatty hump provides substantial water for transdesert caravans.

7. Dilutes waste matter. When the body removes a nitrogen group from an amino acid, the ammonia formed is a highly toxic water-soluble gas. One microgram (one billionth of a kilogram) in one liter (about a quart) of blood can kill a person. The diluting power of water keeps us alive amidst this and other deadly toxins. The diabetic excretes large amounts of water in the urine as the body tries to dilute the excess sugar being removed from the blood by the kidneys.

8. Regulates body temperature. The body needs to maintain a constant internal temperature at or very near 98.6⁰ F. Water, through heat retention in the body, and through its cooling effect as sweat evaporates, does a magnificent job of holding body temperature constant. We sweat constantly (insensible). Sometimes sweat becomes noticeable (sensible). Sweat is excreted through skin pores to lower the body temperature through evaporation. It is during the cooler parts of the year that people usually find themselves urinating more often. Urine, rather than sweat, becomes the route for the body to expel unwanted fluid. The lungs also lose a considerable amount of body water.

9. Provides lubrication. Your bone joints are lubricated by synovial fluid, a substance so slippery that even space technology cannot surpass its lubrication qualities. Swallowing food is easier because mucous and saliva "grease" the esophagus. Eyes move easily in their sockets from the lubrication of tears. All of these fluids are primarily water.

10. Provides traction. Small amounts of sweat on the fingertips provide a much better grip, as when people lick their fingertips when thumbing through a phone book.

11. Protects exposed areas of the body. There are nine avenues through which invading microorganisms can enter your body. Mucous and tears help keep these areas free from infection, dust, and debris; thanks to water.

12. Keeps the body neutral. Proper acid/base balance in the body is close to neutral (pH of 7). Water is neutral and thus keeps this critical acid/base balance in check.

The Thirst Mechanism

When your body has lost a certain amount of fluid, the blood draws on its fluid reserves, including saliva. This makes the mouth feel dry and causes thirst. Also, when the blood becomes salty from fluid loss, the brain reacts to encourage fluid intake through the thirst mechanism. Unless you are losing fluid at a rapid rate, the thirst drive will keep you from dying of dehydration as long as fluid is available. But thirst does not always maintain ideal fluid levels in the body. Some dehydrated people do not experience thirst,

TABLE 15: Sources of Daily Intake and Output of Water
(In Milliliters)

Intake		
drinking fluids (water, soup, etc.)		500-2,000
water in solid foods (fruits and vegetables are up to 90 percent water)		600-1,200
metabolic water (produced internally)		300-400
	Total (average)	2,000-2,500
Output and Loss		
urine		400-2,000
feces		80-200
water vapor from lungs		300-600
visible sweat		0-2,000
insensible sweat		300-500
	Total (average)	2,000-2,500

perhaps because their bodies have adapted to low fluid levels. Yet these people can have many of the symptoms of dehydration, including dry skin, constipation, and muddled thinking. New data shows that animals exposed to air pollution drink less fluid because of the reduced effectiveness of their thirst mechanism. It is necessary for many people to make a concerted effort to drink five to ten glasses of clean fluids daily to maintain optimal body fluid content.

However, in spite of the incredible value of high fluid intake, you can even overdose on water. One woman was told to drink fluids before a medical test. She thought more would also be better. After thirty glasses of water she was delirious and nearly died from overdiluting her body's electrolyte solution.[1]

Water Deficiency

Only a few days without water is enough to kill most people. A large adult working briskly in a hot dry sunny climate could lose ten quarts of water in one day. Without regular fluid replenishment, this person could die before the day is out. Athletes are at serious risk for water deficiency. A half dozen high school football players die each year from dehydration as the myth continues among some coaches that withholding fluid from players makes them tougher. Many amateur athletes risk death or injury when working out on hot days without regular water intake. More on this subject in the chapter on athletes.

Given all the critical functions of water in the body, deficiency symptoms become equally extensive and impressive. Early sub-clinical symptoms are lowered disease resistance, confusion, weakness, dry skin, constipation, dry mucous membranes, and low blood pressure.

Later clinical symptoms are cramps, heat retention, and rapid heart beat. Heat exhaustion incorporates weakness, cramps, and serious disorientation. Heat stroke involves the inability to sweat, shock, unconsciousness, bluish lips and fingertips, rapid and shallow breathing and other life-threatening symptoms. People suffering heat stroke need to be cooled and hydrated immediately.[2]

Water Quality

More than 300 different organic chemicals have been found in the municipal drinking water in the United States, of which 22 have been found to cause cancer.[3] Lake Erie near Cleveland and the Columbia River near Portland were known to catch fire in the 1970s. Small towns in Missouri and New England have recently been evacuated because their underground water supplies contained everything from dioxin to gasoline. In 1982, seven of the twelve municipal wells in Atlantic City, New Jersey, were closed because of a nearby toxic dump site.[4] Nine million gallons of PCB, arsenic, and other deadly chemicals had been haphazardly poured into pits, from which they seeped into the well water. Each year American industry produces 90 billion pounds of toxic waste, most of which is irresponsibly disposed of. In 1980, the Surgeon General's office called the toxic waste mess an environmental emergency. The Environmental Protection Agency called it "a ticking time bomb, ready to go off."[5]

In addition to chemicals, there are dozens of bacteria that commonly inhabit water supplies throughout the world. Prior to 1908, there were numerous outbreaks in the United States of typhoid, dysentery, cholera, and other water-borne diseases. In 1908, Jersey City, New Jersey, was the first to add chlorine to the municipal water supply in 1908 to seriously slow down these deadly diseases. A recent nationwide survey found that most cities do not test their water often enough for contamination, and about 10 percent of those that do test find their water exceeds federal standards for bacteria count.

The chlorine that is added to city water supplies combines with other pollutants to create chloroform, which is potentially a cancer-causing substance. The Environmental Protection Agency has found that death from colon cancer is far more common in people exposed to chlorinated water for twenty years or more.[6] Chlorine is bleach. If you have ever accidently touched bleach and found your skin dead and peeling within days, then you have an appreciation of its lethal effect.

In 1974, New Orleans's water was found to have liberal amounts of numerous dangerous and cancer-causing agents. Trihalomethanes (including chloroform and carbon tetrachloride) are a group of potent by-products from the interraction of chlorine with other pollutants. Not surprisingly, New Orleans residents have a higher incidence of various types of kidney, bladder, and urinary tract cancer. These are the areas of the body trying to purge the system of these potent toxins. Surely some people who have inexplicably encountered certain diseases may have the water to blame. Yet how pure should tap water be when about 95 percent of it is used to cool industrial machines, water lawns, and wash cars? Perhaps we should separate drinking water from water for industry and agriculture.

Other problems with water pollution include:

Cadmium (dangerous to heart and blood pressure) from galvanized pipes.

Lead from auto exhaust, lead-soldered water pipes, and industrial pollution.

Mercury from industry.

Nitrates (from agricultural fertilizers), which turn into nitrosamines in the stomach and are carcinogenic. The San Joaquin Valley in California must post signs on public drinking fountains warning children and pregnant women to avoid the water because of its high nitrate content.

Asbestos from industry. This is deadly in even trace amounts.

PCB (polychlorinated biphenyl) from industry, found in everybody and everywhere on earth. It is lethal.

Sodium from highway salt; can cause hypertension.

Pesticides and herbicides aplenty, mostly of unproven safety.

Radioactive wastes and acid rain.

Varieties of Water

Hard water contains a lot of calcium and magnesium salts. It has been proved that people who drink hard water run a lower risk of heart disease.[7] "Hardening" of the arteries is rarely from too much calcium but rather from an imbalance or deficiency of calcium and magnesium. Yet the reduced cleaning power of hard water can frustrate some people, so they buy water softeners. This is fine for cleaning clothes and dishes. But water softeners remove the calcium and magnesium salts and replace them with sodium salts in a procedure called "ion exchange." Large bags of rock salt end up being used in water softeners. If this water is consumed, there could be a major risk for hypertension. Don't drink softened water.

Natural spring water varies in its mineral content, depending on the spring itself. Most have some calcuim, magnesium, sodium, and potassium. Some even contain lithium, a substance used in pharmaceutical levels to treat clinical depression. Club soda is processed tap water with heavier carbonation and more sodium from various additives. Seltzer is multifiltered water with added carbonation; it is anecdotally known as a digestive aid and provides a healthy, refreshing beverage.

Recommendations

You need water. And lots of it. Regularly. Your city water supply is possibly substandard or even dangerous. You cannot wait for the government to clean up the underground aquifers and rivers. With over fifty-five thousand

TABLE 16: Water Purifying Techniques

	Advantages	*Disadvantages*
Bottled water	Low initial cost; usually pure and tasty; provides emergency store of drinking water.	higher cost in long run; some companies merely flavor city water, so you must demand chemical analysis; bulky in storage; difficult for some people to change the large bottles; may not remove all the impurities.
Multistage home filter units	Less expensive in long run; never a shortage or excess of water; convenient to use; usuallly keep valuable substances (calcium, magnesium, fluoride) in water; require no electricity.	High initial cost; take space on counter or under sink; require some installation; may not remove all of the impurities; filter must be changed regularly.
Home distillation units	Remove nearly all the impurities; can be less expensive in long run.	May leave certain petrochemicals in water since they have a low boiling point; high initial cost; require electricity; work slowly; water has no flavor.

chemical dump sites in the United States, according to the Environmental Protection Agency, this could take decades.

Table 16 shows the advantages and disadvantages of various water purification techniques. Choose one according to your needs and budget. But do choose—your life is at stake.

Two-thirds of the earth's surface is covered with water, yet 99 percent of this is either seawater or locked into the polar ice masses. Europeans have learned to live with conserving water and scrutinizing their drinking water. Americans are only beginning their education in these areas. Your body is likely experiencing a water shortage, both in quality and quantity of fluids given to it. Alcohol and caffeine are diuretics and thus do not count as fluid intake. Do your body a favor and drink five to ten eight ounce glasses of clean water daily.

Find out what *you* can do about cleaning up water pollution. Write to: Safe Drinking Water for All: What You Can Do, League of Women Voters Education Fund, 1730 M Street, N.W., Washington, D.C. 20036. Also write to: Manual for Evaluating Public Drinking Water Supplies, Water Supply Division, Environmental Protection Agency, Washington, D.C. 20460.

11
VITAMINS

"Vitamins, if properly understood and applied, will help us to reduce human suffering to an extent which the most fantastic mind would fail to imagine."
— DR. ALBERT SZENT-GYORGI,
NOBEL LAUREATE AND DISCOVERER OF VITAMINS C AND B_6, 1937

The English physician Lind was able to prevent and cure scurvy with lime juice. The Dutch physician Eijkman found that rice polishings cured the dreaded beri-beri. In both instances, tiny amounts of certain parts of food substances were able to cure dastardly and fatal conditions. Evidence continues to accumulate that vitamins could fulfill Dr. Gyorgi's statement.

Some consider vitamins to be a cure for nearly everything. Others say that very few people in the United States need to worry about their vitamin intake. Somewhere in between lies the truth.

Vitamins are a group of potent organic compounds required in the diet in minute quantities to perform specific metabolic functions of growth, maintenance, and reproduction. This definition is worth analyzing.

They are indeed potent. One milligram of vitamin B_{12}, evenly distributed, will supply one healthy adult for one full year.

They are organic, that is, based upon the element carbon ("inorganic" would adequately describe minerals).

They are required in the diet. Other substances are found in the body but are manufactured from other dietary factors—for instance, orotic acid is found in the body but not required in the diet, since it is made internally. These are not true vitamins. Later we will discuss substances that may be considered vitamins for some people.

Table 17 describes the difference between the two basic categories of vitamins: water soluble, such as ascorbic acid, thiamin, riboflavin, niacin, pyridoxine, B_{12}, folacin, biotin, pantothenic acid; and fat soluble, such as A, D, E, K, which dissolve in solvents like ether, alcohol and benzene.

Some vitamins, such as niacin, D, and A, can be consumed in their ready-to-use format (preformed) or in a raw material state (precursor), which the body then uses to make that vitamin internally.

TABLE 17: Differences Between Fat and Water-Soluble Vitamins

Water Soluble	*Fat Soluble*
Minimal body stores	Body can store considerable amount (primarily in the liver)
Required on regular basis	Not necessary on daily basis
Absorbed into bloodstream	Absorbed into lymph system with other fatty substances

Since vitamins are required in such small amounts, most are measured in milligrams per day, some in micrograms (one-thousandth of a milligram) per day. A few are expressed in international units (I.U.), which are a measurement of biological activity.

In the following detailed discussions of individual vitamins, deficiency symptoms are classified as subclinical (subtle, less obvious, may not be perceived as anything worth worrying about by some people) and clinical (a blatant and severe symptom, something that might keep you home from work). Note how, for some vitamins, toxicity symptoms may be very similar to deficiency symptoms. Foods are listed in descending order of concentration (richest sources first); especially concentrated sources are marked with an asterisk (*). Note also that a question mark (?) by any statement or number indicates that there is some but not substantial evidence of that effect.

Fat-soluble Vitamins

Vitamin A

Vitamin A (retinol, carotene) is as multifunctional a nutrient as any that exists. Green plants are the beginning of the food chain on earth, with beta-carotene being the invaluable assistant helping chlorophyll to capture the sun's energy in the process of photosynthesis. The importance of A is shown in our ability to either consume it directly (from animal sources) or make it from the raw materials of carotene (in plants). Think of the various earth-tone pigments that emerge as leaves turn in the autumn; some of these colors are versions of carotene.

Functions. Works in three separate ways in the body. This is somewhat baffling to scientists.[1] Combines with the protein opsin to form visual purple (rhodopsin). Light strikes this compound and causes it to split. The nerves in the retina sense this splitting and vision is transmitted to the brain. Involved in all mucous membranes, including the eyes, nose, throat, and genitourinary passage. Thus it is integral to disease resistance. Maintains all skin tissue, including the cornea of the eye. Important in cell division, especially cell differentiation, which is the poorly understood process that occurs during fetal development. One cell splits to form two. One of these cells may become a liver cell and the other may become a kidney cell. Important in growth, as in the normal spacing of teeth and the proper lengthening of bones. Necessary in sperm production. Essential for the fertilized egg to develop properly. Essential for normal cancer prevention but has been misused as a cancer cure.[2] Works together with zinc in many functions.[3]

Deficiency symptoms. Subclinical: Poor night vision. Increased frequency and severity of illnesses.[4] Greater vulnerability to cancer.[5] Acne; bumpy or hardened skin. Reduced tearing ability, making for dry and red eyes.[6] Mildly stunted growth. Less than ideal fetal development. Low sperm count. Anemia and loss of taste and smell.[7] Clinical: Night blindness. Keratinization (hardening) and follicular hyperkerotosis (bumps) of the skin surface. Frequent and severe infections. Stunted growth. Improper development, such as bone malformation or tooth misalignment. Severe acne. Male sterility. Severe deformities of the fetus. Cancer. Xerosis of the eyes, with spots on eye and tissue becoming translucent and sagging out of socket.

Toxicity symptoms. Does not occur until the vitamin A carrier, retinol binding protein, is saturated with absorbed A. Thus, a protein deficiency interferes with normal A metabolism and increases the risk for A toxicity.[8] Pain in joints. Vomiting and nausea. Headache similar to that from brain lesions. Stunted growth. Irritability, hair loss, liver enlargement, and fetal deformities. Toxicity has been produced only with the preformed animal version of vitamin A. Plant beta-carotene produces a yellowing of the palms, eyes, and skin but is less toxic than preformed A. No toxicity was observed in humans consuming 500,000 international units of beta-carotene for long periods of time.[9]

Characteristics. Fat soluble. Destroyed by oxygen or sunlight. Lost in feces when mineral oil is consumed. Higher needs for alcoholics. Body's ability to use A increases sixfold when vitamin E is taken along with it.[10] Diabetics may not be able to convert beta-carotene easily to vitamin A, so they may need preformed A. Animal sources (especially liver) more potent than plant sources. One I.U. equals 0.3 mcg retinol.[11] Oral contraceptives increase blood levels of retinol binding protein. The significance of this is still not understood.[12]

Sources. Liver,* fish liver oil, vitamin-A-fortified milk, butter, margarine, egg yolk, dark green vegetables (such as broccoli, peas, kale, spinach), yellow vegetables (such as squash, carrots, pumpkin, sweet potatoes), orange fruits (such as apricots, cantaloupe, papayas, peaches), watermelon, and cherries. In plant products, the beta-carotene content varies with the intensity of the color; thus dark green spinach is higher in vitamin A than pale green spinach. Dark yellow carrots are higher in A than faded-looking carrots. Studies show that people with diets high in beta-carotene (a strong anticancer nutrient) tend to eat fewer foods that might promote cancer (such as burned meats and nitrates).[13]

People at risk. Those working in bright light most of the day (painters, lifeguards, skiers, office workers). Post-teen acne syndrome strikes people who read under bright fluorescent lights all day, thus using more vitamin A for vision needs and leaving less for skin maintenance. Because of reduced absorption, patients who have recently undergone intestinal surgery.[14] Alcoholics, who often suffer night blindness without supplemental vitamin A. Diabetics, since their ability to convert beta-carotene may be stunted. Smokers. Preterm infants with low levels of beta-carotene have a high risk for lung problems.[15] Those who do not consume fresh produce regularly. Millions of people throughout Africa and Asia suffer clinical vitamin A deficiency, since they culturally do not include foods with vitamin A. At least a half million children each year go permanently blind from vitamin A deficiency (xerosis), which causes deterioration of the eye tissue. Vitamin A deficiency and the use of MSG in food are both very common in the Philippines. Authorities have recommended supplementing MSG with vitamin A.[16] Levels of vitamin A in the body drop off sharply after burns, wounds, cancer, and other illnesses,[17] indicating an increased need.

Daily intake:

USRDA: 5,000 I.U. (1,000 retinol equivalents).
Supplemental: 2,500 to 25,000 I.U.
Preferred form: Beta-carotene.
Toxicity: As low as 20,000 I.U. for children, or 30,000 I.U. for pregnant women. For healthy adults the body must saturate its vitamin A carrier before toxicity occurs.[18] This usually means about 2 million I.U. total (or 50,000 I.U. each day for several weeks). If the person is suffering from protein deficiency, the toxicity level is lower. Beta-carotene is much less toxic than the preformed animal version of A. Possible toxicity problems include bone disease for those with kidney failure,[19] birth defects (150,000 I.U./day),[20] high levels of calcium in the blood,[21] headache or pseudo-tumor,[22] nausea,[23] weight loss, weakness, dermatitis, psychosis,[24] loss of menstruation.[25]

Vitamin D

Vitamin D (cholecalciferol, ergocalciferol) is the ultimate escort of calcium. With too little or too much D, calcium (and, indirectly, magnesium) metabolism goes awry. If this happens, the nerve and muscle systems suffer first and most. Vitamin D is considered a hormone by some biochemists. Vitamin D can be produced internally with minimal exposure to sunshine. People who are native to sun-drenched equatorial areas usually are darker pigmented than those from temperate climates. The brown tanning pigment melanin is a protective mechanism for the body to avoid both excess ultraviolet radiation and vitamin D toxicity.

Research into the epidemic levels of bone disease in older adults has found that low vitamin D levels are at least partly responsible. Perhaps an inefficient kidney and liver could be responsible for not activating D to its full potency.

Functions. Anything to do with calcium metabolism. The absorption, transport, deposition, and usage of calcium. Since magnesium works in harmony with calcium, it too can be affected.

Deficiency symptoms. Subclinical: Poor bone growth and formation, muscle cramps, heart palpitations, irritability. Clinical: Hollowed bones (osteoporosis) or softened bones (osteomalacia), increased risk for colon cancer, hip fractures, bowed legs and pigeon chest if occurring during growth years. May result in deafness,[26] rickets.

Toxicity symptoms. Nausea, anorexia, weakness, headache, high urine output, mental retardation, digestive disturbances, kidney damage, calcification of soft tissue, higher risk for heart disease,[27] high blood pressure, and palpitations. Even workers in a vitamin D factory have shown signs of toxicity from touching and breathing the vitamin.[28]

Characteristics. Fat soluble. The body can produce its own D through sunlight exposure (ultraviolet light) on the skin. Smog, makeup, clothes, clouds, dark skin, and the distant rays of the winter sun can all mean less vitamin D in the body. Vitamin D formed in the skin from sunlight must be activated by both the kidneys and the liver before it becomes usable. The increasingly polluted atmosphere reduces sunlight penetration and has lowered vitamin D from sun by 15 percent in the last two decades.[29]

Sources. Fish liver oil,* fortified milk, salmon, herring, sardines, sunshine on skin (fifteen to thirty minutes per day, depending on intensity of the sun), butter, milk, eggs.

People at risk. Those living in cloudy or smoggy climates or who do not get much sun exposure. People who wear a lot of makeup. Darker-skinned individuals.[30] Vitamin D supplements or sun exposure are essential for long-term breast-feeding of infants.[31] Pregnant and lactating women probably need D supplements.[32, 33] Those who do not drink D-fortified milk. People taking drugs for epilepsy.[34] Postmenopausal women, because of changes in hormones, have a critical need to keep calcium in the bones via vitamin D. Forty percent of older adults are low in D[35] and may need 500 I.U. to keep normal, healthy body levels of the vitamin.[36] Growing children and adolescents have unusually high needs and so are very vulnerable to low levels of D. Asians living in northern climates are common victims of rickets.[37] Rickets is also common in the sun-drenched Middle East, where overprotective mothers have recently begun to keep their infants indoors.[38] Those with cystic fibrosis and others with poor fat absorption.[39]

Daily intake:

USRDA: 400 I.U.
Supplemental: 200 to 400 I.U.
Preferred form: Ergocalciferol.
Toxicity: 2,000 I.U.

Vitamin E

Vitamin E (tocopherol) has been called "the vitamin in search of a disease." It is also called the unicorn among vitamins, because of the many promises early research held for E. Tocopherol is Greek for "to carry and bear babies," a name that came from the importance of E in the fertility of rats. So far, E does not appear to be critically tied to fertility in humans. (So much for applying animal studies to humans.) Deficiencies are widespread in animals but less noticeable in humans. The RDA board lowered its recommendation for vitamin E from 30 to 10 I.U. when it found no glaring deficiency syndromes among Americans consuming less than 30 I.U. per day.

A condition similar to muscular dystrophy is found in animals with vitamin E deficiency, yet supplementation in humans failed to cure muscular dystrophy victims. Rat studies showed vitamin E to be essential for sex drive, yet this did not hold true in humans. Vitamin E has been an elusive nutrient to study, yet it still holds great promise as a preventive and curative nutrient.

Functions. Primarily as an antioxidant. Vitamin E is the sacrificial lamb the body feeds to the destructive free radicals in lieu of cells. E prevents the destructive effects of oxygen on all tissues in the body, especially polyunsaturated fats, which are more prone to free radical attack. Encourages the production of prostacyclin, a substance that helps prevent heart disease.[40] Works with other antioxidants (vitamin C and selenium) and enzyme systems (glutathione peroxidase, catalase, superoxide dismutase) to protect against free radical destruction.[41] E and C together reduce the oxidation of fats (lipid peroxidation).[42] E stabilizes membranes, protects the lungs from effects of pollutants, and prevents tumor growth (via free radical destruction). Plays a crucial role in the normal functioning of the nervous system.[43] Also protects skin, eyes (especially the retina), liver, breast, and calf muscle, and maintains vitamin A potency.[44] E is the only fat-soluble antioxidant in the blood.[45] It is involved in energy metabolism, especially with protecting coenzyme Q,[46] and the synthesis of DNA, RNA, and red blood cells. Influences prostaglandin synthesis. In biochemical theory, E may be an antiaging, anticancer, anti-heart-disease nutrient, but such a statement may be difficult to prove irrefutably.

Deficiency symptoms. Subclinical: Brown spots on the skin as one ages (ceroid pigmentation from free radical destruction of polyunsaturated fats). Fatigue (hemolytic anemia from premature destruction of red blood cells). Muscle degeneration. Premature aging(?). Autoimmune (self-destructive) diseases may be encouraged.[47] Clinical: Reproductive failure (spontaneous abortion in females, sterility in males). Calcification and poor circulation in skeletal muscles. Brain damage, spasms, paralysis. Blindness in premature infants. Fivefold increased risk for breast cancer.[48] Lumps in the breasts (fibrocystic breast disease). Long-term low intake of E can lead to nerve and muscle degeneration.[49] Cancer(?). Heart disease(?). Early death(?).

Toxicity symptoms. May cause behavioral changes.[50] Megadoses may lower output of thyroid hormone.[51] Elevated blood pressure(?). May alter fat and hormone functions in body(?). For those with problems in blood clotting mechanisms, more than 400 I.U. daily could lead to serious bleeding.[52] Does not interfere with blood clotting in normal healthy individuals.[53] Topical vitamin E may cause a rash on wounds in some individuals.[54]

Characteristics. Fat soluble. Easily destroyed by sunlight, time, oxygen exposure. Higher needs in those consuming diets with much polyunsaturated fats. May be destroyed in heat processing of vegetable oils (we recommend cold processed or unprocessed oils). Wheat germ is a rich source of E and is lost in the milling of flour. Large doses of E (an antioxidant) taken with large doses of iron (an oxidizing metal) could neutralize some of the E. One milligram of E equals 1.49 I.U.[55] Still a poorly understood vitamin.

Sources. Wheat germ oil,* wheat germ, corn, soy, cottonseed, safflower, and sunflower oils, mayonnaise, margarine, egg yolk, butter, liver, nuts.

People at risk. Premature infants born with low levels of E, then exposed to the oxygen-rich atmosphere of an intensive care unit; 1500 of these infants go permanently blind each year. Vitamin E (100 milligrams per kilogram of body weight per day) can seriously lower this risk.[56] The higher one's intake of polyunsaturated fats, the higher the requirement for E. Residents of smoggy communities, since E is used up by the lungs more quickly in smog. Cystic fibrosis patients have 25 percent lower serum E.[57] Those who habitually consume saturated or processed fats, or white flour. People with fat malabsorption (i.e., cystic fibrosis, steatorrhea, older adults).[58] NASA astronauts have taken E with them to counteract the anemia-inducing effect of their oxygen-rich environment.

Daily intake:

USRDA: 30 I.U.
Supplemental: 30 to 400 I.U.
Preferred form: d-alpha tocopherol acetate.
Toxicity: 1,200 I.U.(?).

Vitamin K

Vitamin K (menadione) was discovered by a Danish researcher and thus abbreviated K for "koagulation" (Danish for clotting).

Functions. Takes part in making at least two of the proteins involved in blood clotting.

Deficiency symptoms. Subclinical: Prolonged bleeding time when cut. Excessive bruising. Clinical: Hemorrhaging, perhaps bleeding to death, or even internal hemorrhaging from bruises.

Toxicity symptoms. Accelerated breakdown of red blood cells (hemolytic anemia) and liver damage. Vitamin K_1 (phylloquinone) does not appear to produce this problem.

Characteristics. Fat soluble. Since it is produced by bacteria in the intestines, anything that interferes with those bacteria can be harmful to vitamin K production (e.g., oral antibiotics). Infants are born with no bacteria in their intestines, thus usually receive a dose of K soon after birth. Mineral oil carries K out with the feces. Malabsorption conditions caused by disease, old age, surgery, or infections can reduce K production. Several chemicals, including the rodent-killing agent Warfarin, coumarin (from sweet clover), and aspirin can increase the need for K.[59] Requires the normal presence of bile and pancreatic juice for proper absorption.

Sources. Internal production by intestinal bacteria. Yogurt and other cultured milk products help stimulate these bacteria. Also found in liver and dark green leafy vegetables.

People at risk. Those taking long-term oral antibiotics. Newborn infants. Mothers who nurse can pass on extra vitamin K to their infants by taking K supplements.[60] People exposed to pesticides, drugs, and other potential interfering agents. People with diseased or poorly functioning gastrointestinal systems.

Daily intake:

USRDA: None stated.
Supplemental: 30 to 140 micrograms.
Preferred form: Phylloquinone.
Toxicity: 800 micrograms(?).

Water Soluble Vitamins

Vitamin C

Ascorbic acid (vitamin C) has become a central forum for discussing the values and limitations of the RDA. C has many known functions, and there is a growing wealth of information that shows the benefits of taking greater-than-RDA levels.

Vitamin C is no stranger to the limelight. An Egyptian treatise on medicine dating back to 1550 B.C. described the symptoms of scurvy, a deficiency of C. Throughout the world, a method of maintaining vitamin C intake was perpetuated from generation to generation. Scandinavians valued their onion patch the way a cowboy valued his horse. Onions are a decent source of C, and one of the few sources that can grow in northern climates and keep fresh throughout the long winter in a cool root cellar. Canadian Indians showed explorers how to cure scurvy by brewing pine needles and drinking the solution.

It was in the era of world exploration of the sixteenth through eighteenth century that scurvy really took its toll. Deaths from scurvy became so rampant on these long sea voyages that a ship line owner would bring twice the needed men because about half of them would die from scurvy en route. In 1747 Dr. Lind discovered that lime juice cured scurvy. It was a half century later before the English navy mandated the use of limes aboard all ships (hence the nickname "limeys").

Vitamin C is unique in many ways. Humans are among the few creatures on earth that cannot synthesize their own C. Primates, guinea pigs, fruit bats, and Indian bulbul birds are the others with this dubious honor. Those creatures that do make their own vitamin C create awesome quantities relative to our human RDA and are able to use simple glucose as the raw material. There is some evidence that a select few humans may have retained the ability to make their own C,[61] thus being a link to our evolutionary heritage.

Functions. C is as multitalented a vitamin as vitamin A. It is involved in the synthesis of collagen, a tough connective protein, also called the glue that holds the body together. Deficiency symptoms of C have the body literally falling apart since the glue is no longer being manufactured. C is therefore important in wound healing. Involved in several reactions to create important brain chemicals (tryptophan to serotonin, tyrosine to dopamine). Helps activate folic acid to its potent form. Critical in keeping serum cholesterol levels normal because it helps convert cholesterol to bile salts used for fat digestion. Changes cholesterol to a sulfate form that can be excreted in the urine. Keeps triacylglycerols (fats) in the fat cells rather than having them dumped into the blood.[62] Understandably, the level of C is lower in patients with heart disease compared to the normal population. Involved in the making of carnitine, a substance crucial to the proper burning of fats, and in disease resistance through its role in the immune system, in leukocyte formation, and as a scavenger. Shown to reduce the carcinogenic effect of nitrates in the intestines. Helps create epinephrine, the body's "flight or fight" stress chemical. Makes a steroid that prevents the inflammation of skin and joints. Increases iron absorption as much as fourfold.[63] Involved in the release of iron from its escort in the blood so that tissue can use iron. Enhances absorption efficiency of calcium. C is an antioxidant, protecting vitamins E and A and polyunsaturated fats from oxidation, or a slow "rusting" within. In tissue culture, promotes the production of prostacyclin, a valuable aid against heart disease.[64]

Deficiency symptoms. Subclinical: Poor wound healing and excessive bruising. Long-term low intake of C may encourage heart disease.[65] Increased incidence and severity of infections. Irritability and confused thought. The National Cancer Institute has observed that residents of the Sunbelt, where vitamin-C-rich citrus fruits are available year round, have half the cancer mortality rate of the nation at large. Premature wrinkling and aging of the skin. Anemia and fatigue; 75 percent of scurvy patients are anemic.[66] Poor athletic endurance. Poor stress tolerance. Reduced memory and problem-solving ability.[67] Women with intake of less than 30 milligrams daily have ten times the risk for cervical dysplasia (abnormal growth in cervix).[68] Clinical: Severe pain in joints. Swelling, infected, and bleeding gums. Loose teeth. Skin easily bruised or cut, and underskin blood spots (petechia). Labored breathing (dyspnea). Increased risk for cancer and heart disease(?). Scurvy.

Toxicity symptoms. Gastric distress—gas, cramps, diarrhea. May affect copper status.[69] Chewable C erodes tooth enamel.[70] In those with poorly functioning kidneys, excess C may produce kidney stones.[71, 72] Megadoses may impair immunity.[73] Physiological dependence; people who consume large amounts of C, then suddenly cease megadosing, can create scurvylike symptoms in spite of a "normal" intake of C.[74] This "rebound scurvy" is becoming especially common in infants of women who took large doses of C while pregnant.[75] The body becomes used to abnormally high intake and then is unable to adjust to the drastically lower level. Inhibits the effectiveness of blood clotting agents.[76]

Characteristics. Water soluble. Alcohol impairs absorption.[77] Lost in light, heat, storage time, exposure to oxidizing metals (iron and copper), when cooking water is poured out, or when an alkaline ingredient (like sodium bicarbonate) is used in cooking. Daily intake of 200 milligrams maintains saturation of C in most healthy people.[78] Smokers bind up to 500 milligrams of C per pack of cigarettes, making the many health dilemmas of smokers more explainable.[79] High concentrations found in adrenal glands and lenses of eyes. Bioflavonoids aid in the absorption of C.[80] Oral contraceptive users have lower blood levels of C.[81]

Sources. Terminalia ferdinandiana* (a fruit found only in tropical Australia; looks and tastes like an English gooseberry) contains about 2,500 milligrams per 100 edible grams[82] compared with 100 milligrams per 100 edible grams for fresh citrus, Barbados cherry* (from the Caribbean area), rosehips,* sweet peppers,* broccoli, cauliflower, kale, lemons, strawberries, papaya, asparagus, spinach, cantaloupe, oranges, grapefruit, tomato. Most fruits and vegetables contain some C. Liver is the only significant animal source.

People at risk. Smokers and alcohol abusers. Men may have twice the need that women have.[83] Those who do not regularly consume fresh produce. Crohn's patients. Rapidly growing children, adolescents, pregnant and lactating women.[84] Older adults may need greater than RDA levels.[85] People exposed to many carcinogens, like nitrate and burned proteins. Those under great stress. Men living alone.[86] People who eat mostly processed food or who pour off the water when cooking fruit and vegetables.

Daily intake:

USRDA: 60 milligrams.
Supplemental: 50 to 1,000 milligrams.
Preferred form: Ascorbic acid.
Toxicity: Rebound scurvy could occur when going from 5,000 milligrams to normal daily intake (about 50 mg). Gastric distress may set in at 2,000 milligrams for sensitive individuals. Mild diarrhea occurs in many people when consuming more than 20,000 milligrams daily.

Vitamin B₁

Thiamin (B_1) deficiency was discovered when people began refining their food supply. The Indonesians, eager for nineteenth century progress, began eating the refined white rice the Dutch had brought with them, and large numbers contracted beri-beri. The term "vitamine" (as in amino acids) was coined in 1911 by Casimir Funk, who thought it a protein from rice polishings that cured beri-beri. The term was later changed to vitamin when it was found that thiamin was not a protein substance.

Thiamin is a key ingredient in the body's ability to burn fuel, especially carbohydrates. The results of its deficiency are devastating. Beri-beri, which is Indonesian for "I cannot, I cannot," is the deficiency condition of thiamin.

Functions: Energy production, especially carbohydrate burning (thiamin pyrophosphate). Synthesis of RNA, niacin, and fats. Nerve transmission. Deactivating substances that could become oxalates and create kidney stones.

Deficiency symptoms. Subclinical: Fatigue, irritability, loss of appetite, constipation. Weight loss. Tender muscles. Personality changes and reduced attention span. Greater urge for alcohol(?). Clinical: Slowing and enlarging of the heart. Senility. Severe nerve impairment including numbness, increased sensitivity, tingling in the extremities. Depression and perhaps permanent nerve damage. Wet beri-beri involves fluid accumulation in the lower extremities; dry beri-beri does not have the edema but does have severe muscle wasting and emaciation. Cardiovascular problems. Degeneration of optic nerve and blindness.[87]

Toxicity symptoms. Unknown.

Characteristics. Water soluble. Lost in heat, oxidation, baking soda, irradiation, cooking water, coffee, tea, and meat preservation. Alcohol, stress, sugar, and many drugs increase the need for thiamin. Garlic and onion increase the absorption of thiamin. Chlorine from tap water destroys some thiamin.

Sources. Brewer's yeast,* pork,* kidney, liver, peas, wheat germ, macaroni, peanuts, whole grains, beans, nuts.

People at risk. Alcoholics. Older people, especially women.[88] Seventy-five percent of college women were found to be low in B_1.[89] People who consume large amounts of sugar. Pregnant women.[90] Those eating a diet of refined and unenriched grains, still common in the Philippines and elsewhere. People exposed to PCB.

Daily intake:

USRDA: 1.5 milligrams.
Supplemental: 1 to 10 milligrams.
Preferred form: Thiamine hydrochloride.
Toxicity: Unknown through oral intake. Repeated intravenous injections can instigate anaphylactic shock.

Vitamin B_2

Riboflavin (B_2) is a yellow-green pigment that was found to be the reason consumers did not like nonfat milk—the yellow-green color of riboflavin stands out once the fat has been removed. So the dairy industry added nonfat milk solids and was able to mask this unappetizing color. Riboflavin was lost in extensive amounts when the milk man would leave clear glass bottles of milk on the porch in the sun. Amber bottles and opaque wax containers solved this vitamin thievery. There is still speculation that translucent plastic milk bottles allow some riboflavin destruction, even from the fluorescent lighting in grocery stores.

Functions. Energy production (flavin adenine dinucleotide). Involved in the synthesis and breakdown of fats. Activates vitamin B_6 and folic acid. Involved in making red blood cells, corticosteroids (anti-inflammatory substances), and glycogen (the body's carbohydrate storage form).

Deficiency symptoms. Subclinical: Fatigue. Dry or greasy, scaly skin. Reduced athletic endurance.[91] Mild deformities of fetal development. Higher risk for cataracts.[92] Can shorten lifespan of red blood cells. Clinical: Cracks at the corner of the mouth (cheilosis). Inflammation of the mucous membranes of the mouth with smooth and inflamed purple-looking tongue (glossitis). Depression and hysteria, possibly leading to nerve damage. Eyes may become red, tired, burning, itching, or sensitive to light, all due to increased blood vessel growth in the eyes, since riboflavin is involved in maintaining circulation to the eyes. Vision may be dimmed. Cataracts.

Toxicity symptoms. Unknown.

Characteristics. Water soluble. Exercise increases needs.[93] Unstable upon exposure to light or alkaline solution (like sodium bicarbonate). Oral contraceptives increase the need for riboflavin.

Sources. Brewer's yeast,* kidney,* liver,* heart,* milk,* broccoli, wheat germ, almonds, cottage cheese, yogurt, tuna, salmon, macaroni, Brussels sprouts, asparagus, eggs, green leafy vegetables.

People at risk. Alcoholics. Very active people may need twice the RDA level.[94] Oral contraceptive users.[95] Non-milk consumers. Adolescents, the elderly,[96] and low-income groups.[97] Those dieting or fasting.

Daily intake:

USRDA: 1.7 milligrams.
Supplemental: 1 to 10 milligrams.
Preferred form: Riboflavin.
Toxicity: Unknown.

Vitamin B₃

Vitamin B₃

Niacin (B₃) deficiency was described by a Spanish physician in 1735 and given the name pellagra from the Italian word meaning "rough skin." Pellagra was a primary cause of death and was responsible for 10 percent of all mental illness in the southeastern United States throughout the late nineteenth and early twentieth centuries. Dr. Joseph Goldberger discovered that high-quality proteins cured the disease. He even lived with and swallowed throat samples from pellagra victims to prove to his colleagues that pellagra was not infectious but rather dietary in origin. His efforts were to little avail, as it was two more decades before dietary cure of pellagra became the common medical practice.

Functions. A critical component of energy production. Synthesis of DNA, fatty acids, and cholesterol. Very important in brain functions, since the body can convert tryptophan (an essential amino acid) to either niacin (in a very inefficient 60 to 1 ratio) or to the critical brain component serotonin. Since the body's number one priority is always energy, when tryptophan is diverted to be made into niacin, serious mental disturbances can develop.

Deficiency symptoms. Subclinical: Fatigue, confusion, poor digestion, loss of appetite, insomnia, loss of memory. Fats are elevated in the blood. Clinical: Scaly and dark-pigmented skin that has been exposed to the sun or mild trauma. Diarrhea along with poor fat absorption and consequent deficiencies in the fat-soluble vitamins. Low chlorine in the gastrointestinal system which contributes to intestinal infections and lesions. Tongue becomes swollen, corroded, and brilliant red. Nervous symptoms include headache, emotional instability, dementia, and catatonia (a zombielike state).

Toxicity symptoms. One form of niacin (nicotinic acid) can produce a rapid dilation of the blood vessels and a resulting blushing effect. A sudden high intake (two grams per day) can produce skin disorders, decreased glucose tolerance, high uric acid levels, aggravation of peptic ulcers, and symptoms resembling hepatitis. Liver damage is possible. If supplements are used, a slow and gradual increase of dosages may help avoid these problems.[98]

Characteristics. Water soluble. Relatively stable compared with other vitamins, yet lost when cooking water is discarded. Can be provided by either preformed niacin or the precursor raw material of tryptophan.

Sources. Brewer's yeast,* liver,* peanuts, poultry, fish, meat, whole grains, eggs, milk, and other high-quality proteins.

People at risk. Those on low-protein diets, especially diets high in corn.[99] Those dieting or fasting. From work done on schizophrenics, it appears that some people inherit unusually high needs for niacin that can be met only by supplements.

Daily intake:

USRDA: 20 milligrams.
Supplemental: 20 to 100 milligrams.
Preferred form: Niacinamide.
Toxicity: 3,000 milligrams.[100]

Vitamin B₆

Pyridoxine (B_6) was discovered and named by Dr. Albert Szent-Gyorgi (the same researcher who discovered bioflavonoids and ascorbic acid). Dietary surveys have found that deficiency of this nutrient is common. Pyridoxine is being researched extensively. If protein can be called the elite building material of the body, then B_6 can be termed the master craftsman that assembles the protein complexes.

Functions. Primarily in protein metabolism. B_6 aids in the absorption of amino acids, deaminates and transaminates amino acids. Works with folic acid to activate choline, methionine, and serine. Allows amino acids to be burned for fuel (e.g., cysteine to pyruvic acid). Is an integral component of creating vital brain chemicals (tryptophan to serotonin, making GABA, norepinephrine, acetylcholine). Helps protect against sticky blood vessels (platelet aggregation) and helps regulate serum cholesterol. Helps make histamine, which is a substance that increases capillary permeability and is able to constrict the lung passage. B_6 aids in absorption and metabolism of minerals.[101]

Deficiency symptoms. Subclinical: Protein is everywhere in the human body. And since all protein metabolism requires B_6, deficiency symptoms are diverse: confusion, irritability, nervousness, insomnia, poor coordination, hyperactivity, fatigue, increased incidence of infection. Reduced tear flow with greater risk for eye infections. Fluid retention in pregnancy. Some forms of diabetes may be caused or worsened by B_6 deficiency.[102] Clinical: Anemia and serious fatigue. Emotional instability or depression.[103] Permanent nerve deterioration.[104] Convulsions. Toxemia, which is a serious fluid retention that occurs during pregnancy and jeopardizes both mother and infant. Increased risk for infections. Increased risk for cancer and heart disease(?).

Toxicity symptoms. Extremely high levels of intake can bring on nerve deterioration, characterized by numbness, tingling, and an unsteady walk.[105] It is suspected that these symptoms are caused by the impurities (excipients) used in making vitamins, and thus pure pharmacological-grade B_6 would probably not have these complications.[106]

Characteristics. Water soluble. Many drugs, including oral contraceptives and amphetamines, increase the need for pyridoxine.[107] There are several known inborn errors of metabolism that create an extremely elevated need for B_6. Sensitive to light and alkaline solutions. One of the many nutrients removed in wheat milling and not replaced. Works with zinc in the body in numerous reactions.

Sources. Soybeans,* liver,* bananas,* lamb,* kidney, chicken, steak, poultry, tuna, fish, legumes, potatoes, oatmeal, wheat germ. Since B_6 is required for protein metabolism in the body, it is usually found in decent levels in protein foods.

People at risk. Those using drugs, especially oral contraceptives. People on estrogen therapy may need up to 250 milligrams daily of B_6.[108] Those habitually consuming white flour. Those born with an inborn error of metabolism that necessitates more B_6. Pregnant and lactating women. Older adults.[109] Those consuming protein supplements without B_6. Patients on renal dialysis.[110]

Daily intake:

    USRDA: 2.0 milligrams.
    Supplemental: 1 to 50 milligrams.
    Preferred form: Pyridoxine hydrochloride.
    Toxicity: As low as 100 milligrams in some individuals, 2,000 milligrams
      in others.

Vitamin B_{12}

Cyanocobalamin (B_{12}) is one of the more potent vitamins, since only one one-millionth of a kilogram will satisfy the yearly needs of a healthy adult. It was determined to be the extrinsic factor found in liver that cured the dreaded pernicious anemia that had taken so many lives and caused so much suffering up until the 1950s, when B_{12} was identified. B is unique because it has such a complicated absorption process in the human gut and also because it is found primarily in animal products. In the 1960s, vegetarianism began its popularity rise in America. Without adequate nutrition knowledge, some vegetarians had children with permanent mental and physical deformities due to the lack of B_{12} during critical developmental years.[111] Vegetarians can consume adequate B_{12}, but not as haphazardly as carnivorous people. B_{12} deficiency is a common issue for people as they age, since the efficiency of B_{12} absorption in the intestinal tract seems to deteriorate. Serious deficiencies were also found in the first few patients who underwent intestinal bypass surgery to help their obesity. It was then discovered that there are specific sites of absorption for B_{12}.

Functions. New cell growth. More specifically, for reactions that require single carbon transfers, such as the making of choline and methionine (both substances that, among other things, help prevent fatty infiltration in the liver). Synthesis of DNA and red blood cells. Maintenance of the fatty wrapping (myelin sheath) around the nerve cells. Production of the cells that line the intestinal tract, which prevent the body from digesting itself.

Deficiency symptoms. Subclinical: Fatigue. Poor digestion and loss of appetite. Sore tongue. Confusion, agitation, numbness, tingling, moodiness, dimmed vision. Mental problems are often the first sign of low B_{12}.[112] Clinical: Severe fatigue. Degeneration of the spinal cord. Severe gastrointestinal disturbances. Hallucinations and psychosis (megaloblastic madness). Up to 20% of all senile older adults may actually be suffering from a B_{12} or folacin deficiency. Pernicious anemia.

Toxicity symptoms. Unknown.

Characteristics. B_{12} is just barely water soluble, since it is a large and complex molecule. It is for this reason that such a complicated absorption process is needed to get it into the blood and to the tissues that need it. There is an intrinsic factor produced in the intestines that binds to B_{12}. These two then combine with calcium and nestle into a specific site of absorption, where they move through the intestinal wall to be carried by an escort (transcobalamin) to the tissues. If any of these links is missing or malfunctioning, problems in B_{12} metabolism can develop. Absorption is hindered in many people.[113] Since such small amounts are required and the body is very economical with B_{12}, it may take up to five years for a healthy adult without B_{12} intake to develop the symptoms of deficiency. Pregnant or sick people would deplete their reserves more quickly. B_{12} works intimately with folic acid and methionine in many processes, and deficiency of one is often confused with the other.[114] Alcoholics may have a reduced absorption due to damaged intestinal walls.

Sources. Liver,* oysters,* poultry, fish, beef, pork, clams, eggs (primarily animal sources). B_{12} can be produced by bacterial fermentation and thus is found in adequate levels in tempeh (fermented soybeans), spirulina (blue-green algae), some seaweed, miso (fermented soybean paste), and brewer's yeast grown on B_{12}-rich environments.[115]

People at risk. Uneducated vegetarians. Older adults. A number of older psychiatric patients were found to be B_{12} deficient.[116] Those who have had surgery or ailments of the intestinal tract. Alcoholics. Oral contraceptive users.[117] Cancer patients make less intrinsic factor for B_{12} absorption.[118]

Daily intake:

> USRDA: 6 micrograms.
> Supplemental: 3 to 100 micrograms.
> Preferred form: Cyanocobalamin.
> Toxicity: Unknown.

Folacin

Folacin (folic acid or folate) is a name derived from folium, which is Latin for leaf, since dark-green leafy vegetables are rich sources of this vitamin. Anemia is common in this country, and folacin deficiency may be even more at fault than low iron levels. All nutrients have an increased requirement during pregnancy, but folacin is the only one whose requirement doubles. Pregnant women who were given supplements of folacin had a near zero risk of having infants with neural tube defects, a condition in which the nervous system is improperly formed.

Functions. New cell growth, including the surface of the tongue, lining of the intestinal tract, and in pregnancy. Helps activate niacin to its potent form. Involved in the production of choline and methionine to help prevent fatty infiltration of the liver. Synthesis of red blood cells and immunoglobins for disease resistance. DNA production for cell replication, and therefore involved in every phase of life.

Deficiency symptoms. Subclinical: Very similar to B_{12}, since they are so intimately tied together in their metabolic functions. Fatigue, poor memory, sore tongue, digestive problems, constipation. Weight loss, apathy, headache, hostility, loss of appetite. Minor imperfections in fetal development. Increased risk for preterm and low birth weight infants.[119] Increased risk for cervical cancer.[120] Clinical: Severe fatigue and anemia. Toxemia of pregnancy or severe fetal malformations.[121] Spontaneous abortions. Diarrhea and major digestive disturbances. Palpitations. Paranoid behavior and emotional instability. Megaloblastic anemia, or folacin deficiency.

Toxicity symptoms. Excessive intake may interfere with zinc absorption.[122]

Characteristics. Water soluble. Some food sources of folacin are bound and must be "digested" for the body to use them, such as in brewer's yeast. Some people do not readily activate their dietary folacin.[123] Losses are high in cooking and storage and upon exposure to light and acid. Needs are increased with alcohol and drug use, in wound recovery, and in pregnancy. Works with B_{12}. Folacin is lost in wheat milling.

Sources. Liver,* eggs, asparagus, whole wheat, green leafy vegetables, salmon, beans, broccoli, sweet potatoes.

People at risk. Those who regularly indulge in white flour products. Those who do not consume fresh greens. Pregnant and lactating women. Growing children. The older adult has reduced efficiency at absorbing folacin. Those recovering from surgery, especially intestinal surgery or burns.[124, 125] Those who use drugs or alcohol. Women using oral contraceptives and those with abnormal growth of their cervix have low folacin levels in the blood.[126]

Daily intake:

USRDA: 400 micrograms.
Supplemental: 400 to 800 micrograms.
Preferred form: Folic acid.
Toxicity: 15,000 micrograms.[127] Large levels of folacin can mask pernicious anemia (the deficiency symptom of B_{12}), and nerve damage can result. Although this is extremely unlikely, the FDA has established a legal maximum of 400 micrograms for normal people and 800 micrograms for pregnant women.

Biotin

Biotin (vitamin H or anti-egg white injury factor) was discovered when rats fed large amounts of raw egg white developed baldness around the eyes, paralysis, weight loss, and then died. Since biotin is produced by intestinal bacteria, it is difficult to evaluate the role of dietary biotin.

Functions. Involved in many reactions in the body, including those where a carbon dioxide or an amine group is removed. Thus it is critical in energy production. Involved in the synthesis of pancreatic amylase for carbohydrate digestion, nicotinic acid (a form of niacin), insulin production, fats, and antibodies for disease resistance.

Deficiency symptoms. Subclinical: Loss of hair, muscle tone, and appetite. Common skin rashes.[128] Elevated levels of cholesterol and glucose in the blood. Clinical: Anemia and fatigue. Severe muscle pain and weakness. Enlargement of the liver. Depression.

Toxicity symptoms. Unknown.

Characteristics. Water soluble. Avidin (found in raw egg white and deactivated upon cooking) binds biotin and may create a deficiency if enough raw eggs are consumed. Alcohol and antibiotics increase the need for biotin. It is the most expensive of the vitamins, costing roughly $7,000 per kilogram. It is usually not found in vitamin formulas for financial reasons. Works with zinc in the body. Lost in wheat milling. Some people have an inherited need for high doses.[129]

Sources. Liver,* kidney,* the intestinal bacteria of a healthy gut,* egg yolk, milk, yeast, whole grains, cauliflower, nuts, legumes.

People at risk. Those with intestinal problems, including surgery patients and people on long-term oral antibiotics. Those consuming large quantities of raw eggs. Alcoholics and drug users. Epileptics on medication. The elderly, athletes, pregnant women, infants (especially those with skin rashes).[130]

Daily intake:

USRDA: 300 micrograms.
Supplemental: 100 to 300 micrograms.
Preferred form: Biotin.
Toxicity: Unknown.

Pantothenic acid

Pantothenic acid (pantothenol) was discovered by Dr. Roger Williams in 1938, but it received little attention until chemists found the ubiquitous nature of the substance. Its name is derived from the Greek word *panthos*, meaning "everywhere."

Functions. It is part of a key enzyme in energy metabolism and thus relates to energy needs through its role in coenzyme A. Required for the making of fat. Helps make acetylcholine for brain function. Required to help make porphyrin, a part of red blood cells. Stimulates antibody response to invading organisms. Involved in the synthesis of cholesterol. Required to make adrenal gland products and thus is involved in stress tolerance.

Deficiency symptoms. Subclinical: Lowered disease resistance. Irritability. Insomnia, weakness, cramps. Impaired coordination, fatigue, nausea. Poor stress tolerance. Clinical: Depression, vomiting. In animals, a graying of the hair occurs, but the same effect does not take place in humans. Inflamed nose passages. Atrophy of the adrenal glands. Sexual dysfunction. Increased presence of blood vessels in the eyes.

Toxicity symptoms. Unknown.

Characteristics. Water soluble. Lost in wheat milling. Destroyed by heat, acid, or alkaline solutions. Losses can be high in cooking.

Sources. Royal bee jelly,* liver,* kidney,* heart, egg yolk, bran, fish, whole grain cereals, cauliflower, beans, nuts, cheese, sweet potatoes.

People at risk. Those who regularly indulge in white flour products. Those consuming highly processed and refined food. Arthritics.[131]

Daily intake:

USRDA: 10 milligrams.
Supplemental: 5 to 50 milligrams.
Preferred form: Calcium pantothenate.
Toxicity: Unknown.

12

MINERALS

"Gold is for the mistress—silver for the maid.
Copper for the craftsman, cunning at his trade.
'Good!' said the Baron, sitting in his hall,
But iron—Cold Iron—is the master of them all."
—RUDYARD KIPLING, "COLD IRON"

The tarnished copper of a penny, the zinc coating on a rain gutter, the iron of an engine block, the gleaming chromium of a car bumper, the calcium of a piece of chalk. It is hard to think of these metals as being required in the human body—but they are. Of the sixty minerals found in the earth's surface, about twenty are required for human health. We say "about" because this field is gaining knowledge almost every day. There are several minerals that could soon be proved essential for humans. Minerals constitute about 4 percent of an adult's body weight. There is an incredible range in the amounts of minerals found in the body, from 1.2 kilograms (just over 2½ pounds) of calcium to two parts per trillion of cobalt in the healthy adult body.

Because of the difficulties involved in working with these trace amounts, most of what is known about microminerals has been discovered in the last ten years. Some minerals have an evasive nature, so working with them is like trying to grab a feather as it falls. Chromium, for example, can change its valence and be seemingly "lost" in laboratory research.

Another interesting aspect of essential minerals is that a few can be toxic, while most others need to be in balance with other minerals. The only thing that was known about selenium in 1950 was that it was lethal. A purveyor of nutritional supplies in San Diego was nearly put in jail in the 1960s for making selenium supplements, even though scientists had proved it to be essential to laboratory animals. Some federal regulators had great difficulty changing their minds to regard something as essential when it was recently considered toxic. It is still illegal to sell selenium supplements in Australia. Arsenic is another trace mineral that has recently changed sides from toxic to essential.

TABLE 18: Minerals in the Body

Essential; found in large amounts (macrominerals)

calcium	chlorine	phosphorus	sodium
potassium	magnesium	sulfur	

Essential; found in small amounts (microminerals or trace elements)

zinc	fluorine	iron	molybdenum
copper	selenium	iodine	nickel
manganese	silicon	chromium	tin
cobalt	vanadium	arsenic	

Possibly essential

barium	strontium	bromine	cadmium

May be essential, harmless, or toxic

gold	gallium	silver	lead
aluminum	antimony	mercury	boron
bismuth	lithium		

Plus 20 other minerals

Some minerals become involved in the supportive structure of the body, like calcium and phosphorus in the bones. Most minerals play key roles in enzyme reactions. Some are so multitalented that they serve in many different enzyme reactions, like zinc. All of them are critical to human nutrition.

As in the preceding chapter, food sources are listed in descending order of concentration. Note also that a question mark after a statement or number indicates there is some but not substantial evidence of that effect.

Calcium

Calcium is the essence of the Dolomite mountains in Italy and also the chalk that everyone remembers from school days. It is the most prevalent mineral in the human body, with about 1,160 grams in the average adult. Calcium has been in the spotlight lately with the epidemic proportions of osteoporosis that have been discovered among postmenopausal women.

Functions. Ninety-nine percent of the body's calcium is found in the bones, which are the body's primary structural support. The teeth are largely composed of calcium, too. In addition to these structural roles, calcium is involved in growth, blood clotting, muscle contraction, nerve transmission (aids in releasing neurochemical transmitters into the synapse), cell membrane permeability, vitamin B_{12} absorption, maintaining proper blood pressure, and numerous other enzyme reactions.

Deficiency symptoms. Subclinical: Slow, subtle, and often undetectable demineralization of the bones. Irritability, depression. Muscle cramps. High blood pressure.[1] Severe cramping around menstruation time. Clinical: Rounded spine just below the neck. Loss of height. Pain in the spine. Premature tooth loss, from eroded jaw bone. Serious muscle cramps. Heart palpitations. Brittle bones that break easily. Osteomalacia.[2] In childhood, leads to thin bones and teeth.

Toxicity symptoms. Balance is more the key with minerals. When one is consumed to excess, then an imbalance with other minerals is likely. Since calcium competes for absorption with other minerals, a deficiency of iron, magnesium, and other minerals could result from too much calcium. Though many people are diagnosed with calcification of the soft tissue, this is usually caused by an imbalance of minerals and not by an excess of calcium in the diet. An ideal ratio of calcium to phosphorus to magnesium would be 2 to 2 to 1. Yet the refined diet of Western society often puts this at 1 to 4 to ½. Vitamin D deficiency can compound this matter and cause calcium deposits in soft tissue.

Characteristics. Calcium absorption is reduced by:

1. High fat diet. Grandmother used to make soap by combining lye and animal fat. A similar process can occur in your intestines as calcium combines with fats (especially saturated fats) during digestion to form a soap and then is excreted with the feces.

2. Phytates and oxalates. Found in vegetables and grains, these substances bind to calcium in the intestines to make some of it unavailable for absorption. Yet the body compensates and quickly adjusts to this if the phytates and oxalates are in reasonable levels. Leavening (yeast rising) of bread reduces the phytates in grain.

3. Low vitamin D levels. Since vitamin D aids in calcium absorption and use, there are serious calcium problems when vitamin D is in short supply.

4. Tension and worry. Up to 900 milligrams per day of calcium can be lost through excessive stress.

5. Excessive fiber. Too much fiber moves the food through the intestines too rapidly for proper calcium absorption.

6. High intake of minerals (like phosphorus, aluminum, and magnesium) that compete for intestinal absorption sites.

Factors that increase calcium loss from the body:

1. Excessive protein intake.[3] By influencing the kidneys, high protein causes calcium to be lost in the urine.

2. Sedentary lifestyle.[4] Your body will not maintain a strong skeletal sys-

tem when no stress is being put on it. Long-term space travelers might be seriously jeopardized by the calcium lost in a weightless environment.

3. Smoking and excessive coffee drinking.

4. High phosphorus intake. Phosphoric acid and other phosphorus compounds are commonly used in food processing. Soft drinks have high levels of phosphorus. Meats have a 20 to 1 ratio of phosphorus to calcium. The high meat and refined food diet of the West plays havoc with normal calcium balance.[5]

5. Sweat. In a hot dry climate, an active laborer could lose up to 1,000 milligrams per day.

6. Magnesium balance. There is a crucial balance between calcium and magnesium. Low magnesium can cause calcium loss or deposition in soft tissue.

7. Pregnancy and lactation. These maternal duties of creating and nourishing new life require abundant calcium. The calcium is either found in the diet or robbed from the mother's bone supply.

Sources. Cooked bones,* collards, yogurt, turnip greens, broccoli, milk and dairy products, kale, tempeh and tofu (both soybean products), canned salmon and sardines (from the bones); hard water (contains dissolved calcium and magnesium salts) can provide up to one-fifth or more of the RDA with up to 375 milligrams of calcium per liter of drinking water.[6] Calcium absorption is increased with an increase in vitamin C, lactose, and acid foods such as pineapple, tomatoes, and most citrus fruits.

People at risk. Those at rapid stages of growth—infants, children, and adolescents. Pregnant and lactating women. Older adults, especially postmenopausal women. Those whose diet is high in fat, meat, and processed foods and low in dairy products. Coffee drinkers, smokers, alcoholics, sedentary people, those under constant stress or on long-term antacids. In other words, anyone following the semi-suicidal lifestyle of the West.

Daily intake:

USRDA: 1,000 milligrams.

Supplemental: 200 to 1,500 milligrams.

Preferred form: Calcium carbonate. Though dolomite has a nice 2 to 1 balance of calcium to magnesium, it also contains measurable levels of lead, arsenic, mercury, and aluminum.[7]

Toxicity: 2,000 milligrams will likely create an imbalance of other minerals and, by competing for absorption sites, could create a deficiency of other minerals. In 10 percent of the population, 500 milligrams or more of calcium may cause a rebounding effect of excess stomach acid (hyperacidity).

Phosphorus

Phosphorus is the other primary mineral found in the bones. The average adult body contains 670 grams of phosphorus. Since all forms of life use ATP (adenosine triphosphate) for energy, there is abundant phosphorus in many foods. In spite of the many crucial roles it plays in the human body, there is excess phosphorus in the American diet.

Functions. Structural salts of bones and teeth. Structural component of soft tissue, including the striated muscles. Capturing energy as ATP. Activating energy reactions. Absorption and transportation of nutrients. DNA and RNA synthesis, therefore essential to the growth, repair, and maintenance of all tissues in the body. Part of the phospholipids that carry fatty substances in the water medium of the blood. Maintenance of proper acid-base balance.

Deficiency symptoms. Very unlikely due to prevalence of phosphorus in the diet. Subclinical: Weakness, loss of appetite, stiff joints. Clinical: Weak bones and osteoporosis.

Toxicity symptoms. Calcium irregularities, since the two are so intertwined in their bodily functions.

Characteristics. Must be in balance with calcium, magnesium, and vitamin D. Long-term use of some antacids could interfere with phosphorus absorption and create problems.

Sources. Meat,* soda pop (from the phosphoric acid added),* fish, poultry, eggs, cereal, processed foods (phosphorus compounds often used in processing).

People at risk. Heavy meat eaters and soda pop drinkers, because excessive phosphorus interferes with calcium metabolism. Long-term users of antacids may risk low phosphorus.

Daily intake:

USRDA: 1,000 milligrams.
Supplemental: Unlikely to be needed.
Toxicity: 1,500 milligrams.

Potassium

Potassium is the primary positively charged ion inside all body cells. In the primordial soup from which life began, salty ocean water was outside and potassium became the favored ion to exist within the cell. This balance still exists in all forms of life. The electrical charge of sodium dominant outside the cell and potassium inside is often called the "battery" of life. The body spends an abundance of time and energy keeping these minerals in their respective place. For many years, scientists told the public that excess sodium (salt) caused high blood pressure. New evidence points to a potassium, magnesium, or calcium deficiency as being even more influential in developing high blood pressure. The body has a sodium reserve but very little stored potassium, so potassium lost in sweat, vomit, or diarrhea can become a critical issue. It is interesting to note that most animal foods are higher in sodium, while most plant foods are higher in potassium. Grazing animals use their salty taste buds to seek out sodium to balance their high-potassium diet. Since 98 percent of the body's potassium is found inside the cells, blood tests may be a misleading approach to detecting low levels of potassium. A slight variation in potassium levels in the blood can cause muscle irregularities. Since the heart is a muscle, this can mean death.

Functions.   Acid-base balance. Proper fluid balance. Nerve transmission. Muscle relaxation. Insulin release. Synthesis of glycogen and protein.

Deficiency symptoms.   Subclinical: Weakness, fatigue, nausea, constipation, dizziness, inability to concentrate, insomnia, muscle cramps, heart irregularities, high blood pressure.[8] Clinical: Impaired growth, paralysis, sterility, and bone fragility from long-term low levels. Diminished heart rate. In severe deficiencies death is possible.

Toxicity symptoms.   Since the kidneys excrete excess potassium, toxicity is unlikely unless kidneys were damaged or the person took a sudden high dosage of at least eighteen grams in one day. Irregularities in heart rhythm could be fatal if such were the case.

Characteristics.   About 90 percent of dietary potassium is absorbed by healthy individuals. It is lost in considerable quantities in sweat, vomit, diarrhea, and diuretic use. Much potassium can be lost in cooking, with boiled potatoes losing 50 percent of their potassium in the water while steamed vegetables lose only 6 percent.[9] Since the kidneys are responsible for monitoring potassium levels in the blood, kidney patients need to watch their potassium intake.

Sources.   Salt substitutes, dried apricots,* cantaloupe,* lima beans,* potato, avocado, banana, broccoli, liver, milk, peanut butter, meat, citrus, fruits and vegetables in general.

People at risk.   Those using diuretics probably need supplements.[10] Sick people after vomiting and diarrhea. Those who perspire excessively, especially people not accustomed to exercise or heat, since the body eventually adapts and slows down its potassium loss in sweat. Those who do not eat fresh produce regularly. Older adults. People often eat less potassium-rich foods during the warm summer months when regular perspiration raises the need for potassium.

Daily intake:

> Recommended: 1,875 to 5,625 milligrams (no RDA given).
> Supplemental: 100 to 1,000 milligrams.
> Preferred form: Potassium chloride.
> Toxicity: 10,000 milligrams(?).

Sulfur

Sulfur is a yellow mineral that has the ability to form very strong chemical bonds. The body uses sulfur extensively in tough fibrous connective tissues like joints and hair. Though sulfur is in abundance in the body (112 grams in the average adult) and is known to be essential for human health, there is not much else known about it. There is not even a recommended range of intake for sulfur. Much of the sulfur in your body is found in various amino acids (like cysteine) and vitamins (like biotin).

Functions.   Energy transfer, as part of coenzyme A and biotin. Blood clotting. Works with magnesium as a detoxifier. Part of structural proteins of hair, nails, tendons, and skin.

Deficiency symptoms.   Difficult to assess. Could create pain in joints, high blood glucose (insulin contains sulfur, too), and high blood fat levels(?).

Toxicity symptoms.   Unknown.

Characteristics.   It has been proposed that the high health value of garlic and onions may be due to their sulfur content. Taurine, a sulfur amino acid produced from cysteine and methionine, is found in high levels in breast milk (there is almost none in cow's milk) and is known to be important for proper brain development in the infant. Legumes are high in sulfur amino acids and also have an ability to bind toxic elements (chelate) and carry them out of the system.

Sources.   Egg yolk,* garlic, onion, beans, high-protein foods (from the sulfur amino acids), asparagus.

People at risk.   Unknown. Some people with skeletal joint problems may have a low intake or a higher need for sulfur.

Daily intake:

> USRDA: None stated.

Supplemental: 100 to 500 milligrams.
Toxicity: Unknown.

Chloride

Chloride is found in large levels in the adult body (eighty-five grams on average) and is known to be essential. Yet chloride is rarely discussed among nutritionists since it always accompanies salt (sodium chloride) in the diet. Chloride is found in high concentrations in digestive juices, especially hydrochloric acid in the stomach, and in the cerebrospinal fluids that bathe the central nervous system. Chloride is the primary negative ion found outside the cells throughout all life forms. Some scientists have theorized that the chloride part of salt is even more responsible for high blood pressure than sodium is.

Functions. Stomach acid (hydrochloric acid) for digestion. Acid-base balance. Allows blood to carry carbon dioxide for excretion through the lungs. Growth of bone and connective tissue. Key ion outside of cells.

Deficiency symptoms. Unlikely, unless sodium is also depleted. Weakness, nausea, confusion, memory loss. Long-term low levels could create growth retardation.

Toxicity symptoms. It is possible that the high blood pressure attributed to sodium may also be caused by excess chloride. Since a healthy kidney excretes excess chloride, little is known about this area.

Characteristics. Must balance with sodium and potassium intake, since these are the critical ions inside and outside the cell.

Sources. Table salt,* salted foods,* soy sauce.

People at risk. Those with heavy fluid loss through vomiting, diarrhea, or perspiration. Kidney patients. Those on salt-restricted diets.

Daily intake:

Recommended: 1,700 to 5,100 milligrams (no RDA given).
Supplemental: Unlikely to be needed, 100 to 500 milligrams.
Toxicity: 20,000 milligrams

Sodium

Sodium is the dominant ion in sea water and in the water surrounding all cells throughout nature. As 40 percent of the weight of table salt, sodium has been indicted for its role in the 35 million cases of hypertension that

America has.[11] Sodium carries water with it. In healthy kidneys, the excess sodium from the diet is excreted. Yet some people's kidneys get tired of excreting the extra sodium from the diet and start retaining fluid. A stroke is caused by burst blood vessels from excessive fluid pressure.

Sodium is such an essential mineral that our tongues have an area just to help us find salty foods. Salt used to be the primary food preservative, since it deprives the food-rotting microorganisms of water.

Coal miners at the turn of the century died by the dozens from low body sodium due to perspiration. Mahatma Gandhi used a salt strike to get the attention of the British in India. Yet, for many Americans today, the use of salt has turned from need to addiction. People allow their salt taste to become so bludgeoned that increasing levels of salt are required to get the same effect. The result is that many Americans consume forty times the sodium that they need and five times the recommended upper limit. Thirty percent of our sodium intake is found in the food, 30 percent is added by the consumer, and 40 percent is added by the food processor.[12]

Functions. Fluid balance. Acid-base balance. Nerve transmission. Muscle contraction. Glucose absorption. Nutrient transport. Since it is the primary ion outside cells, it is crucial to all life processes. The body carefully regulates the sodium levels of the blood with the kidneys, the hormone aldosterone, perspiration, and other mechanisms.

Deficiency symptoms. Unlikely. Weakness, dizziness, cramps, fatigue, nausea, confusion. Heart palpitations and death could occur.

Toxicity symptoms. High blood pressure. Fluid retention in ankles or other areas. Could even create dizziness from fluid retention in the inner ear.

Characteristics. Intake should balance with potassium and chloride. Much sodium is lost in sweat, vomiting, and diarrhea. The body has a sodium buffer for reserves, so only those losing considerable body fluids need to take supplementary sodium.

Sources. Salt,* salted foods, soy sauce, monosodium glutamate (MSG), processed cheese, processed meats, milk, most animal foods.

People at risk. People who perspire excessively, especially those who are not accustomed to heat or work. With time, the body adjusts to slow down sodium loss in sweat. After repeated vomiting or diarrhea. Strict vegetarians, since plant foods are rich in potassium but marginal in sodium. Most Americans are at risk for excessive sodium intake.

Daily intake:

Recommended: 1,100 to 3,300 milligrams (no RDA given).

Supplemental: 100 to 1,000 milligrams.
Toxicity: 20,000 milligrams(?).

Magnesium

Magnesium is a metal favored by car racing and aviation enthusiasts for its light weight and nonrusting properties. About one-third of dolomite is magnesium, the other two-thirds are calcium. The average adult body contains about twenty-one grams. One-third to one-half of Americans are seriously low in magnesium intake.

Functions. A cofactor or catalyst in many reactions, including energy metabolism in ATP production. Part of bones and teeth. Involved in nerve transmission. Muscle relaxation. Tooth enamel. Cold adaptation. Helps body maintain proper potassium balance.[13]

Deficiency symptoms. Subclinical: Sensitivity to noise. Irritability. Muscle cramps and weakness. Digestive upset. Higher risk for kidney stones.[14] Clinical: Muscle tremors, loss of appetite, personality changes. Calcification of soft tissue, such as hardening of arteries. Baldness. Swollen gums, skin lesions. Palpitations and deterioration of heart tissue. Sudden muscle contractions of the heart and major arteries. This could be fatal.[15]

Toxicity symptoms. Since blood magnesium levels are carefully controlled by the healthy kidney, this is unlikely. Weakness, drowsiness, and lethargy are possible. If blood levels rose above normal, muscle paralysis, labored breathing, coma, and death could result.

Characteristics. Must balance with calcium, phosphorus, and vitamin D intake. Considerable magnesium is lost in sweat, also through use of certain drug, alcohol, stress, and excess fiber intake. Lost in wheat milling. Blood tests may register normal magnesium levels while body cells can be simultaneously low in magnesium.[16]

Sources. Soybeans,* buckwheat, shrimp, wheat germ, almonds, cashews, Brazil nuts, whole grains, molasses, clams, cornmeal, spinach, oysters, crabs, peas, bananas, potatoes, oatmeal, salmon, milk, liver, beef, green vegetables (chlorophyll contains magnesium).

People at risk. People who eat processed food. (Percent of magnesium lost in refining: whole wheat to white flour, 82 percent; brown rice to polished white rice, 83 percent; corn to corn starch, 97 percent; milk to butter, 98 percent.) Those who do not eat fresh greens. Consumers of alcohol. Dieters. Drug users. Depressed people. Older adults. People who perspire considerably. Diabetics. Those on high-fiber diets. Those with low vitamin D intake, since D aids in magnesium absorption. Those on digitalis or diuretics. Pregnant women. Sudden death heart attack is less likely in regions where people drink hard water (high in magnesium).[17]

Daily intake:

USRDA: 400 milligrams.
Supplemental: 200 to 600 milligrams.
Preferred form: Magnesium oxide.
Toxicity: 2,000 milligrams(?).

Zinc

Zinc is a mineral prized by industry for its ability to coat steel and slow down the corrosion process. Zinc is even more prized by the human body. The two grams of zinc found in the average adult body are involved in at least eighty enzyme systems. Zinc deficiency, which is common even in well-nourished America, can lead to impotence and loss of sex drive. Oysters, which are the richest natural source of zinc, are an ancient Oriental aphrodisiac.

Alcohol creates a great strain on the body's zinc supply. Newborn rats of a zinc-deficient mother and human infants with fetal alcohol syndrome have similar symptoms. All are physically and/or mentally impaired. The drug Thalidomide causes rats to have deformed offspring only if the pregnant mother was zinc deficient. Given the ubiquitous role of zinc in human metabolism, and the low zinc level in the American diet,[18] this is a mineral worthy of special attention.

Functions. DNA synthesis. Thus all cells need zinc, especially those involved in rapid turnover, like the lining of the tongue and the intestinal tract. Protein synthesis. Sperm production. Fetal development. Skin growth and healing. Removal of carbon dioxide. Making immune factors for disease resistance. Processing alcohol in the liver. Digestive enzymes that work on protein. Energy metabolism; allows the body to create energy in spite of insufficient oxygen (anaerobic metabolism). Critical for insulin activity, normal vitamin A activity, and enzymes that regulate skin oil. Many other functions.

Deficiency symptoms. Subclinical: Loss of taste and smell. Low sperm count.[19] Poor wound healing. Higher risk for hypertension of pregnancy,[20] Caesarian delivery and smaller infant,[21] toxemia, and birth defects.[22] Lowered disease resistance. Acne. Higher risk for osteoporosis.[23] Night blindness. Enlarged prostate gland. White spots on fingernails. Fatigue and reduced athletic performance.[24] Dandruff. Impaired glucose tolerance. The zinc to copper ratio is an important risk factor in heart disease.[25] Clinical: Stunted growth. Poor sexual development. Severe acne. Impotence. Infertility. Congenital deformities in pregnancy. Elevated risk for all infectious diseases. Elevated risk for heart disease, kidney and liver ailments, anorexia nervosa,[26] and rheumatoid arthritis.[27] Behavioral and sleep disorders.

Toxicity symptoms. Lowering of the high-density lipoproteins (HDL), which could create a higher risk for heart disease; 28 milligrams daily does not affect HDLs,[28] but 150 milligrams does.[29] Could create an imbalance or deficiency of other minerals, especially copper.[30] Poor muscle coordination, dizziness, drowsiness, vomiting, lethargy, intestinal upset. Could lead to renal failure. Galvanized trash cans (zinc coated), when used to make lemonade at large picnics, have resulted in zinc toxicity.

Characteristics. Foods that lower zinc absorption: soya protein isolates, soya-based milk feeds, coffee, cow's milk, cheese, hamburgers, celery, lemon, brown bread, iron supplements, whole wheat bread, high-fiber diets, bran and the phytates of coffee, colas, and teas.[31] Conditions leading to decreased absorption: celiac disease and other malabsorption problems, low stomach acid, gastrointestinal surgery, alcoholism, excessive folacin supplements,[32] and age. Lost in wheat milling. Much zinc can be lost in sweat.[33] Commonly deficient in the United States and probably responsible, at least in part, for a variety of ailments and suboptimal functioning. Much zinc is stored in the prostate gland. Iron and other minerals compete with zinc for absorption sites in the intestines.[34] Oral contraceptives increase the need for zinc, as do excess fiber, calcium, or copper. Anorectics may have a problem absorbing zinc,[35] which either creates or worsens their condition. Zinc intake should be in a 10 to 1 ratio with copper.

Sources. Oysters,* herring,* clams, wheat germ, bran, oatmeal, liver, nuts, beef, lamb, peas, chicken, carrots, eggs, seafood.

People at risk. Older adults. Preterm infants.[36] Those using many drugs. Vegetarians, anorectics, bulimics, fad dieters. AIDS victims.[37] Pregnant and lactating women. Growing children.[38] Serious athletes.[39] Burn patients and those on parenteral nutrition. Some minority groups, especially Mexican-Americans.[40] Alcohol consumers.[41]

Daily intake:

USRDA: 15 milligrams.
Supplemental: 5 to 30 milligrams.
Preferred form: Zinc gluconate.
Toxicity: 400 milligrams.

Iron

Iron has the ability to rust. That is bad on your car, but it is good in your body. The essence of rusting is that the metal can change its electrical valence, which allows the blood to carry oxygen to the trillions of cells in the body. There is only about one gram of iron in the average adult body. But considering the importance of oxygen, this gram is crucial.

Functions. As part of the hemoglobin molecule, iron is charged with delivering oxygen to the body cells. Since all cells need oxygen, this influences every other process of the body. Also involved in antibody formation and generally essential to the immune system as it wards off foreign invading organisms. Iron activates vitamin A. Helps to synthesize DNA, RNA, and collagen. Aids in drug detoxification. Helps regulate blood fats. Involved in the making of neurochemical transmitters in the brain. Energy production in the cytochrome system. Involved in making carnitine.

Deficiency symptoms. Subclinical: Fatigue, irritability, confusion, and apathy. Muscle weakness and decreased exercise tolerance. Lowered disease resistance, leading to more infections and of greater duration.[42] Behavioral and mood changes.[43] Poor digestion. Infants are less responsive, more tense, less active, and more fearful.[44] Gray or white pallid color to the skin, especially in the corner of the eyes where the tiny blood vessels come to the surface. Higher risk for tumors and cancer,[45] candida yeast infections, and herpes viral infections. Clinical: Serious infections due to reduced immune bodies. Hyperactivity and reduced intelligence quotient, especially in children.[46] Labored breathing. Hypochromic (low in color) microcytic (small red blood cells) anemia.

Toxicity symptoms. Iron's rusting can be both good and bad. Good when it is bound to a protein like hemoglobin. Bad when it is in free form, because it can generate tissue damage by free radical destruction. Free radicals are the great white sharks in the chemical sea of life.[47] Iron toxicity becomes particularly critical in the adult male, since there is no means by which the body can rid itself of the extra iron. The body then deposits the excess iron in the soft tissue, spleen, and liver to begin tissue damage. Adult males of the Bantu tribe of Africa suffer from iron toxicity (hemosiderosis) from their home brewing of beer in cast iron kettles. This can lead to runaway growth of bone marrow cells (hyperplasia) and increased susceptibility to infection. Those who take excess iron supplements will probably feel intestinal cramps and constipation. Prolonged use of iron supplements in reasonable levels rarely causes iron overload.[48] Excess iron stores can elevate the risk for heart disease.[49] More than once, continuous blood transfusions have so saturated a patient's body with iron that the person would set off metal detectors in airports.[50] Another form of iron toxicity, hemochromatosis, is found in people who are genetically incapable of regulating iron absorption. This occurs in less than 0.1 percent of the American population.[51]

Characteristics. Factors that aid in the absorption of iron: High acid in the intestines, such as normal stomach acid, vitamin C, citrus fruits. Lactose (milk sugar) stimulates a higher acid level by encouraging intestinal bacteria. Iron chelated into a protein complex, like heme iron, is four times better absorbed than elemental iron from cast iron cookware or vegetables.[52] Heme iron is found in animal sources such as meat, liver, poultry, and fish. When a healthy person's iron supply is low, the efficiency of absorbing iron is increased.

Factors that increase the need for iron: Menstruation. Pregnancy; fetal growth can seriously deplete a woman's iron supply. Regular aspirin use causes microscopic bleeding in the intestines and could create anemia. Rapid growth stages in infancy through adolescence, as the body adds more blood. Donating blood. Blood loss through wounds or surgery can create anemia. Long-term antacid use negates the acid effect in the intestines and therefore lowers iron absorption. Intensive and regular exercise causes a more rapid destruction of red blood cells, unless well protected by vitamin E and selenium.

Absorption varies from about 1 percent efficiency for plant sources of iron (like rice) to 20 percent efficiency for liver and veal muscle. Iron and zinc compete for intestinal absorption sites, so an excess of one can cause a deficiency of the other.[53] The body is remarkably economical, recycling 90 percent of its iron stores. Coffee with a meal can reduce iron absorption by 39 percent.[54] Tannic acid (which is high in tea) interferes with iron absorption.[55] The calcium of milk competes with iron for intestinal absorption sites. Thus heavy milk drinkers are at greater risk for iron anemia.[56] Since iron is an oxidizing metal and vitamin E is an antioxidant, they have an antagonistic relationship. High-dose supplements of iron and E should not be taken at the same time.

Sources. Pork liver,* liver,* cast iron cookware, cream of wheat, clams, beef, pork, veal, chicken, fish, spinach, asparagus, prunes, raisins, nori seaweed.

People at risk. Menstruating, lactating, or pregnant women. Infants and growing children. Athletes, since iron is lost in sweat and blood cells are destroyed more rapidly with intensive exercise. Aspirin users. Alcoholics. Vegetarians. Those with intestinal disorders that cause poor absorption.[57] Blood donors. Surgery and wound patients.

Daily intake:

USRDA: 18 milligrams.
Supplemental: 2 to 18 milligrams.
Preferred form: Ferrous fumarate.
Toxicity: Greater than 30 milligrams for adult males, greater than 60 milligrams for most others.

Copper

Copper, like iron, has the ability to oxidize. Copper is the key to the final extraction of energy from foodstuffs. The eighty milligrams of copper found in the body work closely with iron in several ways.

Functions. Works with iron in red blood cell formation. Energy release in the cytochrome system. The formation of the fatty wrapping around all nerve cells (myelin sheath). Helps manufacture the tough connective tissues of collagen and elastin. Aids in making the tanning pigment melanin. Involved in making an important enzyme (superoxide dismutase) for the body to thwart the effects of free radicals within. Helps to make vital brain chemicals, DNA, and uric acid.

Deficiency symptoms. Subclinical: Anemia, fatigue, and irritability. Lowered disease resistance.[58] Diminished skin pigmentation. Beginning or worsening of arthritis.[59] Steely or kinky hair. Low HDL[60] and higher cholesterol levels in blood,[61] thus raising the risk for heart disease.[62] Clinical: Bone demineralization. Poor maintenance of tough connective tissue, which leads to easily damaged blood vessels and other tissue. Disintegration of the central nervous system. Deficiency in laboratory animals can produce emphysema.[63]

Toxicity symptoms. Nausea, vomiting, stomach pain, headache, weakness, diarrhea, metallic taste in mouth. Can lead to hypertension, irregular rhythms of the heart, jaundice, and death. No adverse effects were found in humans taking supplements of thirty-five milligrams daily.[64] In the genetic disorder Wilson's disease, abnormal copper accumulation leads to irreversible damage of the brain, liver, and kidneys.

Characteristics. Copper and zinc compete in the intestines for absorption; thus an excess of one can lead to a deficiency of the other.[65] Excess calcium can also lower copper absorption. Absorption efficiency is normally about 30 percent. Since copper and iron work so closely in certain functions, their symptoms of deficiency or excess can be confused. Copper is incorporated into digestive bile, and thus can be excreted with the feces. Excess vitamin C intake lowers the body's circulating levels of copper.[66]

Sources. Shellfish, liver, cherries, nuts, cocoa, gelatin, copper water pipes, whole grain cereals, eggs, poultry, beans and peas.

People at risk. Those who take zinc supplements without a copper balance. Patients on tube feedings or total parenteral nutrition.[67]

Daily intake:

> USRDA: 2 milligrams.
> Supplemental: 2 to 5 milligrams.
> Preferred form: Copper gluconate.
> Toxicity: 50 milligrams(?).

Iodine

Iodine deficiency is one of the most common forms of malnutrition. Adults develop an enlarged throat as the thyroid gland swells up. In some areas of the world, this swollen-throat look is so common that people without goiter are called "bottlenecks." Most of the 400 million people around the world who suffer from iodine deficiency live in interior regions, since iodine is found primarily in the sea. There are groups of people in the Andes of South America who have small leather pouches of dried seaweed slung from their sides. Although they don't know why, these pouches full of iodine-rich seaweed protect them from endemic goiter that haunts mountainous regions of the world. The twenty-five milligrams of iodine in the healthy adult body act to regulate the level at which the body burns fuel.

Functions. An important part of the hormone thyroxin, which is in charge of regulating basal metabolism. Thyroxin establishes the pace for how high your body's "thermostat" will be set.

Deficiency symptoms. Subclinical: Fatigue, malaise, and lethargy. Poor hearing.[68] Very susceptible to feeling cold. Gain weight easily. Clinical: Reduced mental abilities or permanent mental retardation (cretinism) when deficiency exists during pregnancy or early childhood. Swollen throat region in adults (goiter).

Toxicity symptoms. Unknown. The use of iodine-based cleansers in dairy farm equipment has led to a significant increase in the iodine content of milk, yet nowhere near any level of toxicity in even the most avid milk drinker.[69] In some people, iodine supplements may cause skin irritations, such as acne.

Characteristics. Numerous foods contain substances that bind iodine in the intestines to make it unavailable for absorption. These goitrogenic foods include radish, cabbage, turnip, cauliflower, rutabagas, and soybeans. Cooking renders these goitrogens ineffective. In the iodine-rich diet of the West, goitrogens are a minor hazard. Iodide (two atoms of iodine) is added to normal table salt, but not to commercial salt nor to salt used in pickling.

Sources.   Iodine tablets (used to purify drinking water when bacteria may be present), iodized salt, ocean seafood, seaweed, milk (due to the iodized cleansers used in the dairy industry), food grown on high-iodine soil (near the ocean where salt spray may reach).

People at risk.   Those who do not consume seafood, iodized salt or commercial milk. Those who eat an abundance of raw vegetables, some of which may be goitrogenic. Growing children and pregnant women, since basal metabolism is higher during these developmental stages. Those who live in mountainous terrain or glacier belts, where the glaciers have swept away the iodine on the soil surface.

Daily intake:

USRDA: 150 micrograms.
Supplemental: 100 to 500 micrograms.
Preferred form: Potassium iodide.
Toxicity: Unknown.

Manganese

Manganese was a key link in the beginning of life on earth. In the early primordial soup, there was no oxygen. About one and a half billion years ago, blue-green algae appeared in the seas and were able to harness the energy of the sun in the presence of manganese to split water into its component hydrogen and oxygen molecules. With oxygen being produced, life on earth became possible. The ten to fifteen milligrams found in the adult body may play an important role in cancer prevention. Deficiencies in animals have been observed, but little is known about deficiencies in humans.

Functions.   Synthesis of skeletal and connective tissue. Release of energy as part of the structure and function of the energy-creating mitochondria in the cell. Manufacturing of fatty acids and cholesterol. Making of DNA, RNA, and urea as part of protein metabolism. Mobilizing fats from the liver. Antioxidant against free radicals, as part of an important enzyme, superoxide dismutase. Involved in making an important brain chemical, dopamine.

Deficiency symptoms.   Unclear. Loss of muscle tone(?). Greater chance of developing diabetes, heart disease, or cancer(?). All cancerous tumors examined have been found to have an inordinately low level of manganese.

Toxicity symptoms. There are manganese-mining regions in Chile where the miners develop what is called "locura manganica," or craziness from manganese. The symptoms are similar to the radical mood swings of a manic depressive. Initially there is unaccountable laughter, heightened sexuality, inability to sleep, and hallucinations. This is followed by deep depression, impotence, and a catatoniclike state. The final stages are similar to Parkinson's disease and are treated in the same way. Toxicity of manganese from the diet is highly unlikely.

Characteristics. Only about 3 percent of the manganese in the diet is absorbed. Excess calcium stunts manganese absorption. Lost in food refining. Since other minerals compete with manganese for intestinal absorption sites, it is possible that regular use of magnesium-containing antacids could create a manganese deficiency.

Sources. Rice bran,* wheat bran,* corn germ, whole grains and cereals, green vegetables, nuts, legumes, tea, ginger, cloves.

People at risk. Those taking large amounts of mineral supplements without consideration for proper balance. Excessive milk drinkers. Those consuming highly refined diets or on low intake of vegetables and legumes. Those genetically prone to cancer.

Daily intake:

Recommended: 2.5 to 5 milligrams (no RDA given).
Supplemental: 2.5 to 20 milligrams.
Preferred form: Manganese gluconate.
Toxicity: 30 milligrams(?).

Chromium

Chromium deficiency may be responsible for an abundance of death and disease in the developed nations.[70] Chromium is critical for the proper burning of glucose in the cells. The six milligrams found in the adult body are critical to the regulation of fat, carbohydrate, and protein metabolism. It is likely that up to a third of all adult diabetics could have their disease significantly improved (but not necessarily cured) by taking chromium supplements.[71] Because of the great value and almost zero toxicity of chromium, some researchers have recommended an ideal intake of the higher end of the 50 to 200 range stated by the RDA people.

Functions. Chromium is locked into the center of a molecule called glucose tolerance factor. GTF works with insulin and cyclic AMP to allow glucose to pass into the cell and then to be burned.

Deficiency symptoms. Subclinical: Fatigue and irritability. Impaired glucose tolerance.[72] Hypoglycemia and the radical mood and energy swings that accompany that condition. Higher risk for heart and vessel diseases.[73] Clinical: Since glucose is the favored fuel for most cells of the body, a lack of GTF will lead to the burning of more fats and protein. This results in lean tissue wasting as the body begins to burn its protein stores. It also can elevate fats in the bloodstream and thus cause all sorts of vascular diseases. There is an elevated risk for diabetes, heart disease, kidney disease, cataracts, and other diseases of vessel obstruction.

Toxicity symptoms. Unknown. Trivalent chromium taken orally has failed to produce any toxicity symptoms on any animals tested.[74]

Characteristics. From 0.5 to 2 percent of dietary chromium is absorbed.[75] Hair chromium is an excellent indicator of body chromium status over the long run. Much chromium can be lost in sweat.[76] The chromium in brewer's yeast is special in that yeast contains some glucose tolerance factors which may facilitate chromium use in the body. Human subjects fed twenty grams of brewer's yeast daily, containing only forty-eight micrograms of chromium, had significant improvements in the fatty components of their blood.[77] The GTF chromium in yeast is lost in food refining. Excreted from the body during very high fluid and sugar intake,[78] such as soft drink consumption. Strenuous exercise leads to significant chromium loss.[79] Americans have a much lower level of chromium in their bodies than people in the Far East. We also have a much higher rate of heart disease and diabetes. There is likely a link here.

Sources. Brewer's yeast,* liver, meat, cheese, legumes, beans, peas, whole grains, black pepper, molasses. Note that molasses and whole grains are good sources, while their refined counterparts of white flour and sugar contain almost no chromium.

People at risk. Pregnant and lactating women, since these stages of life create such a drain on chromium stores. Women with multiple pregnancies have a much higher risk for developing diabetes later in life, perhaps due to the chromium drain of pregnancy(?). Patients on tube feedings.[80] Those on a high-sugar diet. Those who regularly use white flour products. Serious athletes.

Daily intake:

Recommended: 50 to 200 micrograms (no RDA given).
Supplemental: 100 to 500 micrograms.
Preferred form: GTF from yeast.
Toxicity: Unknown.

Fluorine

Fluorine is one of the most abundant elements in the earth's crust. For centuries it was known that certain isolated communities had very few dental problems. It was suspected that their water was responsible. Indeed, fluoridated water can reduce the incidence of dental caries by at least 50 percent.

Functions. Aids in the hardening of calcium salts throughout the body, including the bones and tooth enamel.

Deficiency symptoms. Subclinical: Increased susceptibility to dental caries. Bones that are not as hard as they could be. Clinical: Excessive dental caries. Softened or hollowed bones. Osteoporosis.

Toxicity symptoms. Brown mottling of the teeth. This is cosmetically unappealing yet there are no other known effects of excess fluoride in the diet.

Characteristics. Since the earth's crust is so abundant in fluoride, water can be an excellent but very unreliable source. Some water is so high in fluoride that it causes mottling. Other water is so low that the people who drink it regularly have excessive dental caries. Fluoridated water helps maintain some control of fluoride intake. In the 1950s a rumor was spread along with the other paranoia of the McCarthy era that fluoridated water was a communist plot to control the minds of Americans. The rumor was untrue and ridiculous yet has stayed in the minds of many taxpayers. This is one reason fluoridated water is not the rule of the day. All major health agencies have sanctioned the fluoridation of water. There are no health risks and only benefits to be derived from fluoride's being added to municipal water supplies.

Sources. Naturally fluoridated water from underground springs,* artificially fluoridated water, crops raised on fluoridated water, food cooked in fluoridated water, mackeral, salmon.

People at risk. Those consuming nonfluoridated water. Pregnant and lactating women. People who have a genetic tendency toward many cavities. Those on a high-sugar diet.

Daily intake:

Recommended: 1.5 to 4 milligrams (no RDA given).
Supplemental: 1 to 10 milligrams.
Preferred form: Any form; should be given early in life, while bones and teeth are developing, to be most effective.
Toxicity: 500 milligrams(?).

Selenium

Selenium, until about twenty years ago, was thought to be toxic for humans. It is now on the cutting edge of nutrition research as being a mineral that can lessen much of the disease and premature death in this country. Seventy micrograms, rather than the currently listed fifty, should be the minimum acceptable intake level.[81]

Functions.   As an antioxidant to neutralize free radicals. Free radicals are the ever-present destructive forces in the body that can induce cancer and premature aging. Selenium works with vitamin E[82] to placate the rampaging free radicals. Prevents tissue inflammation.[83] Prevents heavy-metal toxicity.[84] Bolsters the immune system to help ward off infections and even cancer.[85] Aids in the repair of DNA when it has been damaged by carcinogens or mutagens.[86] May be involved in killing strangely growing precancer cells, which likely occur in many people.[87] E and selenium protect against the effects of radiation.[88] As a protective antioxidant, selenium encourages the production of arachidonic acid and prostacyclin,[89, 90] both of which are champions of good health.

Deficiency symptoms.   Higher risk for heart disease or cancer.[91, 92] Premature aging(?). Animals with selenium deficiency develop the symptoms of muscular dystrophy. One year of selenium therapy has been shown to improve the symptoms found in human muscular dystrophy victims.[93] Greater risk for heavy-metal toxicity (i.e., cadmium, mercury).[94]

Toxicity symptoms.   Selenium is one of the more finely tuned nutrients in the sense that both too little and too much are disastrous. The range between these two limits is not that great. Excess selenium can impair normal sulfur metabolism and thus result in abnormal bone and cartilage development. Degeneration of heart and liver. Higher risk for decayed and missing teeth. Nervous syptoms can include blindness, paralysis, respiratory failure, and abdominal pain. The recommended upper limits of intake, 200 micrograms, are much too low, say some elite scientists.[95]

Characteristics.   Since selenium is not an essential nutrient for plants, those grown on selenium-poor soil thrive just as well as those grown on selenium-rich soil. There is a relationship between selenium levels in the soil and the incidence of cancer in this country. Selenium content in food varies widely. Selenium-grown yeast provides the most active form.[96] Cystic fibrosis patients need high-potency selenium supplements.[97]

Sources.   Brazil nuts (one nut can supply up to 50 micrograms, the minimum acceptable level established by the RDA board),[98] food grown on selenium-rich soil,* selenium-enriched yeast, soybeans, tuna, seafood, meat, whole grains.

People at risk. Many Americans, since few of us know where our food originated. Those with a genetic risk toward cancer. Residents of the South Atlantic seaboard have unusually low selenium levels.[99] This area is sometimes referred to as the "stroke belt." There could be a connection between the two. Of the twenty-seven nations that keep such records, Americans are near the bottom for selenium intake.

Daily intake:

Recommended: 50 to 200 micrograms (no RDA given).
Supplemental: 50 to 500 micrograms.
Preferred form: Yeast.
Toxicity: 3000 micrograms(?).[100]

Molybdenum

Molybdenum is one of the rarest elements in the earth's crust. The world's highest incidence of esophageal cancer is found in an area of China where molybdenum is even more rare in the diet.

Functions. Mobilizing iron from liver stores. Uric acid excretion (gout sufferers experience pain as uric acid builds up in the joints). Works with fluoride in hardening of calcium salts. May be a useful antioxidant.

Deficiency symptoms. Fast heartbeat and breathing rate.[101] Visual problems. May have higher risk for cancer,[102] cavities, sexual impotency, and gout(?).

Toxicity symptoms: Unknown.

Characteristics. May help detoxify hazardous substances, such as sulfites used as produce preservatives. Little is known.

Sources. Buckwheat,* lima beans,* soybeans, wheat germ, liver, barley, oats, lentils, sunflower seeds.

People at risk. Those consuming a highly refined diet, because it is likely that molybdenum is lost in food processing.

Daily intake:

Recommended: 150 to 500 micrograms (no RDA given).
Supplemental: 150 to 500 micrograms.
Preferred form: Sodium molybdate.
Toxicity: 2,000 micrograms(?).

The following micronutrients are known to be essential in human metabolism, but little else is known about them.

Cobalt is an integral part of vitamin B_{12}. There is some evidence that it may function in other enzyme systems of the body. Since its only established function is with B_{12}, deficiency symptoms would be the same as with this vitamin. Sources of cobalt (and B_{12}) include liver, kidney, oysters, clams, meat, fish. Cobalt is used as a foam stabilizer in beer. Some heavy beer drinkers could develop cobalt toxicity. There are no recommended, supplemental or toxicity levels known for cobalt.

Nickel may play a role in iron use, fat metabolism, and RNA and DNA synthesis. There are no known cases of deficiency symptoms, except when laboratory animals are raised in a nickel-free environment. It can be absorbed through the skin. A toxic form of nickel is inhaled in tobacco fumes. Nickel is widely distributed in most foods, especially fruits and vegetables.

Silicon is thought to stimulate normal growth, collagen synthesis, and bone calcification. It is found in whole grains. Recent studies have shown silicon plays a role in protecting against heart disease.[103]

Tin may be involved in maintaining the structure of proteins. Tin cans may cause suspiciously high levels of intake.[104] Little else is known.

Vanadium is probably involved in iron and fat metabolism, growth, reproduction, and bone and tooth development. With its possible role in tooth formation, low vanadium may lead to increased dental caries. A deficiency of vanadium has been found to interfere with the sodium/potassium pump that is vital to each living cell.[105] Low vanadium might also increase the risk for breast cancer.[106] Black pepper, soy, corn, and olive oil, olives, gelatin, and unrefined foods are sources of vanadium. Refined diets are low in this mineral.

Arsenic is known to be essential in rats and may be essential in humans.

Minerals Likely to be Toxic

Aluminum has been implicated in the senility of Alzheimer's disease and osteomalacia in renal dialysis patients. Aluminum is a favorite additive of the food industry, found in everything from table salt (as an anticaking agent) to baking powder to a flour whitener. Aluminum pans and skillets along with food stored in aluminum foil could contribute small amounts to the diet over a lifetime. Some antacids use aluminum as their base. Even some toothpastes and deodorants have substantial aluminum. Since most healthy bodies excrete three-fourths or more of the ingested aluminum, some researchers have proposed that Alzheimer's is the result not of aluminum toxicity but rather of cells gone awry. Nevertheless, we recommend minimizing your aluminum intake.

Cadmium is also potentially toxic and not well excreted by the body.

Found in cigarette smoke, canned foods, urban air pollution, and certain water pipes, this mineral has been named a culprit in the high blood pressure of many individuals.[107]

Mercury is the problem behind the "mad hatter's syndrome," spoken of in *Alice in Wonderland*. The hatters of olden days had to work with mercury compounds. Through pollution and contamination, mercury can accumulate and cause neurological damage. Mercury, a deadly toxin, is used to formulate silver fillings in dentistry. Some dentists have cured patients of untreatable symptoms by removing the silver fillings and replacing them with plastic ones. Subclinical mercury toxicity almost certainly exists throughout developed nations.

Lead is a potent toxin that is not easily expelled by the body. Selenium helps prevent lead buildup, even when we are exposed to lead. Lead toxicity can create general fatigue, headache, lethargy, and personality changes because it interferes with receptor sites in the brain. Since it is found in lead-seamed cans, newsprint, pewter, urban air, paint, ceramic glazes, drinking water, and an abundance of industrial pollutants, there is no shortage of lead exposure for the average American. The sales of leaded gasoline have been shown to directly relate to the levels of lead in the placental blood of newborn infants.[108]

There are other elements found in the human body that may be either essential in trace amounts, harmless trace impurities from the environment, or toxic, including barium, bromine, strontium, gold, silver, bismuth, gallium, antimony, boron, and lithium.

13

QUASI-VITAMINS

"Some of the jury wrote down 'important' and some 'unimportant.'"
—LEWIS CARROLL, ALICE IN WONDERLAND

The substances discussed in this chapter aren't currently considered essential vitamins, since people can survive without them. In order for a nutrient to be considered an essential vitamin, humans must go through predictable stages of deficiency symptoms shortly after removing that nutrient from the diet. A lack of anything in this chapter will not kill you quickly, but some of these substances may be required in the diet for optimal health. Once it was easy to categorize the thousands of substances in the diet. They were either essential, harmless, or harmful. But many of the ones discussed here do not fit any of those categories.

Our diet supplies only the crude precursors of substances that are required in the body. For most healthy people and for survival, that works fine. Yet some people, especially the sick, the old, and the very young, cannot convert enough raw materials to be able to carry out the processes of life efficiently. Quasi-vitamins attempt to bypass some of the in-between conversion steps and give the body a closer semblance of what it really needs.

Some substances in this chapter may provide a little better health for many people. Others may someday be considered essential vitamins for some people. Some of these quasi-vitamins may be essential only for the sick and the very young. Some are fakers of the lowest kind. Many have been mired down in a sea of confusion because impure compounds are used in research. Some are so new and unresearched that no one can really pass judgment on them. A growing constituency of scientists have labeled some of the substances mentioned in this chapter as being "conditionally essential" nutrients, meaning they are required for some people during certain phases of life.

All vitamins and minerals now considered essential started out being called quasi-vitamins. We cannot be naive and overzealous in accepting every bizarre substance with only anecdotal evidence as support. But we should be receptive and open minded to new ideas. This chapter is composed entirely of "new ideas." A few will die the ignominious death they deserve, having flourished briefly in the spotlight and given false hope to some very sick people. And some may well become the Cinderella at the ball, as they take their rightful place in mainstream nutrition and the healing arts.

Choline and Lecithin

Since 1932, choline has been known to be essential for various animals. Choline is essential to humans, but not in our diets, since we are able to make some choline ourselves.[1] Under the guidance of enzymes containing vitamin B_{12} and folacin, the amino acids glycine and methionine contribute some of their parts to form choline. Not every human makes enough choline internally to keep ideally healthy, as shown by the fact that choline is effective in treating fatty liver in alcoholics.[2] Choline has also been shown to lower blood pressure in humans and animals[3] and to improve memory.[4] Choline is probably the most active and effective part of the popular food supplement lecithin, which is why the two are discussed together here.

Choline is part of the vital brain and nerve chemical acetylcholine; is part of brain structure and growth, in the form of sphingomyelin; helps prevent fatty infiltration in the liver, as a lipotrope; and is a valuable methyl donor, a ubiquitous role throughout human metabolism.

The richest sources of choline are egg yolk and lecithin, followed by liver, soybeans, fish, and cereal. The average diet in the United States provides about 500 to 900 milligrams daily of choline. It has been suggested that choline should be provided in tube feedings for hospital patients and in infant formulas.

Lecithin is a phospholipid substance capable of dissolving in both fat and water mediums at the same time. For this reason, lecithin is a favorite additive of the food industry. Lecithin can emulsify ingredients and keep them from separating, as it does with salad dressings, cookies, and candies. It is one of the few food additives that is actually good for you. It appears that the promising claims of lecithin's health-giving properties are primarily derived from its high choline content.

It has been found that lecithin:

- was more effective in treating manic depression than the drug of choice, lithium;[5]
- lowers blood cholesterol levels;[6]
- lowers cholesterol and triglycerides;[7]

- improves the condition of some patients with Alzheimer's disease;[8]
- helps dissolve gallstones (oral cholic acid was also used for a six-month experimental period);[9]
- improves tardive dyskinesia (uncontrolled muscle spasms from age or overmedication);[10]
- has had some success in treating other diseases, including Gilles de la Tourette (a collection of jerky movements with facial and vocal tics), Friedreich's ataxia (poor muscle coordination), Huntington's disease (a genetically transmitted deterioration of the nervous system), and myasthenic syndrome (a muscular disease).[11]

Myoinositol

Here is another substance known to be essential in the diet of various animals, but clear cut deficiency symptoms have not been outlined for humans.[12] Myoinositol is very similar in chemical structure to glucose and is made by the body from glucose. Myoinositol is a constituent of phospholipids, which become an integral part of all cell membranes. It is also important in fat metabolism and perhaps in the maintenance of normal levels of fat in the blood.

In whole grain foods, myoinositol is present in a more complex form, as phytic acid. This is the substance that binds minerals, like calcium and iron, and makes them unavailable for intestinal absorption. Most foods contain some myoinositol. Citrus fruits (except lemons) and cantaloupe are the best sources. Whole grains, beans, and nuts are good sources. The average American diet provides about 300 to 1,000 milligrams of myoinositol daily.[13]

Myoinositol helps protect humans against fatty infiltration of the liver and can improve the fatty liver of the alcoholic. In rats suffering deficiency of this nutrient, baldness is a common symptom. Unfortunately, human studies have not been successful in treating baldness with myoinositol. Studies have shown that myoinositol may play a role in slowing or halting nerve degeneration in diabetics.[14]

Carnitine

Here is a rising star in the field of nutrition. Discovered early in this century and then forgotten for fifty years, L-carnitine has been researched considerably in the past decade. Its role is basically as the shuttle system to pull fats into the mitochondria of the cells for energy production. Though carnitine is essential in the diet of some lower forms of life and possibly some newborn animals (sometimes referred to as vitamin BT),[15] it is not currently considered essential in the diet of humans. We manufacture our own carnitine using the amino acid lysine and requiring methionine, vitamin C, niacin, B_6, and iron to complete the construction.[16] Discovered by Russian scientists in meat extracts in 1905, it was named carnitine from *carnis,* which is Latin for flesh. Indeed, there is no carnitine in plant foods. The richest source of carnitine is mutton, which has three times the carnitine levels of lamb and beef. Chicken contains one-tenth the carnitine of beef. Very few other foods are good sources.

Carnitine helps the body burn fats efficiently. It is found in 100 times greater concentration in the heart than in the blood, which is understandable given the heart's preference for fats as a fuel. Because of its essential role in fat burning, carnitine has been shown to be effective in:

• preventing the oxygen-starvation death (ischemic myocardium) of the heart tissue, which occurs in heart attack victims;[17]

• lowering triglycerides and raising HDLs markedly, thus seriously lowering heart disease risk;[18]

• improving exercise tolerance in heart disease patients;[19]

• reducing frequency and severity of angina attacks in heart disease patients;[20]

• reducing incidence and severity of heart beat irregularities (cardiac arrhythmias) in patients using kidney machines (hemodialysis);[21]

• reducing cardiac arrhythmias in heart disease patients;[22]

• improving the course of patients with cirrhosis of the liver;[23]

• increasing motility and perhaps the fertility of men who are sterile due to low carnitine levels in their sperm;[24]

• improving athletic endurance and energy;[25]

• improving the body's adaptation to fasting and assisting in weight loss through efficient fat burning;[26]

• lowering the heart disease risk for diabetics.[27]

Scientists are sufficiently impressed with carnitine that they recommend its inclusion in infant formulas, hospital tube feedings, and as supplements to heart disease patients and diabetics.[28]

Fatty Acids

Yes, fats are essential for health. And certain categories of fatty acids are drawing an incredible amount of attention for their health-giving properties. Linoleic acid has long been known to be essential in the diet. From linoleic acid, the body makes, among other things, prostaglandins. Prostaglandins are a related family of substances that regulate areas as diverse as the secretion of insulin, gastrointestinal function, neurotransmitter function, blood vessel tone, salt and water balance, blood pressure, and the "stickiness" of the blood cells (platelet aggregation).[29]

Until recently, most scientists assumed that there was enough essential fatty acid (linoleic acid) in the high-fat diet of Americans. It was also assumed that most people possessed healthy systems that could process the linoleic acid into linolenic or arachidonic acid or any other by-product. These assumptions are now being questioned. New research shows some amazing healing properties of fish oil (eicosapentaenoic acid or EPA), docosahexanoic acid (DHA), and gamma-linolenic acid (GLA, or evening primrose oil). The health hazards of the abundant hydrogenated fats (trans-fatty acids) that we eat are becoming more obvious, too. Fatty acids deserve serious consideration in the science of nutrition.

Eicosapentaenoic acid. EPA is found primarily in cold-water fatty fish. Researchers saw that the diet of Greenland Eskimos was high in fat, cholesterol, and protein while being low in fiber, carbohydrates, and vitamin C. According to known principles of cardiovascular health, these people should have been dying of heart attacks in droves. Yet they weren't. Intense investigation isolated a protective factor in their diet: EPA. The best dietary sources of EPA include (best listed first): Chinook salmon, Atlantic mackerel, pink salmon, albacore tuna, sablefish, herring, and rainbow trout. The plant foods spirulina and purslane also contain fats that are very similar to EPA (called omega-3 fats). Most fish have at least some EPA. Residents of the Great Lakes region should avoid consuming too much of their fish because of its dangerous levels of the potent toxin PCB. The benefits of EPA would be far outweighed by the hazards of PCB.

EPA has an impressive record in research laboratories. It is effective at:

• lowering blood pressure;[30]
• stimulating the production of prostaglandin (I-3), which exerts a protective effect against heart disease;[31] heart disease risk is cut in half by eating only two ounces of fish per week for a lifetime;[32]
• preventing the "stickiness" of blood cells that causes many people's blood vessels to become blocked;[33]
• treating certain emotional disorders, including schizophrenia, manic depression, and agoraphobia;[34]
• lowering serum cholesterol and triglycerides by 50 percent or more;[35]
• improving the symptoms of rheumatoid arthritis;[36]
• improving disease resistance;[37]
• inhibiting the body's synthesis of leukotrienes, thus reducing the inflammation in skin and joints;[38]

- protecting against certain kidney problems (proteinuria);[39]
- improving the chances of surviving a heart attack;[40]
- protecting the brain from damage incurred during a stroke;[41]
- producing major improvements in the blood lipid profile of heart attack risk patients (plasma cholesterol was lowered 45 percent, triglycerides 79 percent, and HDLs were raised);[42]
- inhibiting the growth of tumors when used with DHA.[43]

But fish oil follows the pattern of all other nutritional factors—you can have too much of a good thing. Excessive fish oil was shown to slightly lower the body's white blood cell production, which might mean lowered disease resistance.[44] The intake levels necessary to achieve this drop in white corpuscle production was 3.2 grams of EPA. This is about the same amount found in a three-ounce portion of the richest food source of EPA, Chinook salmon. Also, since EPA increases the time required for one's blood to clot, some people may develop excessive bleeding problems. One heroic and foolhardy case was reported in the scientific literature of an Oxford professor who, impressed with the spate of evidence in favor of a high fish diet, went on a near total seafood diet supplemented with vitamin E.[45] This fellow developed anemia, prolonged bleeding time, and his plasma vitamin C level fell to nearly zero. In other words, if a little bit is good, then more is not necessarily better.

Certain patients with hypertension have been shown to have a poor ability to manufacture EPA internally. All of us have the ability to make some EPA within. For some people with high blood pressure, EPA may be considered an essential "vitamin."[46]

Because of the many benefits of EPA, we recommend that you eat a minimum of two to ten ounces of fish weekly.

Docosahexanoic acid. DHA is another omega-3 fatty acid related to EPA. DHA is found primarily in fish oil and human milk. It is virtually nonexistent elsewhere, including commercial infant formulas. The human brain is about 70 percent fatty substances, including significant levels of DHA. Studies have shown that young animals raised without DHA in their diet develop mental and visual problems.[47] Fish should be consumed by pregnant and lactating women for optimal development of their infant's brain. This is just one more argument in favor of the natural way of nourishing infants: human milk.

Linoleic acid. Linoleic acid is a dietary essential. About 60 percent of the fat consumed in this country is at least partially hydrogenated. This process seriously reduces the linoleic acid content of the fat and also lowers the body's ability to make fatty acid by-products like GLA.[48]

There are numerous factors that will lower your body's ability to make its own GLA and arachidonic acid, including:

- high dietary cholesterol intake or high blood cholesterol;
- high intake of saturated or hydrogenated fats;
- stress-released adrenaline;
- excess alcohol intake;
- diabetes;
- atopy, which is a very common nonfatal inherited condition manifested by asthma, skin eczema, or inflammation of the membranes of the nasal passages (rhinitis).

In other words, some people probably suffer an inability to make optimal levels of the various fatty acids required by their body's metabolism. Dietary gammalinolenic acid bypasses these metabolic failings and gives the body a more finished product. Some people's metabolisms can make arachidonic acid, EPA, DHA, and prostaglandins from a small amount of linoleic acid in the diet. Other people may need the GLA prebuilt in the diet in order to maintain health. Seeds of the ribes family (currants and gooseberries) and spirulina contain measurable amounts of GLA. GLA has been shown to:

- improve the symptoms of eczema, a common and difficult-to-treat skin rash;[49]
- reduce hypertension caused by stress;[50]
- reduce the pain and fluid retention of cancer (used along with vitamin C);[51]
- treat pre-eclampsia (fluid retention of pregnancy) and perhaps prevent the life-threatening toxemia;[52]
- improve the symptoms of premenstrual syndrome;[53]
- lower serum cholesterol;[54]
- aid alcoholic withdrawal symptoms and perhaps reduce the cravings for alcohol.[55]

There is some preliminary evidence that GLA supplements may improve the course of hyperactivity, hypertension, and diabetes for some patients,[56] and may prove to be an effective weapon against certain types of cancer[57] and arthritis.[58]

Most healthy people on a balanced healthy diet could exist on the linoleic acid found in plant oils like soy, safflower, corn, sunflower, and linseed. Linseed oil has a unique mixture of fatty acids that has been shown to increase the internal levels of DHA and EPA. Linseed oil is also the richest source of linolenic acid, a fat that is now considered essential for humans.

This field is very new. Most of the data about fatty acids has been elucidated in the past decade. Our recommendations are to lower your intake of fats, especially saturated fats. Eliminate hydrogenated fats. Minimize alcohol intake. Use plant oils, including some dietary linseed oil. (Do not use the artist's version of linseed oil, which is for diluting oil-based paints, not for consumption.)

Bioflavonoids

There are about 500 similar yet different chemicals that fall into the category of bioflavonoids. The more commonly referred to bioflavonoids include rutin and hesperidin. Until recently, the maze of bioflavonoids has caused mixed results in laboratory experiments because researchers were using impure substances. Bioflavonoids are found exclusively in the plant kingdom and are thought to participate in the capturing of the sun's energy in photosynthesis and various other plant functions. The vivid rainbow colors of autumn foliage are due partly to bioflavonoids. Food sources include citrus fruits (especially the outer white pulp), buckwheat, other plant foods, and even honey (since honey is gathered from plants by bees).

Bioflavonoids do not cure colds (although they may help prevent them), do not cure cancer (some types if taken excessively may even cause cancer),[59] nor does vitamin C require bioflavonoids in order to be effective.[60] Bioflavonoids have been shown, however, to have other amazing healing properties:

- improving the blood flow in cardiovascular patients (rutin, hesperidin, and vitamin C were used together in this study);[61]
- killing bacteria and fungus;[62]
- relieving headache pain without irritating the stomach;[63]
- relieving arthritis pain while fortifying the joints;[64]
- reducing the pain of insect bites, stings, and oral surgery (topical use), with a potency comparable to topically applied cocaine;[65]
- helping to prevent the painful and sometimes blinding buildup of fluids in the eyes of diabetics;[66]
- acting as an antihistamine to relieve the symptoms of allergies;[67]
- stopping viral infections;[68]
- killing cancer cells in laboratory tissue cultures;[69]
- helping to detoxify benzopyrenes, a common cancer-causing substance found in burned, smoked, and barbecued meats.[70]

Purified forms of the various bioflavonoids are difficult to find in American health food stores, since even highly skilled laboratory chemists have difficulty purifying bioflavonoids down to just one factor. We recommend that you eat abundant fruits, vegetables, whole grains, legumes, and honey to get a broad spectrum of bioflavonoids in natural form.

Interestingly enough, rutin is a bioflavonoid known to prevent capillary fragility,[71] such as occurs in strokes. One of the richest sources of rutin is buckwheat (also high in magnesium), which is a staple among a select group of Russians who are noted for their impressive longevity.

Another obstacle for bioflavonoids is that they may be inactivated by the liver. Therefore, if they are absorbed into the lymph, they would likely get a chance to work within the body's biochemistry. Otherwise, by being absorbed into the blood, they would be brought directly to the liver for deactivation. Little is known about how they are absorbed, either in the skin or intestines. Problems in obtaining the same results in research may stem from the inability of the bioflavonoids to get to the organ or tissue that needs healing.

Coenzyme Q

In order to extract the maximum amount of energy from food, your body sends the by-products of carbohydrates, fats, protein, and alcohol through a series of enzyme steps. One of the latter steps, called oxidative phosphorylation, requires an interesting substance called coenzyme Q, or ubiquinone. CoQ has been used successfully to treat heart disease patients without the usual barrage of side effects found in synthetic drugs.

For years, researchers wondered why animals with a vitamin E deficiency ended up with problems in energy metabolism, since E seems to have nothing to do with energy production. Then it was discovered that E encourages the production, and prevents the destruction, of CoQ. Hence, CoQ is the bridge that relates vitamin E to energy.[72]

CoQ can be made internally. The amino acids tyrosine and phenylalanine, plus vitamin E, niacin, folacin, pantothenic acid, B_6, and B_{12}, are required for the body to produce CoQ. Thus a deficiency in any of these nutrients can result in a deficiency of CoQ.

Since Q holds such an integral job in the energy-producing mitochondria, it is not surprising that it has also been shown to have impressive therapeutic value:

- stimulates the immune system;[73]
- reduces the toxic effects on the heart of the drug adriamycin;[74]
- enhances the pumping action of the heart and speeds recovery in heart-failure patients;[75]
- enhances healing in various gum (periodontal) diseases;[76]
- lowers blood pressure in certain individuals.[77]

About half of the hypertensive patients treated with CoQ (thirty to sixty milligrams oral dose daily) have had significant reduction in blood pressure. Methodist Hospital in Indianapolis and the Institute for Bio-Medical Research at the University of Texas are using CoQ as normal treatment for heart-failure patients, with 91 percent of the patients reporting some improvement after one month of supplementation.

Lipoic Acid

This substance works with thiamin in energy metabolism to convert pyruvate to acetyl CoA. This process is the bottleneck in the burning of carbohydrates, just as carnitine is the limiting step in the burning of fats. Sometimes called thioctic acid, lipoic acid is found in food substances like liver and yeast and can also be produced internally.

Rabbits fed lipoic acid along with high cholesterol diets ended up with serum cholesterol levels one-fifth as high as the control group.[78] In test-tube studies, lipoic acid improves the tissues' ability to use glucose and oxygen.[79] Its therapeutic value in humans includes reducing the pain and improving the condition of diabetics with nerve degeneration (neuropathy), using 100 to 200 milligrams daily;[80] and improving various liver ailments, including cirrhosis, hepatotoxicity, hepatic dysfunction, and hepatitis.[81]

Nucleosides

Some nucleosides hold the blueprints for growth and repair of the body (DNA). Other members of this group direct and control the production of most substances in the body (RNA). Others act as the "gold currency" of energy exchange (ATP).

Inosine is converted to adenosine, which is then used in making DNA or ATP (adenosine triphosphate). Unfortunately, the gastrointestinal tract destroys any oral nucleosides before they can be absorbed. Thus, oral intake has produced mixed results at best. Yet physicians and researchers in Europe have used injectable forms of nucleotide precursors to help their patients. In this form of delivery, adenosine and inosine have had excellent results at lowering serum lipids, relieving angina pain, combatting viruses, and even improving senility.[82] The American medical establishment has looked upon these results with great apathy.

On a more practical scale, orotic acid, a precursor of RNA and DNA, has shown value as an oral supplement. Bilirubin is a toxic by-product that sometimes builds up in infants and can cause brain damage in the condition called bilirubinemia. In a controlled study, 300 milligrams daily of orotic acid lowered the bilirubin levels significantly; only four of the orotate-treated infants required a blood transfusion while thirty of the control group needed a blood transfusion to avoid brain damage.[83] The Russians have reported good results in using orotic acid for patients recovering from heart attack.[84] Other researchers have used orotic acid to successfully treat gout (elevated uric acid in the blood).[85]

Given what little is known about this substance, we do not think that most healthy adults would benefit by taking supplements of orotic acid. It is essential within your body, but healthy people appear to be able to make enough of it. Orotic acid could be a valuable health supplement for the conditions mentioned.

Glucose Tolerance Factor

GTF is a chromium-containing molecule that assists insulin in permitting glucose into the cells of the body. GTF is very important. The only source of GTF is brewer's yeast grown in a chromium-rich environment. A healthy normal person can take chromium from the diet and manufacture GTF internally. Yet there is evidence that not all people can do this efficiently.[86]

Chromium and GTF overlap considerably, but there appears to be something very special in the chromium available from GTF. It is more efficiently absorbed and more potent in the body. Since it improves the body's ability to handle glucose, GTF has great value in lowering fats in the blood and helping diabetics and heart disease patients. Among the therapeutic values of GTF and brewer's yeast are:

• improving the symptoms and conditions of diabetics;[87]
• lowering serum cholesterol and raising high-density lipoproteins, all of which lowers the risk for heart disease;[88]
• improving acne (2 teaspoons of yeast providing 400 microgram of chromium daily);[89]
• enhancing disease resistance.[90]

If you use brewer's yeast, slowly build up to a maximum of a tablespoon per day. Brewer's yeast can encourage flatulence in people who are not used to it. For people inclined toward heart disease, diabetes, or hypoglycemia, GTF may be an essential vitamin. For others, GTF may be a health booster.

Taurine

Here is a nutrient that could be described as both renegade and superstar. While most other amino acids are actively involved in protein synthesis, taurine is usually involved in other processes. Taurine is completely absent in plant foods, the richest animal sources being human milk, shellfish, and muscle tissue. Taurine works in many different and seemingly unrelated processes throughout the body. For the more vulnerable stages of the human life cycle (infancy, old age, or illness) we may need to consider taurine an essential nutrient. Taurine has sufficiently impressed researchers that it is now included in some infant formulas and has been successfully used to treat a wide variety of ailments.[91]

Taurine has been found in all cells of the body. Some of its functions include:

• the early development of the nervous system, especially the retina of the eye;
• calcium regulation in all cells, including muscle cells, making it of particular interest to the heart;
• being bound to liver bile and thus apparently involved in fat digestion;
• protecting cell membranes from destruction.

Researchers feel that taurine is extremely important in the early developmental phases of growth. Perhaps it is more than coincidental that early human milk (colostrum) is very high in taurine, with levels decreasing as infancy progresses. Presumably, this provides immature infants with a prefabricated source of taurine and weans them once they are able to make it on their own. Since cow's milk is well past the colostrum stage, there is little to no taurine in commercial milk. Infants raised on taurine-deficient formula and patients trying to exist on parenteral feedings are all at risk for a taurine deficiency.

Healthy normal people make their own taurine from the sulfur-containing amino acids methionine and cysteine with the help of vitamin B_6. Since excess alcohol destroys methionine stores[92] and nearly half of all Americans are low in their intake of B_6, the possibilities for low levels of taurine production are great. The greater the taurine intake in the diet, the less the drain on bodily stores of methionine and cysteine, thus allowing these two essential amino acids to do other important work in the body. Taurine supplements are probably not of any value to healthy normal adults. We encourage the consumption of some meat in the diet in order to include taurine.

Taurine has been shown to: have an anticonvulsant effect on epilepsy;[93] lower blood pressure and improve heart muscle tone for patients with congestive heart failure;[94] and protect membranes against peroxide damage.[95]

Ginseng

Ginseng has been used as a medicine since before the pyramids were built. It is as revered in Europe and Asia as it is scorned by the American medical profession. Ginseng was chewed by Russian cosmonauts to prevent infection. Henry Kissinger and Chairman Mao used it. It is standard issue in the backpacks of Chinese and North Vietnamese soldiers.

Ginseng is an herb with fleshy roots. It thrives in cool, damp, shady forests. The favorite variety, rare in the wild, is grown commercially in northeastern Asia, while other varieties grow in the upper Great Lakes region of the United States and Canada. After four to six years of growth, the carrotlike roots of the plant are steamed and dried to produce red ginseng. When the roots are peeled and prepared, the product is called white ginseng, which is the type more commonly used.

Ginseng faces the same problem that bioflavonoids had: impure preparations without any standardized method of processing, yielding mixed results in scientific experiments. Researchers persisted and eventually found the active ingredients in ginseng: triterpene saponins based on the dammaran structure and collectively called ginsenosides. They then developed a strain of ginseng plants with a predictable level of active ingredients. Next, they standardized their method of extraction and processing. The result was a predictable compound, ginsana. Once these steps were taken, laboratory results have shown that ginseng can:

- stimulate the central nervous system;[96]
- stimulate the immune system while either raising or lowering both blood sugar and blood pressure;[97]
- increase stamina and physical endurance;[98]
- improve blood flow, mental abilities, and the elasticity of blood vessels in older adults;[99]
- improve coordination, reflexes, and quicken recovery from physical work;[100]
- improve general well-being, reaction abilities, oxygen capacity of the lungs, and sex hormone production;[101]
- enhance work capacity.[102]

In a significant review of ginseng, the Japanese researcher Dr. O. Tanaka found evidence that, among other benefits, ginseng could decrease heart rate, dilate blood vessels, retard fatigue, stimulate nerve growth, stimulate ATP activity for energy, lower fats in the blood, stimulate the main endocrine glands, lower blood sugar, protect against stress ulcers, increase the muscular contractions of the gastrointestinal tract for better regularity, and reduce inflammations.[103]

On the other hand, women taking excessive doses (3,000 milligrams daily) have reported the appearance of masculine traits, such as a noticeable moustache. Ginseng appears to be able to stimulate or depress various parameters in the body, depending on the person in which it is working.

Among those who feel that "if a little is good, then more is better"—which is not so for ginseng or anything else in nutrition—"ginseng abuse" syndrome has been noticed by American physicians. Their patients consuming 3,000 milligrams daily experienced nervousness, insomnia, skin eruptions, and diarrhea. They also had significant withdrawal symptoms when ginseng intake was abruptly stopped.

Ginseng is neither useless nor essential. Ginseng teas provide a warm social beverage and probably nothing more.

Helpful Bacteria

Microorganisms are everywhere on the planet, from the hottest to the coolest climates, from the cleanest to the newest of humans. We are all hosts to a limitless variety of bacteria, yeasts, and other invisible creatures. It has been estimated that one pound of human fecal matter contains about 50 billion bacteria. Microorganisms can be quite useful. They help us to produce certain foods, like yogurt, wine, cheese, soy sauce, tempeh, and the "seasoned" expensive meats of Europe. Certain bacteria can also be extremely helpful in the human body.

Lactobacillus acidophilus is a culture of bacteria famous for producing yogurt. Yogurt has been shown to help lower cholesterol in the blood.[104] New studies show that the same bacteria from yogurt help guard the intestinal tract from potent carcinogens.[105] Millions of Americans are lactose intolerant and thus excluded from the many nutritional benefits of milk. Yet yogurt, sweet acidophilus milk, and kefir (all bacterially fermented dairy products) help these people to digest the lactose and thus make milk an option in their diet.[106]

An unusual but most helpful use for lactobacillus is in treating vaginal infections. Injections of L. acidophilus cleared up vaginal infections in 93 percent of the women studied.[107] Kefir milk has been used by some women as a douche to treat these same vaginal infections. Lactobacillus fermented dairy products are also useful in clearing up diarrhea, especially for people on oral antibiotics.[108] Lactobacillus protects the gastrointestinal tract against invasion by disease-causing organisms. If you are concerned about the cleanliness of the food you will be eating, consume some acidophilus foods before, during, and after to help insure intestinal dominance of the "friendly bacteria."

There is no need to buy expensive tablets of acidophilus. Merely include at least one of the bacterially fermented dairy products in your diet on a daily basis.

Digestive Enzymes

Nature provides most of us with a chemical bath in our intestines that will kill or disassemble almost anything we eat. Hydrochloric acid is produced in the stomach at levels strong enough to eat a hole in your living room carpet. The stomach protects itself by secreting a layer of mucous. Also, the stomach sloughs off its inner cell lining regularly to provide a fresh surface. The intestines provide an equally impressive chemical show. They produce digestive enzymes that are specific to carbohydrates, fats, and proteins. The intestines also make factors that aid in vitamin and mineral absorption. When all systems are working right, you will digest and absorb as much as 90 percent of the carbohydrates, fats, and proteins you eat.

However, not everyone has a perfectly healthy system. Especially in the sick, the elderly, and those under severe stress, there can be significant changes in the quality and quantity of the digestive juices. Fresh pineapples contain a strong enzyme, bromelin, which will break down protein tissue. Fresh papaya, a tropical fruit with sweet orange-pink flesh, also contains a strong digestive enzyme, papain. For some people, consuming fresh papaya or pineapple may help protein digestion. It will do nothing for the digestion of carbohydrates or fats. We suggest that people with ailing digestive systems lower their fat, spice, and alcohol intake, eat small frequent meals, and consume these particular fruits if they find some relief in them.

Pangamic Acid

Sometimes referred to as vitamin B_{15}, pangamic acid has left a storm of controversy in its trail. Allegedly discovered in the pits of apricots (same hiding place for laetrile, a cyanide compound), pangamic acid has been touted by *New York* magazine with bold headlines that it cured everything from alcoholism to schizophrenia, with a cautiously added "maybe."[109]

Laetrile, or amygdalin, a substance derived from the apricot pit, has been used in maverick treatment of cancer. There have been anecdotal claims by cancer survivors that laetrile cured them. Yet all well-controlled scientific studies have shown laetrile to be useless against cancer.[110]

One German scientist considered pangamic acid a hoax until better laboratory controls were developed to determine its structure and effects.[111] Russian scientists claim to have used pangamic acid (calcium pangamate) to raise the HDL levels of heart disease patients, thus improving their coronary risk factors.[112] A group of Polish scientists found that rabbits fed high levels of cholesterol and then pangamic acid had decreased levels of cholesterol in the intestinal region.[113] Even American researchers have found some value in pangamic acid, as it was shown to significantly enhance the immune system in human subjects.[114]

Actually, pangamic acid is not a vitamin, nor is there any evidence that the body needs it. There is some evidence that two of the major ingredients found in the B_{15} products being marketed may be carcinogenic.

The field is laced with confusion and contradictory results. Given this, the potential harm and the likelihood that pangamic acid supplements are not pure, we suggest that you avoid this compound until more is known.

Chondroiton Sulfate

Chondroiton sulfate is found in the cartilage of most mammals, including humans. It seems to have great potential as a healer in certain forms of heart and bone disease. In a study of forty-six elderly patients with constricting blood vessels (prime candidates for heart attacks), chondroiton sulfate was able to lower blood cholesterol and triglyceride levels while also prolonging clotting time. All of these factors lowered their heart disease risk.[115] Chondroiton sulfate is certainly not a vitamin but may some day prove valuable in treating certain diseases.

SOD

Superoxide dismutase (SOD) is an enzyme produced in the cells of most animals. SOD is a very effective antioxidant that protects the tissues and may even slow the aging process. Yet oral supplements of SOD are chemically torn into unrecognizable shreds in the intestinal tract and absorbed as fragments, so oral SOD is useless.[116]

PART THREE

NONESSENTIAL DIETARY COMPONENTS

WE EAT FOR MORE REASONS THAN JUST BIOCHEMICAL NOUR-
ishment. Food is part of culture, family, comfort, satisfaction, religion, and
the mental "glitches" we harbor in our subconscious. There are many thousands of chemicals found in foodstuff. About fifty of these chemicals are essential to human health and have been discussed in the preceding section.
This section deals with substances that we probably don't need in the diet:
alcohol, caffeine, food additives, and naturally occurring toxins.

14

ALCOHOL

It was discovered by accident. It has been banned by various religious groups. It was, for a brief time, outlawed in America. The Romans revered it, considering it a medicine each soldier was entitled to, as much as food and clothing. It has ruined many a life. Yet its mild sedative effect is useful enough that many hospitals and nursing homes use it regularly. Most important, it won't go away. So we had better learn what effects it has and how to deal with it.

Alcohol is a nutrient by virtue of its seven calories per gram, but it is certainly not nutritious, since it carries almost no vitamins, minerals, or protein. There are somewhere between 6 million and 15 million alcoholics in this country. One out of three drinking adults consumes five drinks at any given sitting.[1] Alcohol constitutes about 10 to 20 percent of an average adult's daily calorie intake. Since this figure can range up to 50 percent and the Senate dietary recommendations are for less than 5 percent, alcohol definitely plays a role in the nutritional status of America.

Alcohol is the product of yeast fermentation on various carbohydrates. Grapes turn into wine, hops and barley into beer, molasses into rum, potatoes into vodka, rice into saki, corn into whiskey, juniper berries into gin, and so on. The concentration of alcohol will reach only about 20 percent (or 40 proof), at which point the yeast begins to die in its own by-product. To produce alcohol of greater strength, it must be heated, then cooled in condensing coils to catch the early vapors of alcohol. This is how distilled spirits are produced. Depending on the caution and care taken in this distillation process, the alcohol purity can go beyond 95 percent (190 proof). Pure alcohol is called "everclear" and is normally used in research or industry. Ethyl alcohol, or ethanol, is consumable liquor. Methyl alcohol, or methanol, should not be consumed because it can cause blindness or death. Isopropyl alcohol is nonconsumable rubbing alcohol.

Since alcohol is such a simple molecule, it requires no digestion. It can be absorbed in as little as five minutes in the stomach. With some food in the stomach to inhibit absorption, about three-quarters of the alcohol will move on to be absorbed in the intestines. The alcohol then moves through the blood to the liver to be processed into something usable. Once converted to a ketone, it is used in preference over other energy sources of protein, carbohydrate, and fat. The average healthy adult of 132 pounds (60 kilograms) can process about a half glass of wine in an hour. Larger people can process more (0.1 grams of alcohol per kilogram of body weight). Any alcohol consumed beyond this limit can create havoc in the system.

Physiological Effects of Alcohol

Digestive System

Alcohol can be quite harmful to ulcer patients, since it causes a greater flow of hydrochloric acid in the stomach. It interferes with the normal muscular contractions of the intestines, reducing the efficiency of digestion and absorption. It causes numerous nutrients to be poorly absorbed,[2] including thiamin (cuts absorption in half),[3] niacin, B12, folacin,[4] calcium, magnesium, sugars, and protein. It increases the need for zinc, magnesium, and other nutrients.[5] Reduces the normal food intake for many people who are more concerned with drinking than eating,[6] thus creating nutritional deficiencies. Thiamin deficiency is so common among heavy drinkers that thiamin fortification of alcohol has been proposed.[7] It increases the risk of cancer to the mouth, esophagus, colon, lungs and stomach,[8] especially in those who smoke as well as drink. By eating food with alcohol, one can minimize the harmful effects on the digestive system. Alcoholic drinks have significant calories and can be the primary cause of a weight problem.[9] Other studies show alcohol to be a poorly used calorie source. Alcohol does not provide its calories' worth in energy to all people. In some individuals, alcohol burning in the cells may be like a car stuck in the mud; although energy is being released, work is not being done.

The liver is the organ that processes alcohol. If alcohol intake is excessive, the liver suffers fatty infiltration leading to deterioration and eventually to death.[10] With its crucial role in processing and storing nutrients, incapacitation of the liver is a serious problem. There is a direct relationship between alcohol intake and cirrhosis of the liver.

Nervous System

Alcohol slowly sedates the brain, often showing in a lowering of social inhibitions.[11] With increased consumption, memory becomes impaired and speech is slurred. Soon, coordination of the muscular system is seriously hampered. The person may be stumbling. Nearly half of all traffic fatalities involve alcohol or drug abuse because of poor judgment and diminished hand-eye coordination. Death of brain cells can occur in serious alcoholics. This may be irreparable. Recent memory loss is common in heavy drinkers, with some people going home to their old house shortly after moving to a new home.

Heavy drinking can play a part in white-collar crime, since it distorts otherwise healthy ethics.[12] Alcohol lowers blood sugar, the preferential fuel of the brain, thus creating more than a few "mean drunks" when they slide into hypoglycemia. Highly sweetened drinks can create a vicious hangover with both the sugar and alcohol lowering blood sugar by morning.

Alcohol is a fat solvent.[13] The fatty wrapping around the nerves can be dissolved by continued abuse with alcohol. Delirium tremens (DTs) is a condition of uncontrollable muscle spasms found in later-stage alcoholics. The DTs are a result of nerve impulses "jumping off the track" and also of insufficient magnesium to allow normal relaxation of muscles.

Alcohol affects the sleep pattern to deter normal rapid eye movement and dreaming. Alcohol prevents the normal action of vitamin A in the eyes. Many alcoholics have poor night vision.[14] Alcohol enhances the action of drugs, so that death from drug overdose can result. Heavy drinkers develop a formidable detoxification system (called MEOS), which makes the calculation of medication and anesthetics a true challenge for physicians.[15]

Reproductive System

Alcohol requires zinc to be processed, thus using up precious zinc stores. Zinc is involved in sex drive, sperm making, and male hormones. Heavy drinkers often lapse into sessions of infertility, impotence, and lack of libido. The irony here is that drinking dissolves the thin veneer of social restraint, thus making sex desires greater, yet physical ability is diminished in the male.

Alcohol can be a serious poison to the developing fetus.[16] Somewhere between 30 and 70 percent of the pregnant women consuming five to six drinks daily give birth to deformed infants.[17] Pregnant women are advised to avoid alcohol. About one out of every 750 infants born in this country suffers from the irremedial damage of fetal alcohol syndrome (FAS), the third leading cause of birth defects in this country, which affects the brain, appearance, and physical abilities. These children may be permanently retarded or just more prone toward hyperactivity and less tolerant of stress. Their physical defects can include everything from poor muscle tone, to strange appearance, to deformed sex organs.

Circulatory System

Alcohol raises the liver's output of high-density lipoproteins (HDL),[18] which are protective factors against heart disease. Moderate drinkers (two drinks or less per day) have a lower rate of heart disease than abstainers.[19] These cardiovascular benefits disappear with high levels of alcohol intake.[20] Alcohol elevates fats in the blood. Heavy drinkers bludgeon the liver, and thus impair its ability to process fats. This can seriously increase the risk of heart disease. Calories in alcohol can encourage obesity, which also increases heart disease risk. By draining the body of thiamin, magnesium, calcium, and other nutrients directly involved in the heart's proper functioning, alcohol elevates risks for palpitations and sudden heart attack.[21]

Through malnutrition, high blood pressure, and the brittle vessels of arteriosclerosis, many alcoholics end up with burst capillaries on the nose and face.

Alcohol is a vasodilator, expanding the blood vessels in the skin region, providing the skier with a warming flushing sensation, while it is actually bringing the internal heat to the surface to be lost. It cools you while you feel warmer and impairs cold adaptation.[22,23] Small amounts of alcohol can lower blood pressure, yet alcoholics generally have higher blood pressure.[24]

Excretory System

As a diuretic, alcohol causes the kidneys to lose excessive water. With this fluid come lost nutrients of all sorts. The brain is very vulnerable to this water loss. Dehydration is a primary cause of hangovers.

Muscular System

When the liver is occupied with processing alcohol, it cannot help regulate blood sugar levels, which the muscles favor. The muscles are weakened, since alcohol must first be processed by the liver before it is useful to the body.[25]

Skeletal System

Alcohol affects the bone marrow[26] and causes calcium loss. A large percentage of alcoholics studied had some measurable degree of bone loss. Osteoporosis is usually more common in postmenopausal women. It was surprising for researchers to find that the level of alcohol intake is directly related to the severity of bone loss, even in young male alcoholics.[27]

Respiratory System

As alcohol slowly sedates the nervous system, the breathing mechanism can be affected. Death from drinking can occur by numbing the autonomic breathing apparatus, which normally allows you to breath even while unconscious. These people just "forget" to breath and so they die. Death from alcohol can also occur by a person's drowning in his own vomit.

Congeners

Congeners are impurities and excipients found in alcoholic beverages. Most of them are harmless to most people. Some can create true discomfort in sensitive individuals. These contaminants are part of the taste and aroma characteristic to each type of alcoholic beverage. Vodka and gin have the least amount of congeners. Blended Scotch has four times the amount of vodka. Pure Scotch and bourbon have even greater amounts of congeners.[28] Wine and beer are also high in congeners. Red wine contains some impurities that are worthy of suspicion. Wines often contain metabisulfite, a preservative used to prevent the browning of grapes. Some asthmatics can be very sensitive to this congener/additive.

Some people naively think that the alcohol industry is so tightly controlled that no harmful agents will enter their drink. Not so. Only a few years ago press reports showed that many beers are filtered with an asbestos material. A recent notice by the Austrian government recalled certain wines, admitting that some wineries had used antifreeze in the fermentation process.[29] Some German wines were found with the same dangerous chemical in them.

When a label says "pure grape wine" it means that grapes were the only fruit used, yet most wineries use massive quantities of white sugar to accelerate fermentation. Most breweries and wineries use the available city water as the basis for their beverage. We don't have to remind you of the disastrous possibilities of municipal drinking water.

One Drink

For the purposes of research, scientists developed a unit of "one drink," which equals: one shot (1½ ounces) of distilled spirits, 86 proof; five ounces of dry table wine; three ounces of sherry or port wine; or twelve ounces of regular beer.

Light beer has had dextrins (short-chained carbohydrates) removed to give it fewer calories. Calories increase in alcoholic beverages as the beer gets darker and more grainy tasting, the alcoholic content increases, the wine is sweeter, or other caloric ingredients are added (such as in mixed drinks).

TABLE 19: Calorie, Alcohol and Carbohydrate Content in Alcoholic Beverages

	Calories	Alcohol (grams)	Carbohydrates (grams)
Ale (12 oz)	225	22	16
Beer (12 oz)	165	15	15
Gin (1 jigger)	126	18	tr
Whiskey (1 jigger)	112	16	tr
Vodka (1 jigger)	135	19	tr
Daiquiri (1½ jiggers rum)	180	22	5
Manhattan (1½ jiggers whiskey)	200	28	1
Martini (1½ jiggers gin)	220	31	1
Dry champagne (135g)	105	13	3
Sweet champagne (135g)	160	13	17
Red wine (120g)	100	12	4
White wine (120g)	95	11	4
Port (30g)	50	5	4
Sherry (30g)	45	5	2

tr: trace amount.

There are certain ethnic groups, among them American Indians and Chinese, that have less capacity to metabolize alcohol, since their distant ancestors had no exposure to it.[30] Therefore, alcohol stays in their systems, longer. Hangovers for these people can be disastrous.

Alcoholism

There are people who simply should not drink alcohol in any amount. Many possible explanations exist about why these people can be enslaved to alcohol. Poor nutrition, the need for higher than normal levels of nutrients, unstable blood glucose, genetic predisposition, and mental problems are all enticing theories. There are between 6 million and 15 million alcoholics in the

United States, depending on which method of assessment is used. A simple question to ask yourself is this: "Would my life be any better without alcohol?" If the answer is yes, then perhaps you should consider yourself a part of this group.

Alcoholism is a disease. It can be treated. Researchers have tried to help alcoholics become social drinkers. It just does not work. Since alcoholics cannot control their drinking, they should not drink at all.

Stabilizing blood glucose will help some people to reduce their desire to drink. When not drinking, many alcoholics are keeping their blood glucose levels on a radical roller-coaster ride with coffee, doughnuts, candy, and soft drinks. Proper levels of nutrients will make a person feel better and thus less likely to seek the shelter of an alcoholic stupor. Professor Roger Williams of the University of Texas found some success in giving high-potency vitamin and mineral supplements plus glutamine to recovering alcoholics.[31] Some of these people may need higher levels of nutrients, so supplements become essential. Interesting work has been on gammalinolenic acid (evening primrose oil) and its role in helping alcoholics to reduce their craving.[32] By following the edicts in the rest of this book, many alcoholics and regular drinkers may find that their desire to drink is diminished.

Hangovers

Germans call it *Katzenjammer*, or "the wailing of cats." To the Italians, it's *stonato*, or "out of tune." The French call it *la guele de bois*, or "woody mouth." The Swedes refer to it as *hont i haret*, or "pain in the roots of the hair."[33] The comedian imitating a hungover person says, "I have two problems. One is that I might die, and the other is that I might not die."

The head is exploding, the stomach is nauseated and churning, the mouth feels like fur is on the tongue. This is the normal hangover. For serious drinking episodes, it will take on new dimensions in horror. For the confirmed alcoholic, it means all of the above and more.

The hangover is caused by a variety of abuses upon the body. Low blood sugar, a dehydrated body and brain, various vitamins and minerals in lower levels, fatigue from abnormal sleeping patterns, guilt from overindulging, intoxication with congener impurities, irritation of the gastrointestinal system, and other hazards combine to make the day after an unenviable one. Too much tobacco, excess junk food, and other affiliates of the drinking evening can enhance the effect of a hangover.

The best remedy is, obviously, to avoid excess indulgence. Barring that, one should eat some high-fat, high-sugar food like ice cream or cheese cake before drinking. This will help coat the stomach. Before going to bed, consume sweet fluids, like apple juice. Take a high-potency vitamin/mineral supplement the next morning and do something to get your mind off your complaints. Though it will not feel good, active games like tennis, basketball, or swimming can shorten the stay of the hangover. Folk remedies include coffee, raw eggs, oyster, chili peppers, heavy cream, cucumber sauce, or even the "hair of the dog that bit you," which means another drink. None of these will speed healing. The drink will merely delay the inevitable sobering process. Coffee doesn't sober a person, but rather makes him a wide-awake drunk. Time and rest are the best healers.

Rational Drinking

Alcoholics, people driving, pregnant women, and certain ethnic groups with low capacity to process alcohol should avoid the stuff. Yet alcohol can raise the heart-protecting HDLs and mildly sedate the jitters of the day. These effects are of some benefit. A scientific study found that nursing home patients improved their vigor, appetite, and self-image when a few glasses of wine were served each night with the meal.[34]

If you do not drink, you should not start for these reasons. If you do drink, keep it within moderation: two to three drinks per day, with some food, not before bedtime. Heavy drinkers should be taking a quality broad spectrum vitamin/mineral supplement to offset the nutrient losses.[35] This supplement should contain 100 percent of the RDA for all vitamins and minerals. Heavy drinkers should also add a gram each daily of choline, myo-inositol, and glutamine, plus three tablets of gammalinolenic acid. Thiamin, ascorbic acid, and L-cysteine have proved rather effective at reducing the health damage done by alcohol.[36] Our recommendations for alcoholic beverages in order of best to worst are: quality dry white wine, other wines, beer, distilled spirits, mixed drinks.

For those people who regularly consume an optimal diet, exercise often, and keep a good mental outlook, moderate intake of alcohol seems to be a longevity factor. Most long-lived societies around the world have their own "home brew." Hermann "Jackrabbit" Smith-Johannson, the 103-year-old cross-country skier, claims that "the secret to a long life is to stay busy, get plenty of exercise and don't drink too much. Then again, don't drink too little."

15

CAFFEINE

"This little bean is the source of happiness and wit."
—ENGLISH PHYSICIAN WILLIAM HARVEY,
DISCOVERER OF BLOOD CIRCULATION, 1657

Legend has it that in 500 B.C. an Arabian goatherd named Kaldi noticed an unusual amount of friskiness in his goats when they ate the little red berries from a certain shrub. He tried the berries himself and found that they helped him stay awake during long stretches on watch. Eventually Muslim leaders were recommending coffee to aid in stamina for religious rites. Coffee appeared in an Arabian medical text written in about the year 900. Gradually, coffee drifted toward Europe, and finally to America by the 17th century.[1]

America has since evolved into the Mecca for coffee drinkers. Though Americans constitute only 5 percent of the world's population, we consume over 50 percent of the world's coffee. We hit our pinnacle of intake in 1946 with twenty pounds of coffee per year for every man, woman, and child, which averages out to about three six-ounce cups every day for every person. Per capita consumption has since fallen to less than half that level.

Caffeine Consumption

Since caffeine is found in so many foods and medicines, most people probably get at least some of this substance daily. Physicians consider 200 milligrams of caffeine to be a pharmacological dosage with potent effects. Eighty-two percent of the adult population consumes 186 milligrams daily, roughly equivalent to two cups of coffee.

Tea contains widely varying amounts of caffeine. When the tea is loose, imported, black, with a longer steeping time, the caffeine is increased compared with tea that is in bags, domestic, green or herbal, and briefly steeped. Weakly brewed Tetley tea contains 18 milligrams of caffeine, while a strong brew of Red Rose contains 90.

Colas are another significant source of caffeine. Today, around the

TABLE 20: Caffeine Content of Foods and Drugs (Milligrams)

Coffee (5 oz)		Tea (instant or	
Regular brewed		5-min brew)	45
Percolated	110		
Drip	150	Cocoa (5 oz)	13
Instant	66		
Decaf brewed	4.5	Milk chocolate	
Decaf instant	2	(1 oz)	6
Soft drinks (12 oz)		Drugs	
Dr Pepper	61	Vivarin tablets	200
Mr. Pibb	57	Nodoz	100
Mountain Dew	49	Excedrin	63
Tab	45	Vanquish	33
Coca-Cola	42	Empirin	32
RC Cola	36	Anacin	32
Pepsi-Cola	35	Dristan	16.2
Diet Pepsi	34		
Pepsi Light	34		

tr: trace amount.
Source: *Nutrition Action* (Aug. 1980), p. 6

world, 80 million servings of cola are consumed daily. It is ironic that, until recently, federal regulations required that there be a certain caffeine content in colas to stop the sale of imitation cola products.

A wide variety of medicines contain caffeine, from sleep inhibitors to aspirin compounds to over-the-counter diet aids.

Chocolate is another source, with six ounces of cocoa or eight ounces of chocolate milk containing 10 milligrams of caffeine.

Caffeine passes through the placenta into the unborn infant and also through the mammary glands into the nursing baby. Thus, many very young people consume measurable quantities of caffeine. The mean intake for a six- to eleven-month-old infant is 4.2 milligrams per day, with some taking in 77 milligrams. Of 800 grade school children studied, 30 were consuming more than 300 milligrams daily of caffeine. Nine of these 30 children were clinically hyperactive.

Caffeine in the Body

Caffeine is absorbed rapidly and completely in the stomach. Within a few minutes after consumption, it has reached all areas of the body. The peak pick-me-up effect occurs about one hour after consumption. It takes about twenty-four hours to metabolize and fully excrete caffeine in the urine. Caffeine does not accumulate in the tissues.

Caffeine stimulates the central nervous system, enhancing alertness, reducing fatigue, and increasing the efficiency of mental and manual tasks, though it does not make one smarter. One cup of coffee triples the adrenaline levels in the blood. Three to four cups of coffee can increase basal metabolism from 10 to 25 percent.

Caffeine dilates the blood vessels and increases heartbeat. This creates an initial warming sensation that quickly turns to a cooling effect because internal body heat is being brought to the surface to be lost in the surroundings. It is a diuretic, relaxing the smooth muscles of the kidneys to increase urine output.

Children, with their much higher metabolism, are more affected by caffeine. A young child drinking one can of cola can get the same caffeine buzz that an adult gets from four cups of coffee.

Harmful Effects

Caffeine is also a drug with the usual list of side effects. By increasing insulin output, caffeine helps force blood sugar into the body cells for an initial outburst of energy. This is soon followed by a fall in energy from the resulting low blood sugar levels. Thus, the coffee-and-doughnut breakfast has a built-in fading period within an hour or two. This roller coaster of mental and physical energy levels could be averted by eating a decent breakfast.

Some people with vulnerable blood sugar levels are affected by even small amounts of caffeine, becoming irritable and anxious; they should not consume caffeine. For most healthy adults, 400 milligrams daily (about five cups of coffee) may cause insomnia, stomach irritation, diarrhea, irritability, and disturbances in heart rhythm (arrhythmia). Many people drinking eight to fifteen cups per day will seek medical help for a variety of physical and emotional symptoms that are brought on by the excess caffeine.

Small amounts of caffeine for the average healthy nonpregnant adult is probably harmless. Yet in excess quantities, for children, for pregnant or lactating women, for those with unstable blood glucose levels, and for vulnerable people, caffeine can be harmful. What is "excess" depends on the individual: for some sensitive children, 10 milligrams is too much; for more tolerant adult systems, 300 milligrams may not be immediately harmful.

Behavioral changes. Children consuming large amounts of colas and chocolate can display irritability and nervousness. Since caffeine passes into breast milk, a mother's coffee drinking may produce an irritable nursing infant. Many adults become temperamental and edgy when drinking coffee.

Excess caffeine can bring on anxiety attacks that mimic real psychotic conditions.

Heart disease. The evidence is partial but not convincing that heavy caffeine consumers have a higher risk for heart disease.[2] Since caffeine influences levels of sugar and fats in the blood, we feel that caffeine abuse may be a risk factor.

Birth defects. Caffeine readily crosses the placenta, thus exposing the vulnerable developing fetus to a potent drug. In animal studies, caffeine has caused reduced fertility and birth defects like cleft palate and bone deformity. Rats fed an equivalent of twelve to twenty-four cups of coffee had partial absence of toes in 20 percent of the pups born. At levels of only two cups per day, the rat pups had retarded bone development.[3] A Belgian study found that 23 percent of the mothers who gave birth to abnormal babies had consumed eight or more cups of coffee daily.[4] Yet human studies have shown no significant relationship between moderate coffee intake (one to two cups daily) and birth problems.[5]

Coffee with cigarettes during pregnancy significantly raises the risk of a lower birth weight infant. Yet researchers have a difficult time separating the effects of caffeine and tobacco, since heavy coffee users also smoke three times as much as those who use no caffeine products. The same women who were heavy coffee users and smokers were also more likely to be overfat.[6] Each factor is definitely a risk.

Cancer. At extremely high intake, coffee may be a potential cancer-causing agent, especially to the bladder and pancreas. Yet studies have shown that one cup per day is no risk for cancer.[7] Anything in between and you take your chances.

Digestive problems. Coffee is famous for its heartburn effect in heavy users. Studies have found that it is not the caffeine that causes this overflow of stomach acid but probably the list of acids it contains.

Breast disease. Lumps and cancer in the breast can result from the family of caffeine-related compounds called methylxanthines. A physician at Ohio State University, Dr. John Minton, studied forty-seven women with breast lumps (fibrocystic breast disease) who consumed an average of four cups of coffee daily. Of the twenty who were able to abstain from all caffeine products, sixteen had complete remission of their problem. Only one of the twenty-seven who did not follow his advice had her problem clear up.[8]

Headache. Caffeine causes dilation of blood vessels. This can cure headaches for some people and create headaches for others. Many people who are regular caffeine users experience a headache from withdrawal of their regular caffeine load.

Body temperature. Caffeine is able to raise the body temperature and thus inhibit the fever-breaking ability of aspirin. Some rather expensive products that contain aspirin and caffeine would probably be less effective at lowering a fever than plain aspirin alone. Fever patients would be wise to avoid caffeine products.

Caffeine Substitutes

Some people may become nearly catatonic without their daily caffeine ritual. If they enjoy it, consume it in reasonable quantities, and it is doing them no harm, then it is doubtful that they need to change their habits. But given both the potential and proven harm of excess caffeine, most of us would be better off with alternatives.

Carob can be used instead of chocolate. Carob, also known as St. John's bread, is a powdered legume product that has no caffeine and is high in protein and complex carbohydrates. It is a bit more expensive than chocolate, but a chocolate cake made with a frosting of carob and low-fat cream cheese and with a whole wheat cake bottom is a complete protein (grains matched with legumes), and thus a fabulous snack or meal. Carob does not dissolve well and thus the electric blender must be pressed into action for simulated chocolate milk and other such goodies. Since carob is milder in flavor, we recommend using three parts carob to one part powdered cocoa to provide better nutrition, less caffeine, and a very acceptable chocolate flavor.

As for decaffeinated coffee, a steam method developed in Switzerland for safely removing the caffeine from coffee beans is preferable to the questionable chemicals used in conventional decaffeination. Grain-based coffeelike products compare nicely with the flavor of coffee, without the caffeine. Chicory is a plant root that is similar in flavor to coffee and may even have some health benefits to the intestinal tract. Postum, made from bran, wheat, and molasses, has only twelve calories per cup. A West German product, Cafix, is made from barley, rye, chicory, and beets. Wilson's Heritage is a barley product that is brewed like coffee and could be used to dilute regular coffee for a reduced caffeine intake.

Teas are generally lower in caffeine than coffee yet still can add up for the heavy tea drinker. Green and herb teas usually have little or no caffeine. Keep in mind that herbs and teas are plant products and thus have the potential of serious medicine effects when taken in excess quantities. Do not pick you own wild teas unless you are well educated on the subject. Although sassafras has been removed from the root beer industry because of its proven cancer risk, sassafras can still be purchased as a tea in health food stores.

Caffeine-free colas are preferable to the high-sugar, high-caffeine conventional colas. Less soda pop overall would be best.

Medicines containing caffeine should be carefully monitored to avoid excess caffeine intake.

Coffee as a Wonder Drug?

Researchers have found some rather amazing properties of caffeine and the coffee bean. Green coffee bean oil is remarkably protective against radioactivity. Coffee bean oil enhances the protective abilities of vitamin E and selenium.[9] Another study found that ground-up coffee beans were quite effective at regenerating liver tissue in rats who had their livers partially removed.[10] Coffee is one of the few proven ergogenic (exercise-enhancing) aids. A study found a 20 percent increase in muscular endurance when a 330-milligram load of caffeine was given one hour before an athletic event.[11] However, coffee is also a diuretic and thus has drawbacks when used for serious athletes.

Recommendations

1. Those who should avoid caffeine include pregnant and lactating women, children, diabetics, heart disease and ulcer patients. At the very least, these people should seriously restrict intake.

2. Some people cannot tolerate caffeine. They should not consume it.

3. Find alternatives such as herbal tea, carob, and caffeine-free soft drinks.

4. Do not consume more than 300 milligrams per day, or the equivalent of about four cups of coffee.

16
FOOD ADDITIVES

"Part of the secret of success in life is to eat what you like and let the food fight it out inside."

—MARK TWAIN

Christopher Columbus happened upon the North American continent while in pursuit of food additives. He was looking for a more direct sea route to spice-laden India. The spices were prized in those days for their ability to bring flavor and aroma to otherwise dull and decaying food. Salt was equally valued for its ability to preserve meats from deterioration.

The use of food additives in modern times has been a compromise. Profit-oriented business interests that wish to produce an appealing food item with an extended shelf life are sometimes at odds with those who see potential hazards in the chemicals used to raise and prepare our foods.[1] There are 2,800 substances intentionally added to the modern food supply. As many as 10,000 others find their way into various foods through some aspect of processing, storage, or packaging and are called "incidental additives."[2]

If food did not deteriorate, and if each town could produce all the food its residents needed in a balanced diet and on a regular basis, there would be no need for additives. But this is not the case. Throughout mankind's history, the food supply has been unpredictable.

Goiter has been effectively eliminated in the United States by adding iodine to table salt. Rickets (vitamin D deficiency) was extremely common in America until vitamin D was added to milk. Few people call for an end to all food additives, because some are obviously necessary. Nor are food additives risk-free, because in certain levels some can be harmful. Therefore, the question becomes: Which additives can be used at safe levels to minimize risks to people?

Antioxidants

Antioxidants prevent oxidative effects on unsaturated fats in foods (lipid rancidity).[3] Vitamin E and vitamin C perform this job in the body and are also on the list of commercial antioxidants. Others include BHT (butylated hydroxytoluene), BHA (butylated hydroxyanisole), various tocopherols (forms of vitamin E), various ascorbate (vitamin C) derivatives, propyl gallate, octyl gallate, and ethoxyquin.

Vitamins C and E are not only safe preservatives but they also add nutritive value to foods. BHT and BHA have had their safety questioned. Anecdotally, BHT and BHA were found to be responsible for untreatable skin rash and inability to lose weight. BHT has been reported to do everything from increasing the lifespan of mice[4] to promoting bladder cancer in rats[5] and causing allergic reactions in even the smallest quantities in the human diet.[6] We recommend that you avoid BHT and BHA whenever possible.

Preservatives

While antioxidants check the spoilage of a food by reducing fat rancidity, preservatives attempt to slow down microbial spoilage. The World Health Organization estimates that 20 percent of the world's food supply is lost by the action of bacteria, yeast, and molds. Current chemicals used in this microscopic war take one of three approaches: (a) attack the cell membrane of the microbe, (b) interfere with its genetic mechanism, (c) interfere with its intracellular enzyme activity.[7] Common examples include benzoic acid (and other compounds containing benzoate), sodium nitrate and nitrite, propionic acid, sorbic acid, sulphur dioxide, metabisulfite or sulfite (attached to sodium or potassium). The food industry has developed a new way to use the accumulating radioactive wastes from nuclear reactors: as a food preservative, Cobalt 60 is used to squelch bacterial growth in food and prolong shelf life.

Sodium nitrite and nitrate have three significant effects on food: (1) They inhibit the growth of the anaerobic organism that causes botulism. Botulism is a condition so deadly that one ounce of this toxin, if evenly distributed, could kill everyone in the United States. (2) They provide a nice bright red color to meats. (3) They combine in the stomach with amino acids to form nitrosamines, known potent carcinogens. They also enhance the carcinogenic effects of alcohol and certain foods.[8] Vitamin C mops up these cancer-causing by-products of nitrites. Nitrates and nitrites should be avoided by pregnant women and young children.

Sulfur dioxide has been known to cause reactions in sensitive individuals. The Food and Drug Administration has proposed a ban on metabisulfite—found in fresh produce, salad bars, potatoes in restaurants, lettuce, wine—because of the lethal reaction that the 500,000 asthmatics in this country could experience.[9] We would only consume Cobalt 60-preserved foods if there were no alternatives.

Emulsifiers and Stabilizers

The food manufacturer often mixes substances that are not partial to one another. Fat and water, for instance, will stay together only under chemical coersion. Emulsifiers and stabilizers attempt to give food a smoother texture and keep it from separating. Lecithin is from soybeans and has both a water-soluble and fat-soluble portion to its chemical structure, which gives it soaplike properties of keeping fat and water together. Many salad dressings and cookies use lecithin. Polysorbate 60 and 80, mono and diglycerides, monosodium phosphates, phosphoric acid and sorbitan monostearate are in this category.

Also in this group are agents that stabilize and thicken a food item. These are often derived from natural food products: agar, alginates, and carrageenan from seaweed; gelatin from animal bones and hides; sorbitol and pectin from fruits and berries; gums from various plants; and sodium carboxymethylcellulose from cellulose and vinegar.

Relative to the other categories of additives, these are among the safest, though they may prompt a consumer to buy a product of inferior nutritional quality just because it is deceptively thick and rich looking.

Coloring Agents

Food manufacturers realize that consumer appeal is often based upon the looks of the food item. If a food is anything but fresh, it usually begins to lose its natural colors. Therefore, great effort is made to develop natural-looking food dyes. Natural dyes often used include chlorophyll (green), beta-carotene (yellow-orange), annato (yellow), anthocyanins (blue at low pH, red at higher pH), caramel (brown), cochineal (also called carmine; crimson). The list of synthetic dyes is extensive yet amorphous, since as one is found harmful and removed from the list, others are developed to replace it. Milk and other dairy products are normally white. Yellow cheese, therefore, has had a dye added to it.

This is one of the more suspicious categories of food additives, with no redeeming quality but window dressing and considerable risks found in those tested.[10] Many synthetic dyes are coal tar derivatives (also found in tobacco smoke), which are known carcinogens . Although the list of FDA-approved dyes continues to shrink as more data are available, there are still six synthetic dyes listed as safe. Among these, FD&C Blue No. 1 and FD&C Green No. 33 have produced cancer in rats at the site of injection, yet the FDA does not consider this valid testing since the dyes were injected rather than ingested. Studies have shown a relationship between excessive food dye intake and hyperactivity in children. Red dye No. 3 affects the brain's ability to produce and accept the vital chemical transmitters between brain cells. Synthetic dyes seem to be potent enough to serve as insecticides. Avoid them whenever possible.

Flavoring Agents

Salt was prized for many centuries for its ability to flavor and preserve meats. Flavoring agents still are the prized possession of any good chef or food manufacturer. Of the 2,000 flavoring agents, 500 are natural and the balance are synthetic. Salt, sugar (discussed below), fat, and spices are the most common of the natural flavorings. There are also natural but deadly flavoring substances, including safrole (root-beer flavoring from sassafras; it is now banned), nutmeg (can cause hallucinations in anything but minute portions), pomegranate roots, slippery elm bark, and hepatica herb. Synthetic flavoring additives include vanillin, limonene, and l-malic acid. Monosodium glutamate (MSG) is a flavor enhancer, which means that it heightens the action of food on the tongue. MSG is the synthetic version of the original flavor enhancer from the Orient, glutamic acid from seaweed, although MSG is much less expensive to produce.

Most of the approved flavor additives are relatively harmless. Sugar, salt, or fat used as a spice is generally innocuous, yet if used as a staple is probably harmful. MSG has been shown to cause partial paralysis of the breathing muscles, also known as the "Chinese restaurant syndrome," since Oriental foods rely so heavily on this flavor enhancer. There is reason to believe that MSG might cause brain damage in developing young animals and may affect the fertility of both males and females. Because of this possible link, MSG has been purged from all infant food. Avoid MSG.

Sequestrants

Many metals are reactive compounds, such as iron reacting with oxygen to form rust. Iron and copper in food would change the flavor, texture, or even create needlelike crystals if allowed to react unchecked. Sequestrants check these reactive metals by creating a molecular cage to prevent their activity. EDTA (ethylene diamine tetracetic acid) is a common sequestrant in food and also an agent used to treat metal poisoning in humans. Citric acid, tartaric acid, various derivatives of phosphates, and even the simplest amino acid in nature (glycine) are in this category of additives. Compared with the other categories, this one is relatively safe.

Anti-Caking Agents

Anti-caking agents absorb moisture so that a powdered mix avoids the clumping that would occur if exposed to a humid climate. Common chemicals in this category include aluminum, ammonium, calcium, potassium, and sodium salts of the long-chain fatty acids myristic, stearic, and palmitic acid; calcium phosphates; potassium and sodium ferrocyanide; magnesium oxide; and various forms of silicic acid.

These are valuable for consumer appeal (although clumping does not harm a food product) and probably relatively safe in the quantities used. Beware of ingesting too much aluminum, though, since aluminum toxicty has been related to Alzheimer's disease.

Humectants

Whereas anti-caking agents absorb moisture to prevent the product from clumping, humectants retain moisture to prevent the product from drying out, such as might occur in breads and cakes. These include glycerol; sodium and potassium lactate; propane-1,2-diol; and sorbitol. These additives are relatively safe in the small quantities used.

Acid-Base Balancers

The acid base level (pH) of a food product greatly influences its taste, texture, cooking characteristics, and shelf life. Acid-base balancers are widely used in dairy products, as well as to flavor soft drinks, prevent discoloration in canned vegetables, and on peeled fruits and vegetables before canning. Phosphoric, citric, acetic (vinegar), tartaric, malic, lactic and other acids are used to make a product more acidic. Sodium sesquicarbonate, ammonium and sodium bicarbonate, ammonium, potassium, and sodium hydroxides, calcium and magnesium hydroxides, and the carbonate versions of each will make a product more alkaline. These are probably harmless in low levels of intake.

Firming and Crisping Agents

Firming and crisping agents maintain the texture of vegetables by keeping the fluid inside the cells. This cell turgor is preserved by such substances as aluminum potassium sulfate, calcium hydroxide, common table salt, and calcium versions of hydroxide, citrate, lactate, phosphate, gluconate, and heptonate. These, too, are relatively harmless in the quantities used, except the aluminum version.

Sweeteners

The human tongue has a sensitive and separate section for detecting sweet foods. This must have evolved from the need for foraging humans to be able to tell bitter foods (often harmful or nutritionally useless) from sweet (often useful in providing carbohydrates, the body's preferential fuel source). Additives make up about 10 percent of our daily food supply, and the vast majority of these additives are sweeteners. Sugar is found in many forms: levulose, mannose, dextrose, sucrose, corn syrup, etc. Artificial sweeteners have been the focal point of much research and public attention. Cyclamates, with 30 times the sweetness of refined sugar, were being consumed in massive quantities by the public until scientific studies showed them to cause bladder cancer in rats. When cyclamates were removed from the market, on September 1, 1969, a presidential inquiry began into the alleged safety of the GRAS (Generally Regarded As Safe) list.

Saccharin, with 300 times the sweetening power of refined sugar, had been used as an artificial sweetener in foods since 1879. On March 9, 1977, the FDA announced that saccharin had been found to produce cancer in the bladder of rats and would be removed from the market. At the time, 5 million pounds of saccharin were being consumed each year in the United States, and a public outcry from weight control and diabetic groups convinced legislatures to leave saccharin on the shelf with a warning label.

Aspartame (a.k.a. NutraSweet, Equal), a derivative of the amino acid aspartic acid, is used extensively now in foods, since it is 180 times sweeter than refined sugar. It tends to deteriorate and lose sweetness after a few months on the shelf. It also breaks down when under high heat for more than twenty minutes and is thus useless for cooking. The Food and Drug Administration has received over 600 complaints from people who consumed too much NutraSweet (more than 2 quarts of sweetened beverages) and developed symptoms ranging from headaches to epileptic-like seizures.

Thaumatin is a natural substance found in a fruit native to central and southwest Africa and is considered the most potent sweetener in existence, yet it breaks down with the least bit of chemical or heat tampering.

Experiments are also proceeding on an L form of natural sugar. Since the body can only metabolize D (right-handed forms) of sugars, the L (left-handed forms) give sweetness without any calories.

The human urge to placate the sweet tooth can make bland but healthy products more palatable. This same urge can become one's demise if taken to excess. The artificial sweeteners cyclamate and saccharin are potentially hazardous, yet saccharin is still used extensively. Aspartame, when used in excessive quantities by sensitive individuals, may have harmful effects. Common refined table sugar, in average portions of 132 pounds per year per person, is also likely to be harmful.

Enzymes

Enzymes are catalysts of a protein nature, thus they speed up the rate of a reaction. In the food industry, the enzymes employed are those that promote changes in a food, such as rennin to allow milk to curdle into cheese, or those that prevent something from happening, such as peroxidase used in the dairy and egg business to prevent the spoilage that would occur from hydrogen peroxide. Large-scale food manufacturing has found it necessary to employ bacteria to make enzymes. Chemical extraction of enzymes, such as natural rennin from cow stomachs, is seriously limited in production volume. Bacillus cereus, Endothia paraciticus, and other bacteria are responsible for making enzymes that stabilize citrus-juice-based soft drinks, stabilize vitamins B_{12} and C, prevent rancidity or oxidation of various products, and prevent the browning of fruit. From various fruitful bacteria has come the enzyme carbohydrase to attack the long-chain carbohydrates in foods and render them into shorter chains, thus producing modified starch.

Most of these are probably harmless in low levels of intake. There is still a controversy about the safety of modified starches.

Nutritive Additives

Four hundred million people around the world suffer from goiter, a gross iodine deficiency. The United States has nearly eliminated this condition by adding iodine to table salt. Vitamin D added to milk has been equally successful in reducing the incidence of rickets. The milling of whole grains causes a signficant reduction in their nutritive value. The replacement of some of the lost nutrients partially compensates for the refining and helps to avoid blatant nutritional deficiencies.

A food is enriched when some of the original nutrients lost in refining are replaced. A food is fortified when a nutrient is added that was not found in the natural food product (like vitamin D to milk or iodine to salt). Vitamin A is added to margarine so that its vitamin A content is similar to that of butter. Many different vitamins, minerals, and amino acids are used in the food industry to improve the nutritive value of various foods.

It is a noble desire to want to improve the nutritional value of any food.

Yet it is somewhat misleading to take a breakfast cereal composed primarily of sugar, add some vitamins and minerals, and then boast of the nutritional superiority of that product. Also, nutritive additives (like zinc, calcium, magnesium, and vitamin B₆) could markedly improve the health of Americans at a very reasonable cost.

Flour and Bread Additives

Though rice sustains most of the Eastern world, wheat is the dietary staple in the West. Thus, bread (especially white bread) has an extensive list of additives approved for use. These fall into distinct categories:

1. Bleaching and improving agents to make white flour very white and improve texture (calcium and potassium bromate, acetone peroxide, and azodicarbonamide).

2. Antioxidants to reduce spoilage (including ascorbic acid).

3. Leavening agents to help the bread rise (yeast, baking powder, baking soda). Baking soda is sodium bicarbonate; double-acting baking powder is generally a combination of baking soda, sodium aluminum sulfate, and calcium phosphate.

There is reason to question the safety of the bromate additives as bleaches. Note that aluminum is found in most double-acting baking powder. Aluminum toxicity may be causing the rising tide of Alzheimer's disease. It would be advisable for the consumer to purchase minimally processed whole grain breads. The blatant superiority of whole wheat bread makes it the nutritionist's choice.

The average person in America consumes 1,500 pounds of food per year, of which 10 percent is food additives. Of the 150 pounds of additives, nearly 93 percent is sugar and salt, leaving about 10 pounds in other food additives. Since some people are not eating their share, that means others are eating much more than theirs. High intake of food coloring and flavoring may cause hyperactivity in children and perhaps mood changes in adults. Some categories of additives are relatively harmless, like humectants and acid-base balancers. Others are probably harmful, such as many of the coloring agents, nitrate, and MSG. Some additives are reasonably innocuous in small amounts, like sugar and other sweeteners. One category, nutritive additives, can either magnificently improve the diet or mislead the consumer.

One cannot categorically indict food additives. Without them, we would not have a regular and palatable food supply. One cannot even make the assumption that all natural additives are better than all synthetic additives, since sassafras and nutmeg are both natural and potentially harmful. The following chapter on naturally occurring toxins in foods will awaken you to the fact that "natural" does not mean a categorical endorsement.

Food companies are usually directed by someone with a business background. Rarely is a nutritionist or other scientist in charge. The chairman is interested in profits, not harming people. The upper echelon of most food corporations know little about nutrition and health. There is significant cost and time involved in getting a new food additive approved by the FDA. So it is the educated consumer, via purchasing power, who can steer the industry in the direction of a healthy food supply.

At a presentation given for the public by a large food corporation, we heard one mother shout angrily at the representative answering questions, "How can you make this junk cereal for our children?" The speaker unctuously replied, "Lady, we'll stop making the stuff when people stop buying it."

Recommendations

1. Select foods in this order: (a) those with no label (fresh produce, meat, fish, dairy, bulk beans); (b) those with a short label (whole wheat bread, frozen vegetables); (c) those with an extensive label as a last resort.

2. Avoid foods with synthetic dyes, MSG, sodium nitrate or nitrite, metabisulfite, and other additives indicted in this chapter.

3. Read food labels. Know what you are consuming.

‒‒‒‒‒‒‒‒‒‒‒‒‒‒‒‒‒ ?➋ ‒‒‒‒‒‒‒‒‒‒‒‒‒‒‒‒‒

17

NATURALLY OCCURRING TOXINS IN FOOD

"If it's natural, it's got to be good for you."

—FAMOUS LAST WORDS OF A FORAGING NATURALIST

It was a very bad idea to act anything but normal in Salem, Massachusetts, in 1692. Twenty people were put to death in various sadistic ways, all on the pretext that they were witches. Religious fanaticism no doubt contributed to this calamity, but historians have found another explanation for this witchcraft hysteria. From examination of tree rings and diaries from that era, it is known that there were two very wet years in that area of the United States. Rye was the staple grain for these people. The mold Claviceps purpurea is known to feed off rye, particularly in damp weather, and produce the toxin ergot. Ergot is a chemical similar in structure to the hallucinogenic drug LSD and will produce intense pain in the extremities, cramps, convulsions, and bizarre behavior. Historians theorize that it was the naturally occurring toxin that led to the erratic behavior of the people who were accused of demonic possession.

The term "natural" has become a key selling point in much of advertising. The assumption is that if it is natural, it has to be good for you. This is not necessarily the case. Soda pop, beer, lipstick, and other products advertise heavily as being "natural" since governmental agencies have no formal definition of the term. Tarantulas, rattle snakes, and the bubonic plague are all natural but hardly good for human health. Although foods in their natural state are generally more nutritious than their refined counterparts, there are some hazards in the common food supply that occasionally even equal the risk of the tarantula.

Food should be a source of enjoyment and biochemical nourishment. For the uneducated, food can be a source of sickness or death. This chapter is dedicated to eliminating that hazard.

Poisons Naturally Found in Food

Cassava (also called yuca or manioc) is a plant with a starchy root that is a popular food item in the tropics. The outer surface contains a glycoside that can cause poisoning of the body's energy metabolism.[1] Processed tapioca does not contain this poison.

West Africa has a particular problem with this toxin, cyanogen, since people there rely heavily on cassava as a staple. Symptoms can include blindness (amblyopia) and nervous degeneration (ataxic neuropathy). Lima beans, sorghum millet, kidney bean, garden pea, sweet potato, Indian gram, and almond also contain certain amounts of this cyanogen. By soaking and washing the food, the risk is reduced. By sprouting the food, risk is considerably reduced. Cassava should be avoided or at least not served as a staple.

Oxalates are substances found in spinach, rhubarb, celery, beetroot, parsley, almond, and tea that bind calcium and other divalent minerals and carry them out of the intestinal tract. Phytates are similar substances with similar action but are found in whole grains like wheat, rye, oats, and barley. In grains, the phytates are reduced considerably by the fermentative action of yeast. Thus unleavened bread is much higher in phytates. Both oxalates and phytates can lead to mineral deficiencies if large amounts are consumed and the diet is low in certain minerals. Residents of the Middle East consume a low-zinc, high-phytate diet that can stunt growth and retard sexual development.

The natural flavor of root beer used to come from sassafras. Sassafras contains copious amounts of saffrole, a cancer-causing agent, and therefore is now banned. Potatoes and a number of spices have harmless amounts of saffrole.

Goitrogens are substances found in plants that interfere with iodine metabolism. Cabbage, turnip, cauliflower, kale, Brussels sprouts, broccoli, and soybeans contain this iodine-binding agent. Regular intake of these vegetables in a raw state combined with a low-iodine diet could produce goiter in those with thyroid problems. Cooking these foods nearly eliminates goitrogens in the diet.

Lathyrogens are substances that are protein in nature and found in the legume plant vetch. The lathyrogens in this pealike plant can cause skeletal deformities or paralysis if consumed to excess. In India, where vetch is usually a small part of the diet, this occurs only when availability of other foods diminishes.

Seeds of the cycad plant, found in the Pacific islands, are susceptible to bacterial attack when consumed and can produce a potent cancer-causing agent, cycasin. These seeds should be soaked, washed, and cooked to minimize the hazard.

Solanine is a deadly chemical found in sprouting potatoes that has an action similar to nerve gas, disabling the central nervous system. All potatoes contain some solanine, but only those exposed to the sun and beginning to sprout contain deadly amounts. Potatoes with green shoots on them should be disposed of.

Trypsin inhibitors are found in soybeans, peanuts, navy beans, and lima beans and will inhibit protein digestion in the intestinal tract. Steaming, cooking, or sprouting will deactivate these potent substances.[2] Lectins are another potent toxin found in legumes and neutralized by cooking or sprouting.

Raw egg whites contain avidin, which binds to the B vitamin biotin. Excessive consumption of raw eggs could create a biotin deficiency. Cooking denatures avidin and renders it harmless.

Hemaglutinins are protein substances that cause the blood cells to clump together, thus impairing their normal function and potentially leading to cardiovascular ailments. Found in soybeans, Guatemalan red bean, Indian red gram, and Philippine mung bean, these substances are inactivated by soaking the beans in water before cooking.

Psoralens are a potent carcinogen found in all parsnips.

Comfrey tea is a favorite among some health enthusiasts. The leaves have been found to be carcinogenic in rats, and the leaves and roots can cause liver damage.[3] Those people trying to pick their own comfrey had best be plant experts. Foxglove, containing the potent heart medicine digitalis, is a dead ringer for comfrey.

Caucasians who are native to the Mediterranean area have an inherited vulnerability to illness when they consume fava beans. Favism causes illness in all people and anemia in young children. Drying and aging of the fava bean reduces the toxicity.

Plantains (a species of banana) contain a substance that induces a common heart condition in the African tribes who consume this food regularly. Cooking significantly lowers the risk. Hypoglycins found in the Ackee fruit of the tropics can seriously lower blood sugar. Djenkolic acid found in a bean popular in Indonesia causes the kidneys to excrete valuable body substances. A purple mint plant found in the United States and Asia (Perilla frutescens) can cause various lung disorders.[4] The Great Plains of America produces some plants that have unusually high levels of selenium from the soil and can induce nervous disorders. Tetradotoxin is found in the ovaries and liver of the pufferfish and is lethal.

Ciguatera is a poison found in tropical fish such as grouper. The Centers for Disease Control in Atlanta estimates that 50,000 people annually are stricken with this toxin. This is the primary condition treated in emergency hospital units near tropical coral reefs. Less than 1 percent of the cases are fatal.[5] Certain fish, clams, and shrimp contain thiaminase, a substance that destroys thiamin in the intestines.[6] Thiaminase is destroyed by cooking. The trendy raw fish (sushi) bars do not make good health sense for this reason and because raw fish may contain larvae of parasitic organisms, which are killed when cooked.

There are many other naturally occurring toxins in food. Certain mushrooms contain deadly poisons. Hemlock, reknowned for its lethal effect on the ancient Greek philosopher Socrates, can also poison humans who eat birds or animals that have consumed hemlock.

Poisons Produced by Microorganisms

The fits and convulsions of ergot poisoning from a mold found on rye plants fit in this category.

Aflatoxins are potent substances produced by the action of the mold Aspergillus flavus on various grains, legumes, and nuts. Aflatoxins can produce cancer of the liver, a most deadly type of cancer, and have been implicated in mental retardation of infants from women exposed to these potent toxins.[7] The best way to avoid this common world problem is to consume grains, legumes, and nuts that are stored in cool and dry conditions.

Improperly stored rice allows a mold (Penicillium islandicum) to produce two carcinogens—luteoskyrin and islandicum.

The Fusarium mold grows abundantly on poorly stored grains and produces the lethal substance tricothecanes, which has been responsible for many deaths in Russia.

Red tide is known to people who live near the ocean. Produced by microorganisms, red tide can become a series of captivating luminescent green waves at night. Yet the dinoflagellates that produce these impressive effects are poisonous and are consumed by various shellfish. The saxitoxin poison is not inactivated by the shellfish nor by cooking, and it can be lethal to humans consuming the shellfish during this time of year.

Poisons Produced in Food Preparation

The backyard barbecue is an American tradition, where food is cooked in the most primitive of all fashions, over a fire. This can be very dangerous for those who like their food well done and for those who use a fatty meat that fuels a continuous flaming fire. The incomplete combustion of animal fat creates potent carcinogens called polycyclic hydrocarbons. Excellent studies have shown that groups of people who eat a lot of smoked food have a higher incidence of cancer of the stomach and other parts of the digestive system.[8]

Enjoy the barbecue custom, but do not cook foods over flames. Low-fat fish and chicken are less likely to cause flaming when barbecued and therefore have double benefits in their nutritive value.

Oleander is an attractive and hearty small tree that grows well in semitropical areas around the world. All parts of the plant are poisonous. Even cooking food over a fire made from ôleander wood is dangerous. There is a substance in oleander that simulates the heart medicine digitalis and thus can cause death from heart failure.

One should also be extremely aware of the type of containers in which food and water are stored. Cadmium, from canned foods or galvanized pipes, can lead to hypertension and cadmium poisoning. Lead—from pewter eatingware, lead-seamed cans, or lead-based ceramic glazing—will cause a general systemic poisoning.[9] Victims of lead toxicity may experience general lethargy, headaches, colic, facial pallor, blood disorders, and a change in the color of the gums.

Space-age technology brought us a nonstick polymer coating for cooking pans. The inexpensive versions of this slippery surface wear away easily and may be consumed. No one knows what the health effects of eating polymer coating may be.

Aluminum is found in higher levels in Alzheimer's disease (a form of senility) victims.[10] It would be wise to avoid eating aluminum, which is found in everything from baking powder to antacid tablets, and to minimize the use of aluminum pans when cooking high-acid foods. Copper water pipes are used in some homes. Excess copper intake can create an imbalance or deficiency of zinc. Zinc toxicity has been brought on by picnicking groups who made lemonade (high acid) in galvanized (contains zinc) trash cans. Lemon and other strong acids can dissolve styrofoam cups and cause the user to consume these hazardous foams. Use stainless steel, glass, cast iron, or other time-tested material for cooking and storing food.

Residual Poisons from Human Intervention

In 1983, the pesticide EDB (ethylene dibromide) was found in potentially lethal levels in the grains on which it was sprayed. EDB use has finally been banned, but modern food contains ever-increasing amounts of other humanly induced toxins.[11]

Humans are in direct competition with other life forms for our food supply. We use poisons to squelch weeds (herbicides), insects (insecticides), fungus (fungicides), and rats (rodenticides) who are vying for crops. In

1962, Rachel Carson wrote the classic *Silent Spring*, which alerted the public to the fact that most poisons touted as being selective in their victims are actually rather general in their toxicity. People began to realize that the same substance that kills the weed or insect may also harm the person who eats the salvaged food crop.

July 4, 1985, the biggest weekend of the year for California's watermelon farmers, had a disastrous end to it as the pesticide aldicarb was found in excessive levels in many watermelons. About 10 million watermelons (a third of the state's crop) were destroyed, although it is likely that only a few of the larger farms were guilty of misusing the product.[12] Regulation of pesticides stipulates that use be discontinued a month before the crop is ready to harvest. For fear of crop loss, many farmers do not comply with this law.

DBCP, a pesticide so potent that its use is now banned, has been found in 2,450 wells across America. The USDA has about 15,000 cases reported each year of acute pesticide poisoning in city regions. Herbicides such as paraquot and dioxin have been extensively used in American fields, but are no longer approved because of their blatant toxicity to humans. Paraquot is still used to destroy marijuana fields in Mexico, while dioxin was the essence of the defoliant Agent Orange used in Vietnam and now thought to be responsible for much death and sickness among those people exposed to it. Dioxin is still used in forestry to kill weeds. DDT is still allowed in forestry and rice fields as a last resort. Ships and storage bins use poisons (like warfarin) to keep rats from consuming the stored food.

Pesticides, herbicides, fungicides, and rodenticides have been shown to produce acute symptoms ranging from paralysis to nausea and vomiting in humans. Too much of these poisons will cause blatant sickness or death. But what are the effects of ingesting small amounts for decades? No one really knows.

It is widely accepted that proper use of pesticides would lead to safer levels in food, but that the farmer and his often illiterate helpers are not totally compliant in following the pesticide manufacturers' directions. A recent newspaper article about pesticide abuse showed the workers using the lids of the pesticide containers as dinner plates. Many farmers have the mistaken notion that if a little is good, then more is better. This is as untrue with pesticides as it is with nutrients.

Some food stores around the country offer "organically grown produce," but "organic" has no legal definition. It implies that compost and manure are used as fertilizer and no pesticides are employed. Most organic products are simply more expensive counterparts of ordinary supermarket items. But if you feel that you can trust your local "organic produce" merchant, this may be a wise alternative.

While diesel farm equipment has helped a few farmers feed millions of people, diesel exhaust is known to be laden with potent carcinogens, poly-cyclic hydrocarbons, most of which fall on the nearby food. No one knows how much of these substances enter the food chain, but it would be wise to wash all fresh produce in warm water before consuming it.

Since the earth's beginning, about 4.5 billion years ago, there have been small amounts of radioactivity to contend with. Unless a caveman were un-fortunate enough to burrow underground and live near a uranium mine, the hazards were minimal. Even radon gas, which is constantly emitted from the earth's core and known to be responsible for a certain amount of lung cancer, can be dealt with simply by not living underground and/or provid-ing adequate ventilation in one's living quarters.

Yet since the advent of the atomic bomb and nuclear energy, these prob-lems have become more serious. Radioactive gases from nuclear power sta-tions, nuclear fallout from bomb testing, and the industrial use of radioac-tive material have all created a rather impressive amount of strontium 90 and cessium 137 in our atmosphere. These radioactive substances are ubiq-uitously found in the food supply now, with the highest levels in dairy prod-ucts and various animal tissue. Most pollutants are concentrated as one moves up the chain of life. It is unfortunate that whole grains have three times the concentration of these radioactive agents that refined white flour products have. With a reduction in atmospheric testing of nuclear weapons, it is hoped that these levels of radioactivity will continue to decrease.

Animal husbandry has evolved considerably in the past few decades. Proper hygiene has reduced the incidence of death and illness of domestic animals. Antibiotics prevent the spread of many epidemics that used to dev-astate a herd. Drugs have been developed to increase the size and rate of growth of domestic animals. Perhaps we have gone too far in the use of drugs in our food supply. Antibiotics are now routinely given to many do-mestic animals, especially dairy cows, since an infection can mean the loss of considerable revenue to the farmer. From this abundant use, streptomy-cin, penicillin, and tetracycline are found in rather predictable levels in meat and milk. "The fate of antibiotic residues entering the body from food is also largely unknown," says an expert chemist from the University of Man-chester in England.[13] Antibiotics may lower levels of beneficial bacteria in the intestines that are responsible for producing vitamins like biotin and K and absorbing minerals like calcium.

The principal adverse effects of consuming antibiotics are: (1) allergic re-actions (found in a few sensitive individuals), (2) changes in the levels of bacteria normally found in the intestines, (3) adverse changes in the stem cells of the bone marrow and subsequent changes in the blood. Chloram-phenicol, an antibiotic used in the dairy industry, has been shown to deter normal blood production in bone marrow.

Hormones were found to have dramatic effects on the rate of growth in cattle. Diethyl stilbestrol (DES) was used for years in rearing cattle until it was found to be carcinogenic, especially for young women and their female offspring. DES is supposedly banned, though there are reports of its continued use. The current status of hormones used in raising animals is an issue of much debate, with health activists claiming abundant misuse and agricultural spokesmen denying these allegations.

Tranquilizers are normally used in the slaughter yards to prevent animals from getting tense and yielding tough meat. How much tranquilizer is used, which kind, and how it could influence human health are all unanswered questions.

It is obvious that some drug use is mandatory for the food to be safe and for the farmer to make some profit, yet how much of this drug use is optional and only to increase profits? The drug residues do end up in the food supply, yet how much or with what effect is still unclear.

We could not leave the subject of food toxins without discussing industrial pollution. In 1985, the lieutenant governor of the state of California, Leo T. McCarthy, predicted that a "toxic time bomb is about to go off," as the public becomes aware of the widespread effect of irresponsible industrial pollution.[14] PCBs were manufactured since the early part of this century for use in paints, plastics, varnishes, transformers, and lubricants. As early as 1919 their toxicity was shown, yet industrial discharge of PCB into the water supply has led to global distribution of this potent toxin. All of us everywhere have some of this now illegal substance in our bodies and food.[15] How much PCB does it take to instigate a harmful reaction? No one really knows.

Residents of the Great Lakes region of the United States are reminded by their public health departments to eat no more than one fresh-caught fish per year, due to the lethal concentration of PCB in these once pristine waters. There is some clinical evidence that PCB adversely effects sperm count and fetal development.

Lead is another issue. Found in paints, roofing material, pesticides, gasoline, and even some water pipes, lead is ever present in the atmosphere and diet of the modern citizen. Lead is found in 500 times the concentration in today's human as in remains of humans who lived in the year 300.[16] Of 79,000 children tested in New York City, 31,000 had significant levels of lead in their bodies, including 4,500 cases of severe lead poisoning. The primary sources of lead today are fumes of vehicles using leaded gasoline and lead in drinking water. Chicago has recently outlawed the sale of leaded gasoline in the city limits. Produce grown near roadsides shows twice the lead concentration of produce grown 1,000 yards from the roadside. Higher levels of lead are found in autistic children. There is an inverse relationship between the levels of lead found in a child's infant teeth and his or her intelligence scores. Lead poisoning, especially among pregnant women and young children, is an issue truly worthy of concern, since it particularly affects humans in stages of rapid growth. What were once thought to be acceptable levels of lead in the body are now considered toxic.

Oil slicks on the ocean yield more polycyclic hydrocarbons. These toxins end up in higher levels in shellfish, since these sea creatures are filter feeders. Nonsmokers exposed to asbestos fiber have five times the risk of developing lung cancer, while smoking people exposed to asbestos have a sixty fold increase in risk. Asbestos was used briefly to make city water pipes. Formaldehyde and other deadly pollutants have been found in water supplies. The use of chemical fertilizers has allowed major increases in crop harvests, yet the nitrates in fertilizers are also found in the water supply. These form the potent carcinogen nitrosamines in the stomach.

The industrial pollutants of the twentieth century are far more potent and ubiquitous than the pollutants of centuries past. Statistics show a correlation between levels of pollution and incidence of many degenerative health problems, including mental illness. Recent congressional efforts point to the seriousness of this situation. The federal government appropriated $3.8 billion for a superfund to clean up toxic waste areas. It is estimated that at least ten times that amount is needed to make the United States a safer and cleaner place to live.

Bacterial Contamination of Food

Each year in the United States about 20,000 cases of food poisoning are reported.[17] No doubt, many more thousands of people suffer symptoms of gastric distress and do not report it, though food may have caused the problem. Bacteria is found everywhere on earth. Some are advantageous, such as those that help us make the biotin in our intestines. Many can be harmful. If given proper conditions these bacteria are capable of producing severe intestinal distress and even death from dehydration. Botulism is particularly lethal. Under ideal conditions, one bacteria could multiply into a colony of 2 million bacteria in seven hours.[18] All food has at least one bacteria present. Therefore, temperature control becomes crucial in preventing food poisoning.

Staphylococcus aureus is found in the skin and mucous membranes of most humans. It is the cause of the skin eruptions we call pimples. Clostridium botulinum is found in soil, water, some animals, and fish. This bacteria grows anaerobically (without oxygen) and thus is the prime suspect in food poisoning involving home-canned products. Recently, an independent hamburger shop was found to be dispensing botulism by keeping fried onions in an oxygen-free environment of grease.[19] Botulism can also occur when infants, with a sterile gut and thus no competitive bacteria, consume foods like wild honey. Clostridium perfringens is found in the intestinal tract of most humans, most animals, and also in the soil.

Salmonella is found in most domestic and wild animals and also in some human carriers.

There are several factors that provide fertile conditions for pathogens to grow on your food:

- Time. One hour or more of bacterial growth can produce intestinal symptoms.
- Temperature. From 60° to 120° F. (15.5 to 48.8° C.), these organisms thrive and reproduce rapidly.
- High fluid content. They do not grow as well on dry foodstuff.
- High protein content. Meats, eggs, dairy, and other protein foods provide ideal nourishment for rapid bacterial growth.
- Surface area. When a food is ground or cut up (i.e., hamburger or potato salad), it exposes more surface area and thus increases the rate of bacterial growth.
- Infestation. Though bacteria are everywhere, certain hygienic standards can help prevent food infection. Food workers should wash their hands regularly and not work when ill.

There are other food-borne pathogens, including hepatitis (a viral infection that seriously hinders the liver), trichinosis (a parasitic worm found primarily in tainted wild meat and pork), and some that are more common in underdeveloped nations. Giardia is a potent microorganism found in pristine mountain springs caused by fecal contamination from humans and wild animals.

Another bacterial contaminant of recent concern is candida albicans. Found in at least 30 percent of all humans[20] and throughout much of the food supply, candida is an opportunistic infection, meaning that it debilitates people who have other health problems.[21] Some health authorities have anecdotally found that otherwise untreatable symptoms disappeared when they were able to rid the patient of candida. A high-sugar diet encourages the candida organism.

Toxins become more concentrated with each level up the food chain. Seaweed, algae, and small fish found in mercury-contaminated water will have less mercury than the largest fish in this food chain. All the more reason to eat lower on the food chain (i.e., more plant food).

Recommendations

1. Avoid the fatty parts of domestic meats. Not only is the fat nutritionally suspect but it is also the depository of much of the fat-soluble pollutants mentioned in this chapter.

2. Do not eat burned, smoked, or scorched meats. Cook food over hot coals, not flames.

3. Eat a wide variety of foods. By concentrating on any one food you may be exposing yourself to a buildup of natural toxins. Small amounts of most of these toxins will not be harmful.

4. Raw food is not necessarily an advantage. Review the foods listed in this chapter. Wash, soak, sprout, and cook them.

5. Wash fresh produce in warm water. This will remove some of the pollutants, both incidental and intentional.

6. Keep your food covered or well wrapped in the refrigerator or on the stove, especially foods high in fluid and protein content. Do not allow food to sit at room temperature for more than one hour. This includes thawing frozen turkeys.

7. Maintain high standards of hygiene in your kitchen, and avoid eating in situations that seem unsanitary.

8. Eat lower on the food chain more often. Large fish are more contaminated than small fish, which are more contaminated than seaweed. Large animals are more contaminated than plant food.

9. Use stainless steel, glass, cast iron, or other time-tested materials to cook and store food. Minimize the use of canned food or remove food immediately from the can upon opening. Do not refrigerate food in its can.

10. Make efforts to help clean up our tainted food supply. Legislation, buying power, voting power, and other means can make a considerable difference in the quality of what we and future generations will consume.

PART FOUR

NUTRITION THROUGHOUT THE LIFE CYCLE

THOUGH INFANTS AND OLDER ADULTS ARE BOTH HUMANS, their nutrient needs vary significantly. Most of this book deals with the nutrient needs of adults. In this section, we discuss the other stages of life.

- Pregnancy—development of the fetus from conception through birth.
- Infancy—the first critical year of life.
- Childhood—ages one through twelve.
- Adolescence—ages thirteen through nineteen.
- Older adulthood—from age fifty-five on.

18

PREGNANCY

"Pregnancy is the only time when you can do nothing at all and still be productive."

—EVAN ESAR

Since the earliest traces of recorded history, humans have assumed there were relationships between diet and pregnancy. Their concepts were more simplistic than true: that sweet foods would produce a sweet-tempered baby, sour a sour-tempered baby, and so on. Modern medicine has had some glaring inaccuracies in relating diet to pregnancy. Only a few decades ago it was considered acceptable practice to have the pregnant woman minimize weight gain, thus producing a smaller baby and an easier delivery. Some physicians even recommended smoking to limit the mother's weight gain. This smaller baby was found to be at much greater risk for a variety of problems that could lead to early infant death. It was thought that toxemia, or the bloating of pregnancy, could be dealt with by restricting sodium and fluid intake. This treatment turned out to be almost as big a risk for both mother and developing fetus as the disease it was trying to prevent. Physicians and nutritionists now have a better grasp of the nutritive needs of the pregnant woman. Restricting calories, sodium, or water does not make sense, considering the increased need for these nutrients during pregnancy.

Nutrition during pregnancy is unique for three very important reasons:

1. The newly developing fetus has no control over its nutrient intake.

2. The phases of fetal development are time-dependent. If the raw materials to carry out a particular phase of construction are not present in the diet at the right time, then the phase will be only partially completed, and may never be finished.

3. The results of diet during this phase of life are irremedial. Children born with neural tube defects, often due to low folacin intake on the mother's part, will never be cured. Infants with low birth weight may have poorly developed organs or even brain stunting. Fetal alcohol syndrome can never be fixed. Animal studies show that even marginal nutrient deficiencies can lead to permanent physical or mental problems. A classic study performed in the late 1940s related diet to the outcome of pregnancy.

Essentially, the better the quality of a woman's diet during pregnancy, the greater the likelihood of having a healthy baby and easy delivery. A few people who followed atrocious dietary practices still had healthy babies, but the odds were very much against them. We still have people tell us that they lived on canned peaches and hot dogs throughout pregnancy and their children are "just fine." Yet how much better could these children have been had they been ideally nourished? Would they be sick less often, more intelligent or more emotionally balanced? These few exceptions of proper fetal development in spite of a mother's lifestyle are examples of the incredible tenacity of the human species. Against all odds, some people manage to survive. This does not mean that these isolated incidences should become examples for others.

There are two key aspects of nutrition in the outcome of pregnancy: (1) current nutrient intake—what a woman eats throughout pregnancy; and (2) nutrient reserves—what a woman has been eating in the past. There is ample evidence to say that pregnant women in this country could have a much lower rate of problems in delivery and prematurity if they paid closer attention to diet and lifestyle.

The study of dietary influences on pregnancy has some inherent problems. One cannot knowingly deprive a group of pregnant women of a needed nutrient just to create a scientific study. For obvious humanitarian reasons, the study of diet-pregnancy relationships has been limited to retrospective observations.

Common Problems of Pregnancy

Low birth weight infants (less than 2,500 grams or 5½ pounds) are at much greater risk for deformities, sickness, and death in the first two years of life. These same small infants are more likely to suffer less obvious problems relating to suboptimal development. Low birth weight infants are brought on by mothers who smoke, drink too much, gain too little weight (less than 15 pounds or 7 kilograms), gain too much weight (more than 28 pounds or 13 kilograms), or have multiple births.[1]

With the burden of excess fluid, blood, and kidney filtration, the pregnant woman is vulnerable to the bloating of edema (also called toxemia or pre-eclampsia). High blood pressure, protein in the urine, headache, and blurred vision are all symptoms of this problem in maintaining proper fluid balance. Some women experience the milder stages of this condition with swollen ankles or wrists. The severely underweight or overweight mother may bring this problem into the delivery room as life-threatening eclampsia. Low calcium intake creates a risk for this bloating, elevated blood pressure, and problems of delivery.[2] Low zinc during pregnancy creates a higher risk for hypertension and edema in the mother,[3] a Caesarian delivery and smaller infant,[4] toxemia and birth defects,[5] and impaired brain development.[6] Optimal intake of protein, B_6, calcium, potassium, zinc, magnesium and all other nutrients helps create a healthy infant and mother. Sunflower oil, probably because of its essential fatty acid content, can help reduce hypertension in pregnancy.[7]

Pica

Pica is the eating of nonfoods, like clay or laundry soap. Sound strange? This condition is common in children and women, and even more common in pregnant women, all of whom are the frequent victims of anemia. Could it be that a low blood cell count alters normal appetite and taste mechanisms? The case studies of pica in pregnant women are fascinating.

In England, a twenty-one-year old woman was hospitalized thirty-eight weeks into pregnancy with severe anemia. She complained of fatigue, dizziness, swollen ankles, and poor appetite. Three weeks of intense iron and folacin therapy failed to improve her symptoms. Upon further questioning, it was found that she had been eating one or two toilet freshener blocks each week throughout her pregnancy. Once she was convinced to stop, she improved rapidly. In another case, a sixteen-year-old woman was about to deliver her baby, when complications arose. It was found that her bowels were almost completely impacted, blocking the infant's descent into the birth canal. Once the fecal matter was removed, birth proceeded normally. It was discovered that the patient had eaten more than a quart of clay per day during her pregnancy. Another patient showed marked wear on her teeth. Her dentist found out that this woman had eaten a shoebox full of clay each week throughout all seven of her pregnancies.

Obviously clay and bars of toilet freshener carry no nutritive value, while they do pose a risk for the pregnant woman. Why pica occurs is not totally understood. We suspect that an unhealthy system, such as from a vitamin or mineral deficiency, gives rise to an unhealthy appetite mechanism.

Stages of Fetal Development

Conception through implantation. Two weeks after conception, the fertilized egg attaches itself near the top of the uterus.[8] Once the uterus begins the placental blood supply, many changes begin to take place in the woman's body.

Organogenesis. The next six weeks are very vulnerable to toxins, alcohol, drugs, and pollutants. This stage (the making of organs) is also vulnerable to low-quality diets in which the vitamins (like folacin, B_{12}, A, and C) and minerals (like zinc) that are involved in cell differentiation may be missing. Experts in this field (embryologists) were able to determine exactly when expectant mothers took the tranquilizer Thalidomide, because of the specific deformity that occurred during a certain phase of organogenesis.

During this stage, the pregnant woman need not be so concerned about eating more food as about avoiding potential toxins and eating a high-quality diet.

Rapid fetal growth. Now that the essential body parts have been formed, fetal growth shifts into high gear. Cells increase in number (hyperplasia) and size (hypertrophy) so that the infant will be able to survive outside the womb after fetal development. This phase is vulnerable to both *quality* and *quantity* of diet. The woman should be eating 300 additional calories and 30 grams of protein per day.

The Brain

The relationship between diet and fetal growth extends beyond the more obvious deformities. Some dentists speculate that a marginal intake of vitamin A might lead to slightly malformed teeth, perhaps forcing the child to wear braces later on. Mild alcohol abuse could cause mild brain problems in the child, like hyperactivity, learning disorders, dyslexia, or even anxiety.

Increases in brain cell number occur almost exclusively during pregnancy and just after birth.[9] If diet is inadequate during these phases, insufficient brain cells are manufactured and the child will never achieve his or her genetic potential for intellect or emotions.

The Placenta

For decades, scientists thought that the infant was a parasite that would steal whatever it needed from the mother's blood supply. This concept would make special diets for the pregnant woman somewhat irrelevant. It is true that the placenta can steal certain nutrients that are available from the mother, such as vitamin C, calcium, and glucose. Yet other nutrients must passively diffuse across the placenta to reach the infant.[10] Thus, for most nutrients, the developing infant can take only what the mother has in surplus.

It was also mistakenly assumed that the placenta would screen out all harmful agents from the fetus. Many drugs, tobacco, alcohol, and other toxins like lead cross the placenta and can harm fetal development.

Diet and Pregnancy

There is a 33 percent increase in maternal blood volume by term. This creates a seriously elevated need for nutrients involved in making red blood cells (iron, copper, folacin, B_6, protein, B_{12}). This added need for blood creates a serious challenge to the mother's diet. Proper nutrition can keep blood levels near normal. The consequences of anemia during pregnancy include fatigue and irritability for the mother, with stunted growth likely for the fetus.

A total of about 300 grams of iron are needed to make the fetal blood supply, with another 500 grams required for the mother's increased blood supply. The iron RDA for the pregnant woman is 18+ milligrams. The "+" means that 30 to 60 milligrams of supplemental iron may be needed.

There is a 50 percent increase in plasma volume (the clear fluid part of blood). An extra five to six liters of fluid between the cells (intercellular) is added to the body, with an additional 50 perent work load on the kidneys to filter this fluid. As a result, many women experience bloating, toxemia, or kidney problems. Aldosterone (the hormone involved in sodium conservation) secretion becomes greater. Well-nourished kidneys will be less likely to retain extra fluid under this additional burden. The needs substantially increase for extra fluid, sodium, and potassium in the diet. Calcium, potassium, and probably other nutrients help keep the kidneys healthy. Protein, magnesium, the essential fatty acid and B_6 help prevent bloating and toxemia by maintaining proper fluid balance.

There is reduced gastric motility. The muscular contractions that massage the food along the intestinal tract begin to slow down. This makes perfect sense because the slower food movement allows for increased efficiency of absorption. The pregnant woman must maintain sufficient fiber and fluid intake to prevent constipation. B_6 supplements and small frequent meals will help prevent the nausea of pregnancy that stems from changes in intestinal movement.

The expanding uterus begins pushing against the mother's internal organs. Pushing against the lungs and elevation of the diaphram will cause shortness of breath. Proper posture and exercise can help. Pressure against the bladder as well as vascular changes there will cause frequent urination. Pushing against the stomach and intestines can also cause nausea and a bloated feeling after eating. Pregnant women can have crackers or other bland food by their beside table and eat these upon waking.

There is an increased output of thyroxin, which causes elevated basal metabolism. All of the woman's systems go into high gear to provide maximum efficiency at serving the developing fetus. Studies find that low calorie intake is a major risk factor during pregnancy. No dieting during pregnancy!

Ideally, 20 to 28 pounds will be gained by term. Of this, there are approximately 7½ pounds are for the infant, 1 pound for the placenta, 4 pounds for the mother's extra blood volume, 2½ pounds for the expanded uterus and muscles to support the fetus, 3 pounds for increased breast size (readying for lactation), 2 pounds of (amniotic) fluid surrounding the fetus, 4 pounds of maternal fat stores to ensure adequate calories for nursing, and more than 2 pounds of protein deposited in the fetus and surrounding tissues.

About 28 grams, or one ounce, of calcium will be pumped into the fetus for its developing skeletal system and other calcium functions. Calcium, phosphorus, magnesium, and vitamin D requirements increase markedly for the pregnant woman. If she does not satisfy these nutrient needs by her diet, then either she, the fetus, or both will suffer by having the mother's bone stores of minerals ransacked.

Hyperplasis (an increase in cell number) is occurring as rapidly as it ever will in a person's life. Hypertrophy (an increase in cell size) is also rapid in the last two trimesters of pregnancy. Hyperplasia has a critical need for nutrients involved in cell differentiation. Cell differentiation is the miraculous process of one undefined cell splitting into two cells, one of which may become a liver cell while the other may become a kidney cell. Nutrient needs include folacin, riboflavin, vitamins A, C, B_{12}, and zinc.

All nutrients are required in higher levels during pregnancy, but only one doubles in need: folacin. Folacin-deficient pregnant women are more likely to have a preterm delivery,[11] while pregnant women taking folacin supplements had an average of one extra week in carrying their infant before delivery.[12] It seems that folacin encourages the birth of a developed and mature infant more capable of thriving in the outside world.

Hypertrophy elevates the need for quantites of nutrients, especially calories and protein. The energy nutrients thiamin, niacin, riboflavin, pantothenic acid, biotin, and chromium are also needed in higher levels. Extra B_6 is required for protein metabolism.

There is an increased demand for glucose to build tissues for the fetus. The fetus has an active pump in the placenta to provide it with glucose, which is the preferential fuel for fetal construction. Insulin and chromium are also required for proper use of glucose. Many women become semidiabetic during pregnancy (gestational diabetes) and lose this malady once they have delivered.[13] Some women do not lose the diabetes with the birth of their child. Multiple births are a risk factor toward adult diabetes for women.

Eat small frequent meals. Increase the intake of complex carbohydrate and fiber. Supplements may help to amend nutrient deficiences. Improve the quality of the diet. Exercise regularly. Minimize coffee, alcohol, and simple refined carbohydrates.

From what is known in this area, it seems likely that nearly any defect or sub-par performance could be due to suboptimal diet during pregnancy. Poor dental health, short adult height, poor disease resistance, low mental capacity, and emotional disorders have all been related to poor diet during pregnancy. Fetal alcohol syndrome has been shown to cause blatant physical and mental defects. About one in every 750 children born in the United States is a victim of this preventable and irremedial disorder.[14] Low folacin has been associated with neural tube defects, a common deformity of the brain or spinal cord. Smoking has been related to small infants, cleft palate, heart defects, and other problems. Protein intake has been linked to brain size and proper development. Blatant malnutrition often yields blatant physical and mental deformities. The list is extensive and well documented.

But what about the finer shades of health that lie between perfection and obvious defects? That, too, has been researched. Not long ago, it was assumed that the infant either developed or it didn't. Lived or died. All or none. Yet new studies show that there are many shades of gray between the black and white of extremes. The infant may develop yet have subtle physical and mental abnormalities. It may even seem reasonably normal yet carry lifetime vulnerabilities toward stress, pollution, disease, and other dilemmas. And the mother's health can suffer later if she was malnourished during pregnancy. Pregnant women with low intakes of vitamin C are more likely to develop gallstones later on.[15]

How many nutrients are in marginal supply in the American diet could retard fetal development? Many. Protein, iron, magnesium, calcium, chromium, copper, selenium, zinc, vitamin A, C, riboflavin, and B_6 are but a few. Would any mother want her baby to fall short of its genetic potential?

Risk Factors During Pregnancy

Diet is critical but it is not the only factor in proper fetal development. Others include:

Smoking. Doubles the risk of having smaller and immaturely formed infants.[16] Prematurity and heart defects are known in this group. Smoking mothers are more likely to give birth to an infant with cleft palate.[17] Smoking with coffee present even further risk to the developing fetus.[18] A host of other problems are suspected.

Alcohol. Fetal alcohol syndrome is common, devastating, and preventable. There are probably many finer shades of problems caused by social-drinking mothers, especially those who are poorly nourished.

Drugs. Only the most essential drugs should be used by pregnant women, and even then only under a physician's direction. The great Thalidomide tragedy showed the scientific world that drugs that can be tolerated by healthy adults may wreak havoc on a fetus. Even excess caffeine (more than two cups of coffee per day) may cause problems.

Age. Immature teenagers have twice the risk for toxemia and problems of delivery. Teen mothers have high nutrient needs themselves due to their biological immaturity, plus high nutrient needs for the infant, combined with bizarre dietary practices commonly associated with this age bracket. Of the over one million teens who become pregnant each year, almost half are under eighteen, and 40,000 are under fifteen. One-fourth of these teens become pregnant again within a year.[19] Older age is also a risk. Expectant women beyond age forty should work closely with their physician. After age forty-five, the risks to fetus and mother increase drastically.

Parity. How well has the woman fared in past pregnancies? If well, then odds increase of the same pattern continuing. The opposite is also true.

Socioeconomic status. Both money (for food and medical care) and education (for proper hygiene and diet) increase the possibilities for an excellent outcome of pregnancy.

Exercise. Exercise improves circulation, blood glucose tolerance, attitude, muscle tone, and may shorten the time spent in delivery and recovery. It should be moderated by common sense.

Stature. Short women can certainly deliver healthy babies. Yet if a woman is short because of malnourishment in her developmental years, there could be problems. The "grandmother effect" means that her eggs may not be properly formed, or her pelvic girth too narrow, or that there are other problems often manifested by short stature. Also, with short and petite women, delivery may be difficult if the father is a much larger person. The infant may be too large for the mother's birth passage and thus require Caesarean delivery.

Genetics. Women whose family lines have a record of giving birth successfully have a greater chance of having an uncomplicated delivery and a healthy infant.

Weight. If the woman is too thin before beginning pregnancy, or she does not gain adequate weight during pregnancy (twenty to twenty-eight pounds),[20] or she gains too much weight, then a risk could be posed to her and the infant.

Attitude. Women under stress are more likely to experience problems. Stress may influence their food intake or their absorption of food, or increase the need for nutrients. The flood of catecholamines (stress hormones) may play havoc with the developing fetus.

Recommended Program for the Pregnant Woman

Work out with your obstetrician your own individual nutrition program, but here are some good general guidelines to follow:

Avoid tobacco and all but the most essential drugs.

Abstain from alcohol.

Minimize caffeine. One or two cups of coffee or tea per day are acceptable. None would be better. Be aware of caffeine in colas, aspirin, and other over-the-counter drugs.

Exercise regularly. Find something enjoyable and nonstressful. Walking and stretching routines are excellent.

Attitude is important. Keep a positive outlook. Get rest. Picture a healthy and happy baby. Talk and sing to the developing fetus. You are what you think.

Diet is uniquely crucial during this phase of life. To a well-balanced non-pregnancy diet, add 30 grams of protein, 300 calories, and make them from high-quality foods. Two servings each from the milk, vegetable, and protein groups will add essential nutrients to the diet. Seventy-eight percent of pregnant women in a study had at least one nutrient deficiency.[21]

Avoid megadoses of nutrients. Excessive levels of vitamins A and D and the minerals selenium, zinc, and iodine could cause serious problems during fetal development. High doses of any nutrient may lead to physiological dependence, which the newborn infant inherits as a vitamin or mineral deficiency. Check the vitamin and mineral chapters in this book and keep nutritional supplementation within the ranges of the levels recommended. This is no time to experiment with excessive levels of nutrients, since optimal nutrition is a question of balance. Too much or too little can cause harm. Pregnant women not using supplements are at higher risk for premature delivery, spontaneous abortion, and having a low birth weight infant.[22] For women recently on oral contraceptives, vitamin supplements are even more important.

19

INFANCY

"I've just learned what makes a newborn babe cry. It's hungry, naked, and already owes the government $1,700."

—ARTHUR GODFREY

The big day finally arrived. After months of anticipation, a healthy infant emerged from its embryonic journey. Now to get about the business of feeding this tiny human being.

Nutrition during infancy is unique for several reasons:

1. It will strongly influence the infant's growth, development, and disease resistance.

2. The results can be irremedial, whether done right or wrong.

3. The infant cannot direct its own nourishment in this crucial phase of its life.

4. The infant's needs are considerably higher (per body weight) than at any other time in the life cycle.

We speak of two separate people now. Both the mother and the infant have nutritive needs to be satisfied in order for both to maintain good health.

Breast-Feeding

How does lactation occur? Throughout pregnancy, the mother was developing her breast size and mammary glands for milk production.[1] The pituitary gland, situated near the center of the brain and about the size of a pea, produces prolactin to encourage breast milk production. Mental outlook can influence the hypothalamus of the brain, which can influence the pituitary, which can seriously affect milk production. Therefore, family support and proper attitude become critical for a woman to be able to breast-feed her infant successfully.

The mother's diet also plays a key role in her ability to nurse. The mammary glands in the breast cannot manufacture their own nutrients but must use what is found in the maternal blood supply. If the diet is high quality, the infant will reap the benefits. The opposite is also true. A scientific study found that nursing mothers required an oral supplement containing ten to twenty milligrams per day of B_6 (four to eight times the RDA) in order to provide acceptable levels of B_6 in breast milk.[2] Ninety-eight percent of nursing mothers who were taking a supplement with some zinc still were consuming less than two-thirds of the RDA for zinc.[3] Zinc is a crucial nutrient for the rapidly growing and vulnerable infant. Zinc supplements are essential for the nursing mother.[4]

For the first few days after birth, the mother's milk will be thin and yellow in color, almost like diluted orange juice. This immature milk is called colostrum. Though it is low in calories and other nutrients, it is rich in the antibodies that help protect the vulnerable infant against infectious organisms. Ten days after birth, the milk will have matured into highly nutritious sustenance for the infant. The milk now looks somewhat bluish in color, almost like nonfat milk.

Advantages of Nursing

Disease resistance. For nine months, the fetus developed in the sterile and semi-weightless environment of the womb. It must now face the rigors of millions of disease-causing organisms; breast milk provides the ideal shield against them.[5]

Lactoferrin is a substance that prevents bacteria from growing in the infant by grabbing the available iron stores and also helping the infant to absorb iron.[6] The bifidus factor encourages the growth of friendly bacteria in the infant's intestines, which then control the growth of unfriendly bacteria. Various antibodies from mother's milk protect the infant from infections in the mouth, throat, and digestive tract. Some of these antibodies leak into the blood stream, since the immature digestive tract cannot screen out all large proteins. Once in the blood, these antibodies donate disease tolerance to the newborn infant. There is a lower incidence of sudden infant death (SID) among breast-fed infants. This fact leads a few scientists to speculate that breast milk contains some very special and yet-to-be-isolated substances.

Less chance of overfatness. Bottle-fed infants are often forced to finish the bottle, while breast-fed infants stop eating when they are full. A breast-feeding mother cannot quantify the exact amount of milk intake, so the infant listens to its own appetite mechanism. The "hindmilk," which comes toward the end of the feeding, is higher in fat (nearly 50 percent) and probably signals the infant to cease feeding. Bottle-fed infants are more likely to start on solid foods earlier; these are higher in calorie density and the infant is encouraged to finish them.

Less risk of allergies. It is known that breast-fed infants have a lower incidence of allergies.[7] There are several possible explanations. Human milk is lower in casein than cow's milk. Casein is a common allergen. The ideal protein ratio found in mother's milk is nearly always well tolerated and probably lowers the sensitivity to other proteins that are introduced later. Also, there is a factor in human milk that helps to coat the intestinal tract and may prevent large proteins from being absorbed into the blood. Breast-fed infants usually do not have other foods introduced as early as bottle-fed infants. Exposing an immature system to a foreign protein may trigger the autoimmune response seen in people with allergies.[8] For more on this, see the chapter on food allergies.

Emotional benefits. There are critical imprinting stages most animals experience, including humans. Many women gain a great deal of confidence from their breast-feeding experience, feeling that they can take care of their child. Close, intimate skin contact encourages a bonding that cannot be simulated with a hand-held bottle. There are many experts in the mental health field who feel that emotional security is gained in the breast-fed infant.

Better formation of mouth and teeth. Sucking involves a considerable muscular effort by the breast-fed infant. The jaw muscles and surrounding vicinity are more likely to develop as they should. Bottle-fed infants have more problems with mouth and tooth formation. Many have the bottle propped up for ease of feeding, which exposes the teeth for long periods of time to the cavity-causing sugars of milk or formula.

Reduced cost. A lactating mother must consume an additional 500 calories per day from food. Food is not free, but the cost of prepared infant formulas is much higher.

Convenience. Bottle-feeding mothers must have bottle, formula, something to heat it on, then allow it to cool, then clean the bottle. Nursing mothers need nothing but themselves.

Sanitation. Mother's milk is clean and hygienic. The same cannot always be said for the water used to dilute infant formulas. Cow's milk and formula must be boiled to kill bacteria, then cooled to a reasonable drinking temperature.

Less chance of mistakes in mixing. Even well-intentioned, well-educated people can create havoc with mistakes in mixing. In a case study, an infant was fed undiluted infant formula. The infant's immature intestinal tract could not handle the concentrated substance and began dumping fluid from the body into the intestines to dilute it. This caused diarrhea and dehydration. The infant died from this tragic mistake.[9] In the 1960s, a manufacturer of infant formulas forgot to add vitamin B_6. Many infants developed convulsions.

Appearance. Oxytocin is a hormone secreted during lactation that causes contraction of the uterus and abdominal muscles. Having been stretched to its limit during pregnancy, the stomach will tighten more quickly for breast-feeding mothers. Also, lactation uses up 700 to 800 calories per day. This is the equivalent of a 120-pound woman's running about ten miles each day. If there is stored fat accumulated from pregnancy, lactation will quickly burn this away. The breasts swell with milk during lactation. Though they do shrink after weaning, many women retain a certain percentage of this added bust size.

Breast health. Women who breast-feed have a lower incidence of breast cancer.

Infant's long-term health. Breast-fed infants have a lower incidence of heart disease. Human milk is also higher in unsaturated fats.

Marginal method of birth control. Though far from infallible, breast-feeding may delay ovulation to help prevent pregnancy. Psychologists have found that a two- to three-year spacing between infants is ideal for both parents and offspring. Physicians say that it takes a woman's body about one year to fully recover from the physical stress of pregnancy.

Nutritional benefits. The overwhelming superiority of breast-milk over cow's milk or even expensive formulas highlights the limited knowledge of the science of nutrition. The more research that is conducted on breast-milk, the more subtle ingredients are found that could markedly influence an infant's growth and development.

Human milk, versus infant formula or cow's milk, has:

• Less protein, but a more digestible protein that more closely matches human needs; enzymes that help the infant digest and assimilate the protein; an ideal ratio of cysteine to methionine, which helps out the immature liver since it is unable to easily convert these amino acids; more taurine, an unusual amino acid found in almost negligible levels in cow's milk. Taurine is known to participate in the development of the central nervous system.

• More lactose. This provides raw materials for brain growth (galactosides). It also stimulates the growth of beneficial bacteria in the intestines to fight off disease-causing bacteria, helps produce vitamins (like biotin and K), and aids in mineral absorption.

• Much higher efficiency of absorbing vitamins and minerals. Approaches 100 percent efficiency.

• Less sodium. This prevents the infant from acquiring an affinity for high-sodium foods.

• More vitamin A and C. If the mother's diet is high quality, then all other nutrients will also be found in higher levels in her breast milk.

• More cholesterol for the fatty wrapping (myelin sheath) that insulates the rapidly growing nervous system.

• More linoleic acid, the essential fatty acid, for cell membranes and prostaglandin production; also, more in gamma-linoleic acid (GLA), eicosapentanoic acid (EPA) and docosahexanoic acid (DHA), all of which may be essential during infancy; less saturated fat; and contains lipase liberating factor, for easier fat digestion.

• Ideal zinc to copper ratio, with better levels of each of these minerals; a special protein to increase the efficiency of zinc absorption.

• Less strontium, the radioactive fallout agent.

• Less phosphorus and twice the efficiency of calcium absorption.

• Fewer trace element impurities. Infant formulas contain much higher levels of aluminum. This could cause toxicity in infants with poor kidney abilities to excrete the aluminum.[10]

• More selenium.

When Mothers Can't/Shouldn't/Won't Breast-Feed

The primary reason today for not breast-feeding is that mothers work out of the home. For some, their companies grant a few months' maternity leave to allow mother and infant to get to know one another and make breast-feeding possible. Other mothers who work out of the home pump their breasts and leave this milk for whomever is caring for their infant, providing all the nutritional and immunological advantages of breast-milk. For some women, however, neither of these options is possible, and infant formula must be used.

Attitude can be an impediment to breast-feeding. Some women think of it as being primitive or messy. Some equate nursing with poverty, since aggressive marketing has made infant formulas seem the obvious improvement of the technological age. Other women do not have the support of their families, especially their husbands. A husband may have felt somewhat neglected during late pregnancy and may want the limelight returned. Or he may want to be more involved in child rearing by bottle-feeding the infant. Some women think that their breasts are too small to properly nurse. Size of breasts has nothing to do with success of lactation. A-cup breasts are as capable of proper nourishment as D-cup breasts.

Illness can be a factor. If the infant is in the hospital, nursing can be impossible. If the mother has an infectious disease, it may not be wise to breast-feed. Check with your physician about this. Some infants are born to alcoholic or drug-addicted mothers, who are unlikely candidates for proper nursing. Diabetes, tuberculosis, or cystic fibrosis may all be reasons not to nurse.

In essence, 85 to 99 percent all healthy women who want to breast-feed and have the support of their families can do so. But when a mother chooses not to nurse for whatever reason, she should realize that quality infant formulas are available.

Nutrient Needs of the Lactating Woman

Although scientists have calculated that lactation costs the woman about 750 calories per day, they recommend an additional intake of 500 calories during this period.[11] The negative balance allows the woman to lose some unwanted fatty deposits acquired during pregnancy. An extra twenty grams daily of protein are needed during lactation. All vitamins and minerals are needed in higher levels, since the mother's diet will be directly reflected in the quality of her breast milk.[12] Calcium, phosphorus, zinc, ascorbic acid, and magnesium requirements are one-third higher. All other requirements are also increased.

We recommend that the lactating women take a high-quality, broad spectrum supplement.[13] Vitamin D supplements or regular sunshine exposure are important for the health of both mother and nursing infant.[14] Fluid intake is important, since she is making about a quart of liquid food for her infant each day. She should avoid strong-tasting foods, such as garlic, coffee, chocolate, cabbage, beans, alcohol, and carbonated beverages, which can pass into her milk and irritate the infant. Some women with colicky babies find that avoiding dairy products helps eliminate the infant's intestinal discomfort. Dairy products are not irreplaceable, but the vitamins, minerals, and protein found in them must be actively pursued in other foods.

Nutritional Weaknesses of Breast Milk

There is no shortage of opinions on this subject. One study concluded that a well-nourished mother can safely use breast milk as exclusive food for her infant for the first year of life.[15] Other experts comment that few mothers are well nourished and thus supplements or other foods need to be introduced at six months or sooner. Still others claim that, regardless of how perfect the mother's diet is, other nutrients are needed by six months.

Iron. A healthy infant born with adequate iron stores via its well nourished mother probably can develop well until six months and then may need extra iron (cereal or egg yolk).[16] In most situations, infants would need extra iron by three months. Both breast-fed and formula-fed infants have a problem here. It is conservatively estimated that at least a third of all infants are anemic.[17] Blatant symptoms are often lacking. Breast milk iron, though not abundant, is much better absorbed than formula iron.[18]

Fluoride. Although mother's intake will improve infant status, the proven benefits of fluoride on tooth and bone formation are impressive. Even if the baby drinks fluoridated water, most municpal fluoride levels are quite low. We recommend the use of liquid fluoride drops beginning shortly after birth.

Vitamin K. This vitamin is in marginal supply in breast milk unless the nursing mother is taking oral supplements of K.[19] The nursing infant begins to make its own K via the bacteria in the gut.

Vitamin E. There are low levels of E in even healthy infants, with premature infants being dangerously low. The multiple vitamin/mineral drops used for the infant should contain about thirty I.U. of vitamin E per day.

Vitamin D. Once thought to be almost absent from breast milk, vitamin D was found in a water-soluble version that had previously escaped researchers. Some exposure to indirect sunlight, ten to thirty minutes daily, will also help the infant produce vitamin D internally. Low-sun areas have a higher incidence of rickets.[20] Sunlight exposure also helps prevent the possibility of bilirubinemia, a buildup of deadly bile in the blood that can cause problems with brain growth.

Food Introduction in the First Year of Life

Biologically, the infant does not have a swallowing ability or mature digestive tract until about three months of age, yet there are still widely used medical texts that allow solid foods to be started as early as six weeks of life.[21] Many experts think that this early introduction of food is a prime suspect for the abundance of food allergies in this country. Despite the proven benefits of avoiding solid foods until later, 20 percent of the infants in the United States are given solid foods by one week of life and 90 percent are started before one month. We recommend avoiding solid foods until six months.

Our program consists of the following:

Birth to six months. Human milk with feedings every two to three hours, except during the night for infants who will sleep through. Liquid supplements with flouride and other vitamins and minerals can make good nutritional insurance.[22] The mother should be well nourished and rested. The premature infant definitely needs nutritional supplements.[23]

Six months. One feeding per day of iron-enriched rice cereal. Rice is least likely to cause an allergic reaction. Mashed potato puddings with milk and juices and live culture yogurt can be served. Avoid frozen orange juice concentrate since this contains the bitter oils from the rind, not to mention the pesticides found on the surface of the peel.

Seven months. Strained or puréed vegetables, preferably dark green or deep orange ones for their vitamin A content.

Eight months. Strained or puréed fruits. These are introduced after the vegetables, because the infant would probably prefer the sweeter of the two and ignore the nutritious vegetables.

Nine months. Puréed meats. Egg yolk cooked into either cereal or mashed potato pudding.

Ten months. Begin serving chopped bread pieces and other finger food. Avoid raisins and other similarly sized food, since the infant can choke on these.

Twelve months. Wean to cup. Many foods may be chopped fresh from the dinner table.

Several points to keep in mind: Do not serve egg white in the first year of life, since this often causes allergic reactions. Allow a one-week introductory period for each new food. This provides a testing phase to see if the infant reacts to the food. If they seem to physically or mentally react, withdraw the food, keep track of these items, and re-introduce after the first year of life, carefully observing the outcome.

Baby foods can be made nutritiously and economically at home. Make extra food when you prepare your meals and purée some of it in the blender. There are also inexpensive hand-held food grinders for this purpose. Pour this mush into ice cube trays and freeze. These small blocks can be thawed to provide ready nutrition that you control.

In the past, baby food manufacturers have used excessive salt, sugar, colorings, additives, and MSG. Some manufacturers still use modified starch. More than a few noted scientists have questioned the use of these modified starches in baby food.

Whenever possible, let infants handle the food to get used to texture, feeding themselves, and hand-eye coordination. Do not force foods. Do not make mealtime a war of wills. Do not use foods as rewards for other deeds. These dubious practices can lead to bizarre food attitudes later in life that promote obesity or eating disorders.

If mother and infant are so inclined, breast-feeding can continue for up to two years, as long as these other foods are being slowly introduced to supplement the nutritive value of mother's milk. Most infants begin tooth formation at around six months. This, more than coincidentally, is the time many mothers cease nursing, since the teething infant may bite the breast. For those mothers who want to continue nursing, if the infant bites, remove it from the breast. The infant quickly learns the results of its behavior.

Your efforts toward proper nutrition will pay off in a healthier, happier, better-looking, more intelligent, and well-adjusted child. Though the child benefits immediately, it also may make the next eighteen years of parenting a lot easier.

20

CHILDHOOD

"The one thing children wear out faster than shoes is parents."
—JOHN J. PLOMP

The infant that slept and ate constantly is now turning into a child. The child can stand, walk, and talk. He is eating his own meals, albeit a bit awkwardly. You are probably aware of some of his food likes and dislikes. A personality is developing. There are several reasons that make the years from one through twelve keenly important in the overall picture of optimal development:

1. The child is very dependent on others to provide decent nourishment and a conducive atmosphere in which to eat and enjoy that food.

2. Growth and maturation of all areas of the body are occurring with amazing speed.

3. Changes taking place during this phase are time-dependent. Damages resulting from inadequate nutrient intake can be irremedial. A well-nourished and secure child is a different human being from the junk-food-reared non-breakfast-eating nutrient-deficient child. The child's eventual body stature is at stake. Overfeeding during the vulnerable phase of childhood can result in excessive fat cell creation. These fat cells act as hungry storage tanks to trigger the appetite of the overfat. Overfat children often become overfat adults.[1]

A child's eating patterns are being trained during these years. Habits involving sugar, salt, fat, texture, subtle flavors, frequency of meals, and speed of eating are being set. Parents who use food as a reward system often create lifetime weight problems for their children.[2]

Optimal nutrition will do more than just allow the child to grow to its genetic potential of physical and intellectual stature. The malnourished child has a greater likelihood of being a poor student and having behavioral disorders.[3] Poor grades and bad attitude can put the child in a rut. The first grader who is sluggish because of a lack of protein or iron can become the disruptive high school student. This "domino effect" could lead to either a life of crime or of contributions to society.

Physical Changes During Childhood

Steady growth in weight and height. By age two, a child has quadrupled its birth weight. The child is also very active and has a high basal metabolism. A seven-year-old has the same calorie needs as his or her adult mother, who has more than twice the body weight, and a 250 percent greater protein need than his or her parents. This incredible growth rate and nutrient demands can create numerous nutrient deficiencies. Zinc deficiency is common in American children, resulting in stunted growth and development of the body and mind.[4]

The ability of children to eat enough food is limited by their small stomachs. Small frequent meals will help this problem. Healthy snacks can be a major asset to the child's growth and will also help stabilize energy and moods. Ice cream, peanut butter, nuts, and meats can be valuable additions to the child's growth, while these same foods should be restricted for the sedentary adult because of their high fat and calorie content.

Brain growth. Interestingly, the brain and body grow together. Studies have found that taller children usually have a higher IQ than shorter children.[5] Fed properly, children grow well in both body and mind. By age four, the child's brain has grown to 90 percent of its adult weight, which accounts for the proportionately larger heads of children. All creatures develop their main survival tool as quickly as possible, and the main survival tool of humans is brain power. The human brain grows so rapidly that proper diet during pregnancy and the first four years of life is vital. Malnutrition in early years can lead to permanent, irreparable stunting of mental abilities along with abnormal behavior.[6, 7] Low-protein diets even stunt the child's ability to adapt to the cold.[8]

Maturing organs and enzyme systems. The child slowly develops the ability to digest and tolerate various foods. Greasy, high-fat, spicy meals are unlikely to be well tolerated by the young child.

Sensitive taste buds. By retirement age, most adults have lost 80 percent of their taste buds. The child has uniquely sensitive taste mechanisms. What tastes good to mom and dad does not necessarily taste good to their child. Strong-flavored foods such as onions, garlic, Brussels sprouts, certain fish, and many other items can all rate a rejection by the heightened taste sensations of the child.

Calcification of the skeleton. The newborn infant is a mass of flexible cartilage, thus facilitating the birthing process. By the end of the first year of life, there is triple the amount of calcium in the skeletal system as there was at birth. The skeletal system is expanding at an amazing pace. A one-year-old child has the same calcium requirements as its parents. Calcium, phosphorus, magnesium, vitamin D, protein, zinc, and vitamin C play a vital direct role in erecting a healthy bone frame for this growing child. Fluoride will help to properly harden the bones and teeth as they are being formed and calcified.

Growing blood supply. While the child doubles in size, so too does the blood volume. This creates awesome needs for nutrients directly involved in making red blood cells—iron, folacin, B_{12}, copper, protein, and B_6. Iron deficiency is as common in affluent America as it is in Third World nations.[9]

Maturing immune system. The breast-fed infant who is sheltered from large gatherings of people may be relatively disease-free. Once the child is brought to day-care centers, birthday parties, friends' homes, and other gatherings where disease-causing microbes can be exchanged, infections may become more common. The immature immune system is being exposed to a variety of new pathogens. It must manufacture the appropriate immune bodies to destroy these invaders. The process of making immune bodies to defend the body from invasion requires high levels of nutrients, including vitamins C, A, B_6, zinc, selenium, and protein.

Food Preferences

The rapid growth of infancy diminishes somewhat during childhood, leaving the young child with appetite fluctuations that can vex the most accommodating parent. Nearly all children go through wild roller-coaster swings in their appetite and food preferences between the ages of six months and seven years.

One of the symptoms of malnutrition is poor appetite, which perpetuates the malnutrition. Most Americans, including children, are low in their intake of zinc, which is a critical nutrient for a healthy appetite. In one study, zinc supplements were given to children who were picky eaters. Within two months, the children were eating much better, with major improvements in their total nutrient intake.[10]

Nearly all children have their own bizarre stages of food preference. They will eat only a peanut butter sandwich or a hamburger or whatever. These stages are usually only a few weeks or months in length. The patient parent will not make a war out of mealtime, but rather provide healthy foods when the child is ready to eat. Children are clever enough to know which of their behaviors will get them the most attention. If a titanic struggle of wills at the dinner table is the only way to receive the undivided attention of their parents, then the child may continue these food games. If the child does not want a food, remove it from the table. If possible, refrigerate, reheat, and re-serve that same food at the next meal. Remember that children are people, too. Just as you do not like all foods, neither do they. Allow them such op-tions. They are developing the skills of independence and choice in some of these tactical "food games." Studies show that food preferences and nutri-tion concepts are rooted in early life.[11] The older a person gets, the more difficult it becomes to change food habits. Get your children started early on the right path to healthy eating.

There are some practical techniques that parents can use to get their kids to eat most foods:

Do not force foods. People are stubborn. If forced into something, they may resist just to maintain their free will. Studies show that young people offered a variety of vegetables will likely eat one of them, while children told to eat one vegetable will often reject it.

Try reverse psychology. Adults often want what is not offered to them. So do children. Prepare the food in question and put it only on your plate and your spouse's plate. Children will notice something different. When they ask, just answer their questions, but do not make an effort to get the food for them, yet. They will soon ask for the food. This stunt works quite often.

Get them involved. Though children may not eat canned green beans, they are very likely to eat fresh beans that they helped grow. Let them work in the garden. It does not have to be a major parcel of land, just something for examples. Let them help prepare foods in the kitchen. Children will of-ten eat even the most atrocious-tasting food if they were involved in prepar-ing it. Let them rip cabbage into the salad bowl, or pour dough for muffins. Sprouts are especially suited to teaching children while feeding them well from your own kitchen garden. For more about sprouting, see the chapter on super foods.

Atmosphere is important. No one likes a tense eating environment. Ob-servations show that children eat better when dining with their peers. So do you. Do not make mealtime the hour for strident accusations and punish-ments. A friendly atmosphere will help them eat enough, digest and absorb better, and develop good mealtime habits.

Be creative with unwanted foods. Raisins and nuts make an interesting face on an oatmeal cookie. Carrot sticks can be logs to be eaten by the forest giant. Broccoli spears may be an orchard. Meat bits may be raised by the crane (arm and spoon) to be loaded into the factory (child's mouth). Children love these games and you will probably appreciate the creative brain play that consumes these happy young people.

Other Nutritional Pitfalls

Finances can be the limiting factor in a child's diet. Federal food stamps, WIC (Women, Infant, and Children) programs, and school breakfasts and lunches are available in most areas.

Many times, it is the parent's misconception about what constitutes good food that creates the problem. Prepared foods, processed meats, soft drinks, snack and candy foods are all very expensive and very nutrient poor. It has been estimated that the average family of four would save about $1,400 per year by having a nourishing diet rather than the usual meals Americans indulge in. Unprocessed foods are relatively cheap and very nourishing.

Stress is becoming an issue in the child's food intake. Poor school performance, divorce of the parents, and fear of being inadequate can create a poor appetite along with reduced digestion and absorption efficiency.

Cultural and social issues can affect proper nutrient intake. Religious beliefs, family status, education of the parents, and cultural background all play a role in what each of us eats, especially the dependent child.

Television plays a formidable role in the child's upbringing. With an average of four to six hours of television watched daily, the child is literally brainwashed by advertisements. TV role models can strongly influence what the child wants to eat.[12] Notice the brightly colored advertisements amidst the Saturday morning cartoons. Notice where these same products are placed in the grocery store—at child height. Notice the influence a three-year-old child can have on a tired mother who is grocery shopping.

Peer pressure becomes increasingly more important as the child enters school and progresses. Although children may like whole wheat bread, if everyone else is eating white bread and they are harassed for their difference, they may give up their uniqueness to be one of the group.

Anemia is all too common among children. The various nutrients required for blood formation, especially iron, are in low levels in the processed diet of the American child. Dental caries are found in over 90 percent of American children, with excess sugar and poor dental hygiene as the primary villains. Obesity may begin this early in life, particularly when there is a genetic tendency and the parents encourage overeating. Overfat children are usually much less active than their normal-weight peers. While females often begin developing overweight problems in childhood, males are often underweight, because of their greater muscle mass and activity level.

Hyperactivity is a growing issue in America. About 10-20 percent of all school age children are considered hyperactive. Symptoms of hyperactivity include one or more of the following: short attention span, excessive activity, distractability, low frustration level, emotional problems, aggressiveness, destructiveness, poor school performance, disruptiveness, poor peer relationships. This condition not only seriously impairs the child's learning process but can be very disruptive to parents and teachers.

Scientists are still carping among themselves about the relative merits of diet therapy for the hyperactive child, but thousands of parents testify to the results. Hyperactivity and other behavioral disorders may be caused by protein allergies, nutrient deficiencies, or sensitivities to substances found in food. After 15 years of controversy, good studies have shown that diet therapy improved the behavior in 62 of 76 hyperactive children tested.[13] Whether it is what we eat or what we don't eat that is at fault, diet therapy with vitamin supplements will significantly help about half of all hyperactive children. The diet should be high in fresh fruits, vegetables, whole grains, and cereals, with no processed foods containing refined sugar or additives. Supplements must have at least 100 percent of the RDA for all essential nutrients. Iron, folacin, protein, calorie, thiamin, niacin, B_6, B_{12}, C, A, magnesium, copper, zinc, and riboflavin deficiencies have all been directly associated with behavioral abnormalities in children.[14] Anemia is common in children; erratic moods are a common symptom of a blood-starved brain. The risk-benefit ratio of feeding the child properly, versus heavy drug sedation for the next decade, strongly favors the diet therapy approach.

Exercise improves about half of all hyperactive cases, with vitamins being 250 percent more likely to help the hyperactive child than the drug of choice (Mellaril).[15]

Nutrition for Optimal Growth

A healthy adult may spend five years indulging in nonfoods and eventually be able to return to old state of health by eating right. The developing child is much more vulnerable to nutritional problems. Poor nutrition can create a permanently sluggish mind. Excess calories can create a permanent war with overfatness. Marginal nutrition can hamper the child's mind, resulting in poor school performance and low self-esteem. Fluoride taken during childhood will help harden teeth and bones, while fluoride in the diet of adults is of marginal value. With an abundance of resilience, the child survives almost any situation, but thrives only on a very carefully chosen diet.

We recommend a diet high in whole grains, fresh fruits, vegetables, legumes, low-fat dairy products (unless their thin frame can use the calories of high-fat dairy products), meat, poultry, fish, and plenty of fresh water.

Avoid refined and processed foods. You may have to slowly wean your children from some of their acquired tastes. Additives, sugar, colorings, flavorings, hydrogenated fats, salt, and other dubious substances found in the refined diet can do no good and may do harm.

Provide healthy snacks at midmorning and midafternoon. Oatmeal or peanut butter cookies, ice cream, fruit, and nuts are all tasty, nourishing snacks for the growing child.

Give them a multiple daily vitamin supplement. It may have to be in chewable, powder or liquid drop form, depending on their age. Be sure to encourage food as the essence of nutrition; the vitamin is for insurance. Supplements should be in addition to good eating, not instead of it.

Provide your children with a proper role model. The "do as I say, not as I do" method of instruction is most ineffective. Give them encouragement for defying the exhortations of the TV commercials and their friends who are junk food addicts. Children are much more intelligent than many people think. By explaining the role of diet in their health, growth, performance, and looks, parents can help their children become nutrition-oriented. This strong foundation will have a major impact on improving the child's life.

There is no finer gift a parent can give a child than habits that will improve the quality and quantity of life. Optimal nutrition will do just that. It would be nice to see our children thrive because of what we feed them rather than survive in spite of what we feed them.

21
ADOLESCENCE

"Adolescence is the age when a youngster starts to eat again even before the dishes have been washed."

—EVAN ESAR

At a certain point in everyone's life, the floodgates are opened and growth and sexual hormones come racing through the body. Neither the young person nor the parents have time to catch their breath. Intense is the key word for adolescence.

Teenagers are not fed, they eat. They feel a need to have complete control over their dietary intake. Physical and emotional changes taking place during adolescence can amaze the parent who observes them each day. The years from thirteen through nineteen are not the easiest stage of life, for teen or parent.

Optimal nutrition can help stave off the "plagues" of teen life: acne, overfat women, underweight men, bizarre eating behavior of bulimia or anorexia, anemia, low energy, radical swings in emotions.

Adolescents, as a group, do not eat well-balanced meals. One-third are biochemically low in B_6.[1] On the average, adolescents consume about half the RDA for pantothenic acid.[2]

Physical Changes

Puberty is the stage of life when secondary sexual characteristics develop. Once a woman's weight approaches 103 pounds (47 kilograms), with fat stores at about 20 to 24 percent, menstruation begins. Thin women may be significantly delayed in this sexual maturation due to their low percent body fat. The monthly menstrual blood loss must be taken into consideration when planning nutrient needs; folacin, B_{12}, iron, copper, protein, and B_6 become particularly important. Also, the menstruating teen is fair game for premenstrual syndrome. See the chapter on sex for more on this issue.

Near the beginning of the growth spurt for men (at about age twelve), sexual maturation begins. It is more than just coincidence that acne, growth, and sexual maturation occur at the same time for many males. Most Americans are low in their zinc intake. Teens are notorious for their bizarre eating habits, thus compounding their zinc deficiency. Physical growth and sperm manufacturing require large amounts of zinc. Low zinc intake plus high zinc requirements can manifest themselves as acne.

Protein needs in the growing adolescent are about 25 to 50 percent higher than in the mature adult on a per weight basis. Because males have very high lean mass, high activity, and rapid growth, they have calorie needs that will stretch the food bill of most parents. A fifteen-year-old active male could easily need 4,000 calories per day, which is roughly twice what he will need as a sedentary full-grown adult. These high nutrient needs provoke almost incomprehensible appetites.

Emotional Changes

All humans are at least somewhat concerned with what others think about them. Teenagers are particularly vulnerable to this peer pressure. They want to belong. To get group acceptance, some will begin using drugs and alcohol and take up bizarre dietary habits.

Sexual development is a powerful and new issue in the teen's life. Most teen men want to be more muscular and most teen women want trimmer hips and waists. Self-image becomes a critical issue as healthy and attractive women often are launched into the nightmare world of bulimia or anorexia. The psychological scars of acne can remain long after the blemish has disappeared.

Sexual maturation often brings oral contraceptives into a teen woman's body. Oral contraceptives elevate the need for folacin, riboflavin, B_{12},[3] B_6,[4] C[5], and probably other nutrients.[6]

Encouraging proper eating habits during these years is more of a psychological issue than just knowing what food should be consumed and putting it in front of teenagers. Parents and educators should be keenly aware of the diplomacy required to nurture the teen through the turbulent years of mind and body growth.

Acne

The skin is the largest organ of the body. It protects us from outside invasion of chemicals, bacteria, and radiation, while it cools us through the evaporation of sweat. It keeps our internal organs in place. The skin has about 3 million pores and many millions of hair follicles that are lubricated by oil glands. The outer layer is a tough collection of tissue called the epidermis. The more delicate inner tissue is the dermis. When dying skin cells clog the opening to a hair follicle, the bacteria inside can create an infection. An acne pustule forms. Acne is typical during the hormonal imbalance years of adolescence and usually disappears by age eighteen. In some cases, acne can be so severe that it causes noticeable pitting in the face region. Acne is not a life-threatening condition, yet there is psychological trauma when a sensitive and vulnerable teenager is trying to impress the opposite sex. There are several techniques that will seriously improve acne.

1. Keep the hands away from the face. There are abundant oils and acids from the hand that will worsen acne when touching the face constantly.

2. Wash each morning and evening with a mildly abrasive washcloth, warm water, and soap. Wash and rinse twice until the skin feels squeaky clean. The abrasive washcloth helps clear away the outer layer of skin cells to prevent them from clogging the pore openings.

3. Keep fat and chocolate levels low in the diet. Though scientific studies have not been able to support the theory, many teens get remarkable relief in their acne when their diet is low in fat and devoid of chocolate. Acne could also be a result of certain food allergies and sensitivities. Be aware of foods that are not well tolerated, especially highly refined ones.

4. Maintain an optimal diet. The body considers skin to be expendable in times of marginal nutrient intake. If there is only enough of a nutrient to keep the essential internal organs functioning, then the skin suffers.

5. Vitamin A and zinc have been shown to be effective in improving acne conditions.[7, 8] We recommend a high-quality diet with a high-potency, broad spectrum vitamin/mineral supplement to be taken daily. This supplement should include 10,000 international units of vitamin A (as beta-carotene) and 30 milligrams of zinc.

Substance Abuse

Over half of all schoolchildren report trying alcohol at least once before age twelve. By early high school years, 90 percent of students have been exposed to alcohol. By college, 90 percent use alcohol regularly. One in twelve will later go on to become a problem drinker and add to the 9 million alcoholics already in this country. There are 3 million problem drinkers between ages fourteen and seventeen in the United States.[9]

Drug abuse is reaching mind-boggling proportions in urban school districts.[10] It is not uncommon to have a twelve-year-old drug addict. Most high school students have at least sampled marijuana or other drugs. One out of eighteen high school students is a regular user of marijuana, and marijuana strength has doubled in the last five years.

Both alcohol and drug abuse have nutritional implications. They can be physically or psychologically addictive. Additionally, most substance abusers have marked changes in their dietary intake. Normal and healthy teens often eat strangely, yet teen substance abusers have even worse dietary habits. Alcohol and drugs create higher than normal nutrient needs as the body attempts to cope with these nonnutritive substances. Many drugs lower the body's level of folacin, which then shows up as nerve disorders.[11] Nutritional deficiencies can create emotional complications, which further worsen the drug-shrouded mind. Radical swings in blood glucose levels from poor eating habits can create depression and other psychological problems that urge the teen to escape into the mental fog of drug abuse.

Weight Control

Women have finished their most rapid growth phase by age thirteen. Because of this, their basal metabolism and energy needs are beginning to taper off. But their appetite isn't. Habits from the past few years of relentless eating still persist. Also, at this phase in life, women develop interests in their appearance and in the opposite sex. Through bombardment in the media, American women are told that a lithe figure in a size six dress is the only way to attract men. These unrealistic expectations create anxiety in teen women's dietary habits. They want to eat but feel that they shouldn't. Occasional forays into the world of junk food seem irresistible, so that many will become bulimic (forcing vomiting after binge eating).

Overfat women are more sedentary than their leaner counterparts. Many of these overfat and sedentary individuals have low iron levels in their muscle tissue (myoglobin). It makes perfect sense that the lethargy of anemia would lead to less exercise, which would bring on overfatness, which would create a serious self-image problem, which could have major impact on what they do and who they do it with. Television viewing hours have been directly related to the incidence and degree of overfatness.[12]

For many female teens, eating can become a stress outlet. In lieu of expressing their emotional and sexual needs, they eat. Parents, friends, family, counselors, and educators can help teens deal with their newly acquired emotions in a more positive outlet than food.

Teen men, with their amazing calorie needs for growth and activity, are often underweight. Obviously, increasing the food and calorie intake will help this situation. Realize that foods that would be taboo during more mature phases of life are acceptable in adolescence. Whole wheat crust pizza, ice cream, hamburgers, nuts, peanut butter, and deep fried chicken and fish are all rich in calories and nutrients. Teens need to be steered away from calorie-rich but nutrient-poor foods like pastries, soft drinks, and candy.

Teens need to be eating and exercising properly in order for their growth to be directed into lean tissue rather than increasing the number of fat cells. Habits acquired during adolescence linger many years after these astronomical calorie requirements have faded. Most adults will testify to the sudden realization that sometime in their twenties they could no longer eat as they did in high school and get away with it. Freshmen at Stanford University were found to gain an average of eight pounds in the first year of college. Teen women need emotional stroking to get a positive image and prevent eating disorders. Teen men need to know that their lanky frame will eventually fill out with flesh. Parents paying the food bill need to be reassured that this phase is a short one, and proper feeding of their teenager will yield a bright energetic adult in only a few years.

Anemia

Up to half of all growing children, teens, and menstruating women in this country are anemic. Fatigue, distress, irritability, poor disease resistance, and even behavioral changes can result from having an oxygen- and nutrient-starved body and brain. Rapid growth requires the body to make new blood. The monthly blood loss that begins for teen women can compound anemia. Anemia could be the cause of a teen's lethargy and irritability. Good food could be part of the solution to the tense atmosphere in a home with a teen.

Stress

The turmoil of adolescence can play havoc with the nutrient status of the teen. The demands of competitive academics, the need to belong, seeking sexual attention, heroics or failure in athletics, friction between parents, breakup of parents at home, anticipating the impending radical changes of life—all these factors can create stress in the teen. Stress can reduce the efficiency of absorbing nutrients in food, lower the ability to recycle nutrients, and cause excessive nutrient loss.

Stress can seriously alter a healthy appetite mechanism. Stressed teens may eat significantly more or less food than usual. Or they may begin craving junk food. People under stress have elevated needs for a variety of nutrients, including protein, calcium, magnesium, thiamin, niacin, vitamin C, zinc, and others. A high-quality diet will help buffer the effects of emotional distress.

Teen Pregnancy

Fifty-three percent of all women between ages fifteen and nineteen are married. One out of four mothers bearing her first child is less than twenty years old. Of all causes of death for older teen women, 6 percent are from complications during pregnancy.[13] The ranks of unmarried pregnant teen women are increasing, with well over 400,000 reported each year.

Given the nutrient demands of her own growth and of pregnancy, plus the low nutrient intake of adolescence, complications for the teen mother are much greater. Teen mothers have a much higher incidence of premature delivery and neonatal death, and four times the incidence of toxemia.[14]

What Can be Done?

Parents, educators, health care professionals, and even probation counselors should be aware of the intimate role nutrition plays in the growth, performance, attitude, and overall health of the adolescent. We should also be realistic in what we expect from teens. This is not the most rational stage of life. There are things we can do to seriously improve the nutrient status of our adolescents:

1. Provide nutritious meals and snacks but do not force teens to eat. Many teens have no one to eat with, and thus are tempted into less nourishing foods. To help the teen resist junk food and eating on the run, provide an attractive and tasty meal with friendly dining companionship. If the house is littered with junk food, then such shall be their diet. Parents should keep in mind that healthy food does not cost more. In the long run, it costs much less.

2. Educators should try to have some nutrition studies within the scope of junior high and high school classes. Instead of counting irrelevant numbers in math class, calculate calories in foods and exercises. Instead of just reading about botany, plant a garden and examine the nutrients commonly found in domestic vegetables. Biology class could discuss the effects of nutrient deficiencies. Teens are intelligent enough to be swayed with facts.

3. Lead by example. Mothers, fathers, teachers, uncles, aunts, grandparents, and anyone else the teen might look up to should be encouraged to set a good role model. Teens are keenly aware of the hypocrisy portrayed by "do as I say, not as I do."

22

OLDER ADULTHOOD

"Youth thinks nothing of health, and age thinks of nothing but."

—EVAN ESAR

Aging and death are inevitable. But how these two enter your life is negotiable. In 1900, only 4 percent of the American population was over sixty-five years of age. With improved health care, that percentage has tripled today to 12 percent.[1] Yet a sixty-five-year old man today has the same life expectancy as a sixty-five-year old man in 1900.[2] We feel that, with improved diet, exercise, attitude, and health care, older persons can be more healthy and active contributors to life.

Nutrition and the Older Adult

Nutrition in older adulthood is unique for several reasons:

1. The cumulative effect of lifetime abuses finally settles in. Decades of seemingly harmless hangovers culminate in an eroded stomach and malfunctioning liver. Eating an extra two peanuts, or ten calories per day, will result in one pound gained each year, which adds up to fifty extra pounds by retirement age. Marginal nutrient deficiencies that slightly hampered health before now have mushroomed into full blown deficiency conditions to seriously impair life.

2. As health appears to be slipping away, an obsession with health begins. Older adults are the primary users of medical services. The thought of health problems, aches, pains, constipation, medication, and other issues can become a consuming passion.

3. The older adult is much less efficient at digesting, absorbing, and recycling nutrients. While there is a lowered basal metabolism that calls for less food intake, there is a need for more nutrients. The reduced output of stomach acid in the elderly can seriously lower mineral absorption.[3]

4. Food does not taste or look as good, due to declines in sensory equipment. Though there is a need for regular nutrient intake, the desire to eat is often missing. Loneliness, fear, and other psychological issues can overwhelm the older adult just when nourishment is so crucial.

Good News About Aging

The debilitated older person is a definite minority of America's senior citizens. Two-thirds of the people over sixty-five are in decent health. Only 5 percent live in nursing homes.[4]

For years scientists have been telling the public that brain cells begin dying in early adulthood, leaving the older adult with the inescapable fate of a shrunken and useless brain. This is not so! A sixty-year-old person has lost 10 percent of his brain volume compared to the early adult years, yet this shrinkage may be due to a loss in the spaces between brain cells. A Baltimore study showed that healthy elderly people have as effective memories as younger people.[5] The National Institute of Mental Health found that oxygen flow throughout the brain of healthy older adults was comparable to oxygen flow in people fifty years younger. Only about 15 percent of all people over sixty-five suffer from Alzheimer's disease, the common type of senility. Several prominent researchers have concluded that mental powers and memory are retained well into old age if a person is healthy and continually uses his mind.

The Baltimore study also found that sexual capacity does not markedly diminish with age. Healthy older men produced hormone quantities equal to those of younger men. Researchers found that the most sexually active older adults were the ones who had been sexually active throughout their lives.

An article about aging in the *Journal of the American Medical Association* found that "dis-use" of the body through sedentary lifestyle was largely responsible for the many "dis-eases" of old age.[6] The sedentary adult often has the same health problems as the older adult. There is abundant evidence that aging can be slowed through an active lifestyle. "Use it or lose it" takes on even more powerful meanings in the context of these findings.

The term "healthy" older adults refers to active, happy individuals who are optimally nourished. Optimal nourishment for older adults can be a unique challenge.

Physical Changes and Their Nutritional Considerations

On the basis of statistical compilation, these "common" changes are not necessarily inescapable but are more a result of the typically disastrous American lifestyle.[7]

Cardiovascular system. The pumping efficiency of the heart decreases by about 30 percent. The ability to diffuse oxygen throughout the body is reduced by 50 to 70 percent. The need for exercise is very high, since exercise improves the oxygen uptake and insulin response.[8] The arteries become stiff and rigid, so the value of vitamin C, bioflavonoids, rutin, proper mineral balance, and avoiding smoking becomes more important. Blood pressure increases, so sodium and cadmium should be restricted, and there is a need for adequate potassium and calcium intake. Fats and cholesterol increase in the blood; reduce fat and cholesterol intake and increase nutrients that allow the body to keep blood fats controlled, such as vitamin C and chromium. Glucose tolerance is diminished.[9] Restrict refined sugar intake, while increasing fiber and complex or naturally occurring carbohydrates.

Nervous system. The tissue that envelopes the brain and spinal cord (the meninges) thickens. Brain volume is reduced by 10 percent from age thirty to seventy. Older adults need to "use" the brain in a stimulating setting. Moods of depression, withdrawal, rigidity of outlook and dementia occur more often as people age. These are often found to be related to poor nutrient intake or a starving brain from vascular disease. Deficiencies of many different nutrients can lead to emotional instability. Short-term memory and learning abilities are reduced. Velocity of nerve transmissions declines by 15 percent. Neurochemical transmitter production decreases. This increases the importance of regular nourishing meals to provide the raw materials for these neurochemical transmitters. Reflexes are slowed. Muscular coordination is diminished, so eating utensils must be easy to manage, and food needs to be easy to cut and serve.

Basal metabolism. Declines about 20 percent between age twenty and ninety.[10] Calorie needs decrease 5 percent each decade after forty, and 10 percent each decade after age sixty. Older adults should seriously control calorie intake yet maintain high-quality diet to avoid vitamin and mineral deficiencies. Also, they should keep active to avoid overfatness.

Kidney filtration. At age eighty, the kidneys have about 50 percent of their efficiency compared to age twenty-five.[11] With a declining ability to regenerate kidney cells, the remaining cells are taxed to their limit. To reduce the concentration of the body's waste matter, much more fluid should be consumed. Yet too much fluid can overwhelm the marginally functional kidneys.

Skeletal system. Sometime in the third or fourth decade of life, the skeletal system becomes less efficient at maintaining its mass. Some loss of bone calcium is inevitable, but it need not be as drastic as the commonly occurring osteoporosis. A study in Utah found that, from adolescence to older adulthood, men lost an average of two inches while women lost eight inches in height.[12] Older adults must be keenly aware of the risk factors involved in osteoporosis, including calcium, phosphorus, protein, magnesium, vitamin D, alcohol, smoking, sedentary lifestyle, and stress. Many experts have called for a 50 percent increase in the RDA for calcium for the older adult.

Gastrointestinal tract. Output of hydrochloric acid and digestive enzymes is diminished. Need to consider that nutrients are not as well absorbed due to inefficiency. B_{12} status is often low in the elderly. Folacin is one of the vitamins that require digestive action to be liberated for absorption. Folacin levels commonly deteriorate with age.[13] The efficiency of digestion and absorption is lower. Avoid difficult-to-digest foods, including high-fat, very spicy, and high-fat cheese items. Motility of intestinal muscles is poor, leading to frequent constipation. Fiber intake needs to be forty to fifty grams per day to provide regularity without drugs. Lactose intolerance is common. The exclusion of milk from the diet will require great nutritional effort to maintain ideal calcium, vitamin D, and riboflavin intake.

Dentition. Eighty percent of the elderly have no teeth.[14] Sore gums or ill-fitting dentures can seriously impair eating. Callousing of the gums allows some elderly to eat without any teeth. Food must be soft in consistency; avoid crisp and sticky foods.

Lean mass. From age twenty on, most people lose muscle tissue and concurrently gain fatty tissue, for a double-edged sword. According to a study of 400 elderly in Missouri, 22 percent of the males and 59 percent of the females were obese by weight standards.[15] By percent body fat measurements, this number would be much higher. Calorie intake should be carefully monitored. Protein intake should be increased in those who are deficient.

Sensory organs. Vision in dim light is diminished. The ability to focus on objects at different distances is worse. A yellow-white opaque ring (known as arcus senilis) around the iris occurs in about 40 percent of the elderly.[16] The lens of the eye takes on an opaque, waxy appearance as cataracts become more common. Glare tolerance is diminished with cataracts. Glaucoma, cataracts, and other severe visual impairments occur in about 15 percent of the elderly.

The skin often becomes dry and cracked, especially in women. Similar skin problems are found in both the malnourished and the elderly;[17] there is probably a relationship there.

About one-third of the elderly suffer hearing loss, especially for high tones and the ability to distinguish speech patterns from background noise. Since men are more likely to have this hearing loss, one can be suspicious that vascular disease, also more common in men, plays a role.

Eighty percent of the taste buds are gone;[18] coupled with a likely zinc deficiency, this makes the elderly have poor taste acuity. Food often tastes bitter or sour. Olfactory abilities are also diminished. Food does not smell or taste as good as it once did. Appetites can be poor and nutrient intake can suffer. Food must be attractively presented to encourage good eating habits.

Psychosocial aspects of eating. One-third of all people over age sixty-five are living below the poverty level.[19] Many will keep the "front" of normal living while sacrificing on their grocery bill. Fear of death and loss of mate or family can influence health and eating patterns. Fear of becoming a burden to society or their children is keen with many elderly. Fear can cause a loss of appetite, while stress can impair digestion and absorption. There is a loss of mobility both in walking and driving, and they may not be able to get to the store regularly for fresh produce. There is loss of self-esteem and independence. In a society that judges people by their working position and income, unemployment and poverty can be devastating to the ego. Many are living alone, and thus may be uninterested in preparing meals or eating. Dr. Jack Weinberg of the University of Illinois observes, "It is not what the older person eats but with whom that will be the deciding factor in proper care for him."[20] Moving away for retirement, scattering of family across the country, and new routines to adjust to can all make nutrient intake a low priority for the elderly.

Is Old Age a Disease?

It is obvious to researchers that aging is dependent on your genes and what you do with them throughout your life. Sandy Shaw, coauthor of *Life Extension,* writes, "Actually, for somebody who is careful, the average lifespan might be 1,000 or even 2,000 years." This is a bit optimistic for today's science. More realistically, 80 years of exuberant living is possible for most people today. Many younger folks can anticipate living zestfully beyond 100 if their lifestyle is optimal. Old age may not be curable, but it can be slowed down.

Recommendations

The older adult needs to be very conscious of balancing calorie intake with needs, since overfatness seems to be the launching point for many maladies of old age.[21] Exercise is imperative to prevent the "dis-eases" caused by "dis-use" of the body.

Cholesterol should be less than 300 milligrams per day and sodium intake kept to less than 5 grams daily, with a serious effort at meeting or exceeding the recommended intake for potassium and calcium. Fat should be 20 to 30 percent of the total calories. Protein intake should be 12 to 20 percent of the calories. The diet needs to be high in fiber and complex carbohydrates. The quality of the diet (nutrient density) is a critical factor.[22] Lowered calorie needs and poor appetite limit nutrient intake. Reduced efficiency of digestion increases the demand for vitamins, minerals, and protein. Water intake should be five to ten glasses per day. We encourage a high-potency vitamin and mineral supplement to be taken daily. Foods (or supplements) rich in the proven antioxidants of vitamin A (as beta-carotene), C, E, selenium, and manganese may help slow the aging process while protecting against cancer.

Studies have shown that taking 1,000 milligrams daily of vitamin C helps older adults toward more vigor.[23] Chromium will help stabilize the semi-diabetic blood glucose curves of the older adult. Try to get two hours total of sunshine each week to improve vitamin D and calcium metabolism.[24] Though alcohol abuse can be an obvious deterrent to good health, one or two glasses of wine with dinner have been shown to improve the health and outlook of the older adult.[25] Choline and lecithin can improve mental performance and reduce the muscular trembling commonly found in the elderly.[26] Carnitine supplements help the body to burn fat and can unclog fat-blocked vessels.[27] B_{12} injections may be needed, since the ability to absorb B_{12} diminishes as we age. Choline, inositol, B_{12}, and folacin help to prevent a fatty and debilitated liver. Niacin (100 milligrams daily as niacinamide) can dilate tiny blood vessels to improve circulation and perhaps even remove opaque deposits in the eye region. Zinc supplements improve all functions in both sexes and may stimulate a renewed sexual interest in males.[28] Garlic, capsicum, and ginger should be in the diet often since they are proven aids to the circulatory system. Ginsana (standardized ginseng) may increase vigor, stamina, and sense of well-being.[29] Fish or EPA should be in the diet often. Gamma linolenic acid supplements may improve many body functions, since the ability to internally produce GLA may decrease as we age. Optimal diet should be the foundation of the older adult's nutrition program. Study the chapters on dietary components for inexpensive, good food sources of all the nutrients discussed here. And nutritional supplements can be a valuable addition.

There should be small frequent meals. Care needs to be taken to consider older adults' background in food and the need to perpetuate some of their traditions.[30] Nutritional supplements and a keen awareness of quality of food intake can help make diet an asset in old age, not a hindrance.

PART FIVE

NUTRITION AND DISEASE

THE PLAGUES OF THE PAST ARE BASICALLY GONE. NEONATAL death is down dramatically. Few people bleed to death or suffer miserably without some pharmaceutical comforts. Yet many of the diseases of the twentieth century have shown a remarkable resistance to being treated even with the most modern medical approaches. Obesity, heart disease, cancer, diabetes, osteoporosis, arthritis, food allergies, smoking, mental health, sexual and athletes' issues now confront the health care professional. Nutrition has an integral role in preventive, supportive, and even curative medicine. Food and nutrients are gentle healers. They work slowly, gradually, and with few or no side effects.

23
OBESITY

"Never eat any more than you can lift."

—*THE NEW WEIGHTLIFTER'S DIET*

Obesity has been called "the easiest disease to diagnose and the most difficult one to treat." America is at least 2 billion pounds overweight. In order to lose that weight, we would have to eat 7 trillion calories less than we burn. There is a long list of health detriments that should concern the overweight individual. Obesity is a major risk factor toward numerous diseases and early death.

Assessing Overweight

The bathroom scale tells you how much you weigh. What it does not tell you is the quality of that weight. For decades, life insurance companies have kept accurate records of the height and weight of their customers and compiled those into tables which told them the weight and height that allowed people to live the longest. Yet these numbers are from the principal clients of life insurance companies, Caucasians of northern European extraction, making them somewhat inaccurate for other races with different builds. Because muscle mass is denser than fat, many athletes, according to these tables, would be considered overweight. Yet the firm and toned body of the athlete would hardly be considered a health risk.

According to these tables, a six-foot-tall male could weigh anywhere from 149 to 188 pounds, depending on his frame, and still be considered normal. Some people, rather than admitting a weight problem, claim to have a "heavy frame," though they may actually have a light frame with excess fat clinging to it.

Excess body fat is more crucial than the amount of body weight, which is why we refer to overweight as overfat. There are several techniques of determining percent body fat.

Underwater weighing. Since fat floats and muscle doesn't, the relative weight of a person on land versus in the water is an accurate determiner of percent body fat. This requires a large water tank, expensive equipment, and someone willing to exhale all of their air as they go under water for a ten second reading. Not very practical. Inaccuracy can stem from residual air in the lungs and gas pockets in the intestines.

Circumference measurements. Scientists found that there is a relationship between the circumference of various bodily parts and the percent body fat. Abdomen, thigh, forearm, calf, buttocks, and upper arm are measured, depending on age and sex. Though the only equipment required is a tape measure, this technique is difficult to master and does not work for certain body builds.

Skinfold calipers. The human body stores about half of its total fat in the skin region to insulate against changes in environmental temperature. Thus, measuring the thickness of skinfolds at specific sites can accurately determine percent body fat. This method requires an expensive caliper for measuring skinfold thickness with a certain pressure. Hundreds of practice sessions are necessary to be considered really accurate at skinfold measuring.

A more practical method for lay people to keep track of their fitness level is the "pinch-an-inch" method, which says that if you can pinch an inch of skinfold thickness either above the hipbone, the back of the arms, or midway on the thigh, then there is likely a weight problem. If the skinfold thickness is two inches or more, then there is likely an overfat problem.

Electrical resistance of fat. One of the purposes of fat in the body is to provide insulation around nerve cells to prevent electrical impulses from "jumping the track." Electrical wiring uses rubber insulation for the same purpose. A device has been developed in which electrodes are connected to the finger and toes and the electrical resistance through the body is then measured. The less resistance, the less the fat content, the greater the lean mass. This technique is accurate and easy to learn, but it requires a rather expensive device. This is the method we use at La Costa.

We strongly encourage you to keep the bathroom scale in its place. The scale can tell the physician or nurse of major weight fluctuations that can be important. Yet the scale can be a fatal blow to the dieter's efforts. You can actually *gain* weight on a reducing program. Once you have lost that initial water weight and some fat, you would eventually find a plateau of very slow weight loss. If you were following the exercise plan and as you neared your best weight, you could gain weight from the heavier muscle tissue replacing the lighter fat tissue. Even though you felt better, looked better, and were

TABLE 21: Percent Body Fat

Females: average—25% (under 30 years), 31% (over 30)
       excellent—10%-15%
       good—16%-19%
       acceptable—20%-24%
       overfat—25%-29%
       obese—30% and up

Males: average—20% (under 30 years), 25% (over 30)
       excellent—5%-10%
       good—11%-14%
       acceptable—15%-17%
       overfat—18%-19%
       obese—20% and up (using skin calipers)

healthier, the scales could deceive you into thinking that your efforts were in vain.

According to the Metropolitan Life Insurance tables, about 40 percent of the population is overweight. Using the techniques of percent body fat, it is estimated that as much as 80 percent of this country is overfat.

Complications of Obesity

Overfat individuals have double the risk of heart disease and four times the risk for diabetes. They are also at higher risk for cancer, kidney and liver ailments, gout, gallstones,[1] arthritis, complications in child delivery, car accidents, and back problems. Glucose tolerance curves improve almost in direct proportion to one's level of fitness.[2] Fat on the abdomen is at a right angle to the spine. Using the same mechanical advantage principle that sailors use when leaning away from their boat, 10 pounds of excess weight around the abdomen puts 100 pounds of stress on the lower back. The image of the jolly corpulent person is inaccurate.[3] Overfat people are actually more prone to depression. Social obstacles confront the overfat individual, like bus seats, turnstyles, and shopping for clothes. The overfat person is less likely to get the job or the promotion. When a Los Angeles dating service asked its clients "Who do you not want to date?" it received the overwhelming reply "a fat person." Even overfat individuals said the same thing.

Types of Overfatness

There are both physical and emotional differences among types of overfatness. People acquire a lean or heavy frame from their ancestors. From that inherited frame, their lifestyle can create a fat or thin physique. The person with an inherited thin frame who has billowed his body with fat has the greatest chance of developing heart disease since he has long since saturated the few fat cells available and is using the bloodstream for fat storage.

Obese people do not have the same increased metabolism after consuming fatty meals that is found in lean individuals.[4] We have actually had people on 600 calories per day at La Costa who, after an initial loss, could not lose more weight. These are primarily overfat women past menopause who have been very sedentary. Also, many people drastically underestimate the amount of food they think they eat. One study found that men misguessed their food intake by 500 calories per day, while women were off by 900.[5]

There is a continued slowing of basal metabolism that is normal with aging. The sodium potassium pump is a primary avenue of calorie expenditure in all resting individuals. The more efficient this pump, the lower the calorie needs and the greater the difficulty will be in weight loss.[6] A continuous parade of diets throughout one's life can further lower metabolism. People with the dubious distinction of having all of the above factors for low basal metabolism have become proverbial marvels of energy efficiency. However, few people have their "system" to blame. Scientists have proved that the majority of overfat individuals are not energy efficient but rather suffering the results of too much eating and/or too little exercise.[7]

During earlier stages of life, when cells are developing rapidly, overfed individuals can increase their fat cell number (hyperplasia). During adulthood, overfed individuals merely increase the size of their existing fat cells (hypertrophy). It is the hyperplastic obesity that is so difficult to treat, since these people have a legion of hungry fat cell storage tanks. The old myth of a "fat baby is a healthy baby" can be the beginning of a lifelong struggle with the waistline. Some bariatric specialists (physicians who deal with overfat patients) feel that even adults might add fat cell numbers when they ride their roller coasters of weight loss and gain.

Women and Weight Problems

Women in America experience more frequent weight problems than men, for a variety of reasons. Women have been the cultural feeder of the household. Many women spend most of their days planning meals, preparing them, shopping for food, and cleaning up. The media creates an exceedingly

TABLE 22: **Weight Loss**

Easiest	More difficult
brown fat	white fat
thin frame	heavy frame
male	female
high muscle mass	low muscle mass
younger	older
activity oriented	sedentary oriented
non-food oriented	food oriented
lean ancestry	heavy ancestry
lean as a child	heavy as a child

gaunt model as the image that all women must live up to. Soap opera role models eat constantly in front of the camera, yet somehow maintain remarkable figures. These unrealistic goals create havoc in some women. Many have a seriously distorted self-image.[8] Many see themselves as fat when they are not.

Physiologically and biochemically, women are different than men. Women, by nature's design, have about twice the percent body fat that men do. These extra stored calories allow woman to bear children even in times of marginal food availability. Because of lower lean mass, women have a lower basal metabolism, which means that they are more fuel efficient with their calories consumed.

Emotional Aspects of Eating

Food is far more than just a means of staying alive. Food can mean comfort, satisfaction, security, family times together, a reward, memories, a glue for social occasions, something to do when bored or depressed. For some people, eating becomes an outlet for emotional problems. It is estimated that somewhere around 25 percent of this country is in need of some psychological counseling.[9] There is also a large percentage of the American population that suffers from eating disorders.

Bulimia is a condition of obsessive eating, sometimes until death. This condition is rare. *Bulimarexia* is an eating disorder in which the person binges on up to 40,000 calories per day, then forcibly purges the system by vomiting.[10] Up to 30 percent of high school and college-age females participate in this deadly technique of weight control. Up to 10 percent cannot control their gorge-then-purge habits, even when urged to do so by family or professionals. These people have a distorted self-image and an intense fear of becoming overweight.

Bulimarectics have the following symptoms: frequent and recurring episodes of binge eating; an awareness that their habits are abnormal; a fear that they cannot control this habit; depression and self-berating following sessions of binge eating. Some of these people can stop their habits with the support of family and friends. Many of them will require professional counseling to deal with the emotional problems that initiated the bulimarexia.

The hazards of this condition are many. Repeated vomiting will result in the darkening of the teeth from strong stomach acid. Loss of electrolytes in vomiting can create weakness, confusion, palpitations, and even death. Protein, vitamins, minerals and other nutrients are missing in the body and health will gradually deteriorate. Many of these people take diuretics and laxatives, further worsening the problem. These drugs all have side effects, including drug-nutrient interactions. Some of these people will become so conditioned to the eat-then-vomit routine that their stomachs will do it automatically, without any prompting.

In addition to the many physical problems of the bulimarectic, about 50 percent are judged to have a borderline personality disturbance with some of the following traits: impulsiveness (gambling, drugs, spending, shoplifting, sex, physical self-abuse); unstable and intense relationships with others; frequent displays of temper or constant anger; identity disturbance with questions of self-image, gender, goals, values, and radical changes in moods; inability to be alone; consistently feeling empty or bored.

There are some scientists who theorize that binging is due to a blatant vitamin or mineral deficiency in the body that triggers abnormal appetite impulses. It is known that the bulimarectic has an intense urge to eat sweet foods. For this reason, it is vital to have the bulimarectic begin optimal nutrient intake.

Anorexia nervosa is a condition of self-starvation. Its victims have an intense fear of becoming obese that does not lessen as they lose weight. Most of them have a disturbed body image and will lose 25 percent or more of their original body weight. Some anorectics eat very little, while others choose excessive exercise to reduce themselves into a gaunt ghost of a figure.[11] There are multiple physical and nutritional complications of anorexia. One-third of anorectics will die if they don't get proper medical and psychological attention.

Weight Loss Gimmicks

Desperately overfat people are especially vulnerable to all kinds of strange—and often dangerous—weight loss gimmicks.

Drugs.   Anorectants to blunt the appetite. Amphetamines to speed up the otherwise phlegmatic individual. Thyroid pills to race up the basal metabolism. Diuretics to cause unnatural water loss. Cathartics to curtail the normal absorption of foods. All are to be avoided.

Surgery.   Wiring of the jaws, which has no lasting effect on weight control.[12] Stapling off a section of the stomach. Removing several feet of the intestines. Lately, a technique of fat suctioning (lipectomy) has been developed by plastic surgeons. These are all drastic and expensive and do nothing to keep you thin in the long run.

Fad diets.   The favorite is the high-protein, low-carbohydrate diet (Stillman, Atkins, Last Chance, Air Force, etc.). This program creates inefficiency in the kidneys, causing fluid loss for a gleefully received but deceiving initial weight loss.[13] The macrobiotic diet, in its initial phase, is a harmless form of vegetarianism; in its final phase it is a dangerous form of malnutrition. Many of these diets have been shown to cause loss of body calcium stores and could bring on osteoporosis.[14]

Some fad diets may have worked, but most were from books that should have been listed in the fiction section of the library. The Lover's Diet: "Reach for your mate, not your plate." The Down Blanket diet played on the physiological trick that a hot person has less of an appetite. Thus "if you are hungry, get under a down blanket." Acupuncture earrings, allegedly to block the appetite mechanism, gave more than a few people an ear infection instead.

Psychological approaches.   One weight loss center makes the client eat his favorite food until he gets ill, then has to stare at the vomit. This form of aversion therapy may work in tobacco withdrawal, but it is ineffective in something as essential as eating.

We highlight these methods to point out the futility of these measures. Less than 5 percent of dieters on an unstructured weight loss program will keep their extra weight off forever. About 95 percent of dieters using these techniques will fail at losing weight forever. The only method that has been proved effective in lifetime weight maintenance is a gradual, multifaceted approach that incorporates nutrition, exercise, behavior modification, and attitude. This program works for all who comply with it. And they stay thin forever.

Lifetime Weight Control

Many solutions have been offered to the obese person. Most did not work. All cost money. Some were harmful. In each failure, the obese individual's self-image slides further into a pit. By using a proven multifactor approach to weight control, success is practically assured, and the svelte figure is maintained for a lifetime of healthy and vigorous living.

Nutrition

Excess calories create overfatness. Eat and enjoy your food. Do not skip meals. "Grazers," who eat small frequent meals, are more successful at maintaining a svelte build than the gorgers who eat a few large meals daily.[15] Concentrate on foods high in fiber and fluids (vegetables, fruits, grains, legumes, soups, water), which will slow down the gastric emptying rate and thus delay hunger pangs. Minimize pastries, sugars, alcohol, and high-fat foods. If you feel you must have some junk food, do it on only one day of the week. The body can absorb just so much of a large intake of calories. But if the food is spaced out over the entire week, the calorie absorption becomes much higher. When you feel hungry, drink a tall glass of water first. Fluids may oftentimes be what the body really wants. Calories do count. Become familiar with the chapter on the exchange system to help you become aware of an optimal nutritional program. At 600 calories daily, nearly everyone will lose weight at a reasonable pace without having health suffer.[16]

Eat until satisfied, not stuffed. There is a difference.

Here are some nutritional "gimmicks" that work:

• Hot fluids (like soup) or high-fiber snacks consumed twenty minutes before a meal will seriously blunt the appetite.

• For rapid and permanent weight loss, eat less fat[17]—only 20 to 30 percent of your total calories. Dietary fat is easier for the body to store as body fat than other calorie sources.[18] Carbohydrates and protein require some metabolic conversion to become stored fatty tissue.[19]

• Vegetarians and fish eaters are only one-third as likely to suffer obesity as meat eaters.[20] It is the fat in meat that creates the weight problem.

• Take 500 to 1,000 milligrams per day of L-carnitine. Carnitine aids in efficient fat burning.

• Take a high-quality broad spectrum multiple vitamin and mineral supplement. This will provide health insurance for those dieters who have been consistently fasting. It will also eliminate the possibility that a faulty appetite may be due to a vitamin or mineral deficiency.

Exercise

We are underexercising ourselves to death in this country. Calorie intake has actually declined since the turn of the century, but as machines take over more of our work load, we do less exercise. The result is overfatness. Exercise is essential to successful weight control.[21] Exercise accelerates weight loss, even beyond what a low-calorie diet could produce.[22] Many overfat people do not eat more than their leaner peers.[23] The difference is exercise.

The Set Point Theory. Each of us has a weight that is easy to maintain. Going above or below that weight is not easy. This "set point" is based upon inherited traits, early feeding habits, number of fat cells, and other influences, and probably increases as we age, due to lowered basal metabolism. The best way to lower this set point is through exercise. Many dieters have found that, in spite of Herculean efforts at fasting, they could not lose weight below a certain point. Exercise is the best way to break through this plateau of weight loss.

• Your workout must be fun (or you will not continue with it), vigorous (or it will do no good), and regular (at least three times per week). Strive for flexibility, strength, and cardiovascular fitness (aerobic capacity), and start slowly, with nonstress exercises like brisk walking, biking, and swimming.

• Join supportive exercise groups or find a reliable partner to work out with regularly. Remember that work and play count in the exercise quota.

• To be most efficiently burning stored fat, your exercise should allow you to say a few words while working out. If you can talk continuously during your workout, then the intensity is too low. If you are so out of breath that you can't talk at all, then you are burning more stored glycogen than fat stores.

Behavior modification

For many overfat individuals, bad habits created their weight problem. Behavior modification to change fattening habits is essential for lifetime weight control.[24] Some people always eat in front of the TV, even if they just finished eating a substantial meal. Others snack constantly while in the car, studying, or reading. These particular habits must be broken and other healthier habits formed in order to lose weight forever.

• Eat and chew slowly. "Speed eaters," people who chew less often and eat faster, nearly always have a weight problem.[25] Put the fork down between each bite. Chew the food twenty to thirty times per mouthful. Allow at least twenty minutes to consume any meal, since it takes this long for the appetite control center of the brain (hypothalamus) to shut off after the stomach is full.

• Don't be a plate cleaner; leave a bite on each plate at the meal's end. Use a smaller plate to make your smaller portions look more substantial. (This trick really works!)

• Keep leftovers out of sight. Store food in opaque containers.

- Eat only at the table. Do not eat standing up.
- Plan your meals. Keep snack foods out of the house. Do not grocery shop while hungry.
- If necessary, avoid the television for a few weeks. Good studies have shown a direct relationship between hours spent in front of the TV and probability of overfatness.
- Food provides emotional as well as physical satisfaction. You must allow for this emotional satisfaction. Enjoy your meals. Use music, candles, nice clothes, and other tricks—not more food—to make your mealtime more pleasant.
- Write down everything that you eat for at least one week. From this diet history, you can observe eating behavior, trends, and other problems that need to be dealt with.

Attitude adjustment

Your attitude is crucial. This is a lifetime program for permanently lean and healthy bodies. If you consider this a temporary weight loss program until you can return to your old habits, then it will be nothing more than another cycle of failure. Think thin. "Thin within" is an effective technique that creates an internal image of a thin person. We spend our energies to fulfill whatever image we hold of ourselves. If you think of yourself as an overfat person, you will eat and exercise accordingly to bring this image to fruition. If you think of yourself as a lean and healthy individual, you will spend your energies to fulfill that image.

Do not berate yourself for occasionally falling off course with this program. Pick yourself up and continue. Do not criticize that image in the mirror. You would not criticize children in first grade for their lack of knowledge, because you know that they are trying and will eventually get there. The same applies to weight loss. You may not be there yet, but you are going in the right direction. Be good to yourself.

Set realistic goals for weight loss within a given time frame. Reward yourself when you reach these goals, with clothes, records, trips, but not food. Learn to cope with the moods (e.g., depression, boredom) that instigate overeating. Seek counseling if necessary.

Seek the support of your friends and family. No one can sabotage your efforts if you are truly sincere. Be prepared for the better but not perfect world of thinness. Lean people are healthier, more energetic, and happier than overfat individuals, but their world is not perfect. There will still be disappointments, taxes, jobs, and unpleasant people to deal with once you are thin. Spouses should work together on these fitness programs. The odds of divorce are much higher when only one of the partners decides to deal with a weight problem.

Know the difference between biological hunger and psychological appetite. Accept total personal responsibility for your weight. There are some things in life we may feel unable to control. Your waistline and general health are entirely up to you.

24

HEART DISEASE

"Thanks to the human heart by which we live. . . ."
—WILLIAM WORDSWORTH

Today half of all Americans die from cardiovascular ailments. More Americans will die of cardiovascular ailments this year than all American soldiers lost in all U.S. wars combined.[1] Yet there is good news. Up to 90 percent of all heart disease is preventable. Even limited efforts at health education have lowered heart disease risks by 20 percent.

Medical science has made great bounds in treating heart disease, from heart transplants, to electronic pacemakers, to heart bypass surgery, artificial hearts. Deaths from sudden heart attack have dropped, thanks to the widespread knowledge of cardiopulmonary resuscitation. Yet bypass surgery, costing $25,000 and up and requiring months of recuperation, has been shown to temporarily alleviate angina pain but does nothing to extend lifespan.[2] The impressive quiver of weapons used against heart disease are neither cure nor prevention. They are even only marginally effective at treating symptoms.

Heart disease was almost unknown before this century. It is still unknown in the underdeveloped nations of the world. Since it is likely to be caused by lifestyle,[3] the most likely cures and preventive techniques will be lifestyle.

The Risk Factors for Vascular Diseases

Age. The chances increase for sediment accumulating or vessels hardening.

Males and postmenopausal women. The male hormone androgen encourages fatty accumulation in the blood vessels. This excludes most women until after menopause, when a hormone change puts them into the risk category. Yet men have quite a head start on heart disease. This is obvious to anyone who has visited a retirement home where the vast majority of survivors beyond eighty years of age are women.

Sedentary lifestyle. Exercise burns fats to prevent them from clogging the arteries. Exercise accelerates the flow of blood through the vessels to prevent sedimentation. It lowers stress levels and prevents overfatness. Indeed, exercise is a near panacea in preventing or even curing heart disease.

Poor diet. High fat, high saturated fat, high hydrogenated fat, high cholesterol, high sodium, high animal protein, high sugar, low fiber, low magnesium, low calcium, low chromium, low selenium, low essential fatty acids, low B_6, low C, low E, high protein, large meals (gorging), and overfatness are all dietary risk factors that may lead to plugged up or hardened vessels. Diet is now considered as important a coronary risk factor as smoking.[4]

Stress. When a person is angry, frustrated, worried, or pushed to the limit, the stressor hormones (catecholamines) flow in the blood stream. They will elevate blood pressure, increase the flow of fats into the blood stream, and perform other tasks that would be valuable if the person were trying to outrun a tiger, but not so valuable for someone sitting at a desk for forty years.

Environmental pollutants. Noise is known to increase heart disease risk as it stresses the central nervous system. Air pollution binds up vitamin E, thus leaving less E to help keep the blood vessels clear. Smoking is a major risk factor. Lead in our air and water is known to be a major risk to the vascular system. There are probably other relationships between the myriad of toxicants we are exposed to and the onset of hardened or plugged vessels.

Genetics. This one is important, but, alas, cannot be modified. Avid runners were shocked when one of their gurus, Jim Fixx, died while running at age fifty-two. Yet he was obese and a chain smoker until his thirty-sixth birthday. He then realized that his genes were not conducive to long life. His father died at thirty-seven of a heart attack. Jim Fixx began running earnestly and outlived his father by fifteen years, in spite of his earlier risk factors. Some people had very long-lived ancestors, while others are not so blessed. All should follow the advice of this chapter. Those with a family tendency toward heart disease should be especially attentive.

How Vascular Diseases Begin

There are three basic problem that can lead to the demise of your blood vessels.

Fatty blockage, or atherosclerosis. Fats are a potential sabboteur from within. Fat is essential for many bodily processes yet does not mingle well with the water medium of the blood. Thus, all fatty substances must have an escort through the vascular network. These escorts, called lipoproteins, are of various types. Some help prevent fatty blockage (the HDL, or high density lipoproteins) while others instigate the problem (LDL, or low density lipoproteins).

Platelet aggregation (or "stickiness" of blood cells). In this situation, particles of the blood begin to stick together and form a clotting network around themselves. This group of clumping blood cells may then sediment to the floor of the vessel and continue the clotting process, just as when you are cut and a scab forms. The clot may begin accumulating fats that are flowing by. This process (thrombosis) may be the beginning of a fatty occlusion (plaque).

Hardening of the arteries, or arteriosclerosis. Calcium may combine with cholesterol in the blood stream and begin collecting along the vessel walls. Calcium deposits can harden the vessels, and thus increase blood pressure since the once flexible vessel walls no longer stretch well. A person with high blood pressure could have these brittle vessels burst. The bursting could happen anywhere along the vessel network. Thus, high blood pressure is a crucial issue in discussing vascular diseases. Ironically, it is not excess calcium intake that leads to calcification of the vessels. Low calcium, high phosphorus, low magnesium, low vitamin D, and other factors contribute to calcification. Potassium, calcium, and magnesium supplements along with a regular exercise program would probably "cure" hypertension for millions of Americans.[5]

Chelation therapy attempts to create an ion exchange process, similar to what occurs in a home water softener. A sodium solution is injected into the patient will in the hope that it will slowly dissolve the calcium and cholesterol deposits.[6] This procedure is very controversial, with those for and against it polarized into near extremist views.

Program to Prevent or Cure Vascular Disease[7]

Exercise. At least three times per week. Motion should be continuous (thus keeping the heart rate up), flowing (like dancing, biking, or swimming), and allow you to just barely talk (this ensures that fats, rather than carbohydrates, are being burned). Target heart rate should be about 220 minus your age, multiplied by .8. Thus a fifty-year old person would need to work out until the heart rate reached 130 to 150 beats per minute for twenty minutes in order for the heart to get a good workout. Overfatness is strongly tied to heart disease and high blood pressure. Exercise "cures" obesity.

Attitude. The "Type A" personality is prone to heart disease. This person is demanding, rushed, intense, and volatile. Venting of emotions is important, but not when it is destructive. Try to relax and enjoy life more. Meditation raises HDLs and stabilizes catecholamine stress hormones.

Smoking. A major risk factor. Binds vitamin C. Raises fats in the blood. Lowers the body's ability to resist clots in the blood. Raises blood pressure and heart rate.

Diet. High priority—fat should be less than 30 percent of total calories. Reduce saturated animal fats and substitute unsaturated plant oils, like soy and safflower oil.

Fiber should be increased until stools are soft and float. Pectin (from fruits and vegetables) may aid this cause.[8]

Cholesterol intake should be cut in half. This means less red meat, dairy products, eggs, fried foods.

Sodium (salt) and sugar intake should be cut at least in half. Studies show that people quickly adjust to low-salt food patterns.[9]

Eat more plant proteins, such as legumes and vegetables, and less animal proteins.

Get an extra 200 micrograms of chromium per day, preferably from brewer's yeast, since only 1 percent of supplements are absorbed. Patients with blocked coronary arteries had one-third to one-eighth of normal levels of chromium.[10] Low chromium in the diet has been intimately linked to heart disease.[11]

Take a well-balanced broad spectrum multiple vitamin and mineral supplement daily. This should contain adequate levels of nutrients that help metabolize fat, including choline, inositol, B_{12}, and folacin. This supplement should also contain adequate levels of antioxidant nutrients like beta-carotene (vitamin A), C, E, manganese, and selenium to help prevent destruction of prostacyclin (a hero in preventing the clumping of blood cells). People with low selenium levels in their diet had a threefold jump in the incidence of heart disease.[12]

Eat garlic often since it lowers blood pressure and fats in the blood while also raising the protective HDL levels.

Eat fish often since studies show that having only two ounces of fish per week cuts the heart attack rate in half.[13]

To help control blood pressure, eat plenty of plant foods, such as whole grains, citrus fruits, and beans, to keep potassium levels up. Use a salt substitute that is half potassium and half sodium.

Keep magnesium intake at 500 to 600 milligrams daily, since low magnesium levels have been associated with sudden muscle spasms, like heart attack. Eat plenty of leafy green vegetables, nuts, soybeans, seeds, and whole grains.

Keep calcium intake at 1,000 milligrams daily. Studies have shown calcium supplements (1,500 milligrams daily as calcium carbonate) reduce blood pressure in hypertensive patients more effectively than medication.[14] There is an elevated risk for heart disease with deficiencies or imbalances in trace minerals like copper, chromium, and even silicon.[15]

It may also be helpful to include the following foods regularly in your diet: Red hot peppers because the capsicum in them lowers the stickiness of fats in the bloodstream. Onions and fresh ginger root. Brewer's yeast (one teaspoon daily), wheat germ (half cup daily), lecithin (two tablespoons daily), yogurt (one cup daily), and apples for their pectin content (two fresh ones daily). Maximize intake of fresh vegetables, fruit, whole grains, and legumes.

Nathan Pritikin was an engineer who suffered a heart attack in 1958. His logical mind deduced that, since heart disease is endemic only to the developed nations of the world, something in our lifestyle caused the problem. After considerable reading, Pritikin developed a low-fat, high-fiber, and exercise (walking) program to treat heart disease. In spite of the scorn he was subjected to, droves of "incurable" patients entered his heart disease reversal program in Santa Monica, California. The success of his diet was impressive. Compliance on his rigid low-fat diet was quite difficult for all but the most motivated people. When Pritikin died in 1985 at age sixty-nine, twenty-seven years after having severely blocked arteries, his vessels were found in an autopsy to be completely free of obstruction.[16]

Heart disease and other vascular ailments have proved amazingly resilient to the drug and surgical approach of modern medicine. You need not complacently accept the fate of plugged or hardened plumbing. You can do something about it. By following the recommendations in this chapter, your odds of getting vascular disease are lowered to one-tenth that of the average person. Your fate is in your hands.

 è▲

25

CANCER

"Spread the word that cancer is not as inevitable as death and taxes."
—DR. THOMAS MAUGH II, NATIONAL ACADEMY OF SCIENCES

A heart attack may be painful and lethal, but cancer is a deep, gut-wrenching fear of the unknown for many people. It shouldn't be. Research in this field is constantly revealing new techniques to deal with cancer. One in three cancer victims will beat the disease through medical treatment. An even more important statistic is that up to nine out of ten cases of cancer are provoked by lifestyle, and thus are also preventable.[1] Diet causes about 35 percent of cancer cases,[2] and stress, sun, chemicals, smoking, and other malleable aspects of lifestyle are also prime contributors. Right now, one out of four Americans will die of cancer.[3] Follow the edicts of this chapter and your risks will be cut to one-tenth that number.

Causes

What is cancer? Briefly stated: cells growing so rapidly that they are out of control. Cancerous tissue grows until it strangles normal functions in the human body.[4]

Cancer may have a variety of causes—including chemicals, radiation from sunlight or radioactive metals, an invading virus, or electromagnetic fields—all of which affect the DNA of the cell nucleus to instigate radical growth. Some experts suggest that all people have minor cancer growth within them at some time in their life. Healthy people are able to squelch the radical growth via their immune system.

Stress seems to interfere with the normal functioning of the immune system, including the production of interferon. People with an external veneer of tranquility and insides of bubbling turmoil are more likely to get cancer. People who are poorly nourished, and thus have a subpar immune system, are more likely to get cancer.

Commonly used chemicals known to cause cancer in laboratory animals include many food dyes, nitrates and nitrites (used as preservatives and color enhancers in foods), formaldehyde (used in plastics, particle board, glues, and many other areas), benzpyrene (found in smoked and burned meats and the exhaust from diesel and jet engines), asbestos (used in ceilings for sound proofing, on car brakes, hot pads for cooking and in fire-retardant materials), tobacco (whether smoked or chewed), and various naturally occurring toxins in foods such as the psoralens found in turnips. Coffee enthusiasts are at risk for certain types of cancer. Some pesticides and insecticides may cause cancer. Reports are only now beginning to surface of cancer deaths related to exposure on the job. Twenty employees who were exposed to the carcinogen benzene in their oil refinery work died of leukemia.[5] Agent Orange, the defoliant used in Vietnam, may have caused cancer and other ailments in the people exposed to this deadly substance. Dioxin, the active ingredient in Agent Orange, is still used in forestry and agriculture in America.

Sunlight is another cancer-inducing agents. Fair-skinned individuals should be especially aware of their exposure. Use sunscreen, limit time in the sun (particularly in the tropics, at higher elevations, and midday in the summer), and slowly increase time to provide a gradual tan. The weekend warrior who continually burns is an excellent candidate for skin cancer. People exposed to fluorescent lighting throughout the day have a greater risk for skin cancer than those who spend much time outdoors.[6]

Radiation from medical X rays or from radioactive wastes can stealthily alter the delicate DNA pattern in the cell nucleus. Madam Curie, discoverer of X rays, died of leukemia, which was probably caused by overexposure to radiation. The National Council on Radiation Protection and Measurements has estimated that 9,000 Americans die each year from lung cancer caused by radon gas. Radon is emitted from the earth in the natural disintegration of radioactive components. Certain areas have more radon gas, but all places have some. As much as one out of five fatal lung cancers involving nonsmokers may be caused by radon gas.

Nutrition and Cancer

With the incidence of cancer swelling for the last four decades in this country and some victims having little chance for survival, many people turned to alternative healing therapies. Some have worked. Many haven't. Yet cancer and cancer therapy can cause clinical malnutrition,[7] which accelerates the course of the disease. There is solid evidence that proves the value of nutrition for the prevention and even treatment of cancer.[8] In 1983, the prestigious National Academy of Sciences published its findings in the very technical book *Diet, Nutrition, and Cancer,* which advocated diet as a preventive factor in cancer. Health authorities estimate that diet alone could prevent one-third of all cancer cases.[9] Obesity increases the risk for cancer of the colon, breast, prostate, and endometrium (vaginal region).[10]

Nutrients Related to Cancer Prevention or Treatment

For all of the following, check the chapters on dietary components for food sources of these nutrients.

Beta-carotene is the plant version of vitamin A. People who have diets high in beta-carotene have significantly lower rates of cancer.[11] Many Americans are low in their intake of vitamin A.

Ascorbic acid helps reduce the likelihood of many types of cancer, even skin cancer from excess exposure to the sun.[12] Once again, many Americans are low in their intake of this valuable nutrient. Vitamin C has been shown to lower the risk of intestinal cancer for those consuming carcinogenic agents like nitrate and burned foods.

Vitamin E is a potent antioxidant. E can help to lower cancer risks. Diets that are high in polyunsaturated fats are more vulnerable to cancer, though these same fats are widely recommended for lowering the risk of heart disease. Polyunsaturated fats, if not protected by vitamin E, have unstable bonds that can become involved in free radical oxidation. Raise your E intake and the risk for polyunsaturated fats probably disappears.

Selenium is a trace element that is undoubtedly low in the American diet. Humans with body selenium levels in the lowest one-third of the population had three times the risk of cancer.[13] Regions of America where there is less selenium in the soil (and thus in the diet) have a higher risk of cancer.[14] Selenium and vitamin E work together in a potent anticancer enzyme system called glutathione peroxidase. Optimal levels of selenium seem to provide a much higher tolerance of toxins and heavy metals like cadmium and mercury.

Manganese is a mineral found in the potent anticancer enzyme system superoxide dismutase. All cancerous tumors studied to date have been low in manganese levels.[15]

Zinc plays an important role in the natural immunity of the human body. Zinc-deficient animals have a higher rate of certain types of cancer. Since most Americans are consuming one-half to two-thirds of the recommended intake of zinc, it is likely that this may relate to high cancer levels. Be aware that too much zinc may encourage cancer, since excess zinc interferes with the anticancer mineral selenium.

Vitamin B_6 has been shown to lend cancer resistance to experimental animals. B_6 is notably missing in the American diet.

Fiber is a tenacious binder of toxic elements in the intestinal tract, where about one-third of all cancer cases originate. Fiber, especially from cruciferous vegetables like cabbage, broccoli, cauliflower, and Brussels sprouts, can seriously reduce cancer risks.

Fat in the diet and in the body can magnify cancer risks.[16] Overfat individuals are more likely to get many types of cancer. High-fat diets elevate the risk fivefold for getting cancer of the intestinal tract, breasts, and other areas.[17]

Other substances that are potentially anticancerous agents include thiamin (works against cancers induced by smoking and drinking), vitamin D (works against cancers of the intestinal tract), superoxide dismutase (probably useless when taken internally), BHA and BHT (food preservatives with possible value and equally possible harm), and L-cysteine and L-methionine, two sulfur-containing amino acids that seem to have potent anticancer abilities.[18] Cancer of the esophagus is more likely with lower intakes of niacin, magnesium, and zinc.[19]

Recommended Program

We are exposed to numerous potent carcinogens ranging from industrial wastes to agricultural pesticides. With a starving immune system attempting to fight off cancer, and the abundance of cancer-causing agents found in our everyday life, it is not surprising that cancer kills one out of four Americans. You can cut your risks by following this program:

• Reduce fat intake to less than 30 percent of total calories. Avoid hydrogenated fats. Minimize saturated fats and use cold pressed vegetable oils such as soy and safflower in your kitchen.

• Reduce body fat to less than an inch of skinfold above the hipbone.

• Take a broad spectrum supplement that supplies 100 percent or more of the USRDA for all essential nutrients. Make sure the following antioxidants are present: selenium, beta-carotene, vitamin C, vitamin E, zinc, Vitamin B_6, thiamin, manganese.

• Minimize exposure to carcinogens including tobacco, excess sunlight, food coloring, nitrate, and poisonous chemicals.

• Keep a positive attitude through exercise, meditation, and activity.

One out of three cancer victims may be "cured" through advanced warning and proper medical treatment. But nine out of ten could have avoided the disease altogether if they followed a preventive lifestyle.

26

DIABETES

"There are no such things as incurables; there are only things for which man has not found a cure."

—BERNARD BARUCH

In the federal cause-of-death statistics, diabetes seems to be a rather unimportant disease in America.[1] That is very deceiving. Thirty-four thousand Americans died from diabetes in 1981. However, experts estimate that from three to ten times that many people died from related causes of diabetes. Diabetics have twenty-five times the incidence of blindness that the average healthy person has, seventeen times the rate of kidney disease, twice the heart disease rate, five times the gangrene rate, much higher risk for impotence, skin lesions, infections, and a barrage of other health problems.

Worse yet, the incidence of diabetes is skyrocketing. From 1965 to 1973 there was a 50 percent increase in the number of diabetics in this country. About 5 percent, or nearly 12 million Americans, are clinically diagnosed as diabetic. That number does not take into consideration the millions of undiagnosed cases plus the millions of others that have impaired glucose tolerance. At the current rate of increase of 6 percent per year, diabetes incidence could double every fifteen years. One out of five people born today will become a diabetic.[2]

What is Diabetes?

Simply put: diabetes is poorly regulated blood glucose due to low or ineffective insulin output. Without insulin, glucose builds up in the blood. The body can burn carbohydrates, fats, proteins, and alcohol for fuel. Most body cells prefer glucose as the fuel source. Some body cells, like the lens of the eye, kidneys, lungs, and brain, can burn only glucose.[3] There must be insulin, glucose tolerance factor (containing chromium), and cyclic AMP (a hormone) in order for the glucose to pass through the cell membrane so that the cell furnace within can use it.[4] The diabetic has an overabundance of glucose in the blood but not enough is getting into the cells. Juvenile diabetes (also called insulin dependent or type I) is a complete lack of insulin. Adult diabetes (or non-insulin dependent, type II) is a result of not enough insulin being made by the pancreas. Insulin resistance means enough insulin is being produced but the cells are not responding to it properly.

In juvenile diabetes, lean tissue wasting is a common problem. With insufficient glucose inside the cells, the body will break down its own protein stores (lean tissue) in order to create some glucose. Ironically, overweight adults are four times more likely to develop diabetes,[5] while the juvenile diabetic is more likely to waste away in thinness.

Testing for Diabetes

The way to tell if you have diabetes is to take a glucose tolerance test. For this test, you would not be allowed to eat any food after your evening meal. The next morning, you would drink a glass of very sweet water (glucose solution). Blood samples would be taken at the beginning, thirty minutes later, and each hour thereafter for the next six hours. If the curve showed that the absorbed glucose in the blood stayed high, you might be considered diabetic. When the sugar levels get too high in the blood, the kidneys begin to filter out the excess. At this renal threshold, sugar is being dumped into the urine to try to maintain the normal consistency and volume of the blood. Much body water is lost in an effort to dilute the high concentration of glucose in the urine. Two primary symptoms of diabetes are excessive thirst and frequent urination. Hence the phrase "sweetness running through." Because skin repair requires healthy insulin response, poor wound healing is another common symptom of the diabetic. For more on the glucose tolerance test, see the chapter on carbohydrates.

There are specially treated paper sticks that can be dipped into the urine to determine the level of fat by-products (ketones). Other paper sticks can tell how much sugar is being dumped into the urine. These litmus tests are usually employed only to help monitor the diabetic, rather than in diagnosis.

Causes

Diabetes may be one symptom which has many causes, including:

• Genetics. Families have inherited tendencies for the pancreas to give out, leaving the person diabetic.

• The pancreas is destroyed through a tumor, virus, autoimmune response of the defending white cells, fibrosis infiltration, exposure to a potent toxin, or some other reason.

- The pancreas may just get tired (beta-cell burnout) from excessive use, as may occur with a high-sugar diet.
- One of the many enzyme systems responsible for making insulin may fail.
- Release of insulin may be blocked.
- Something in the body may bind to and destroy the produced insulin.
- The cells of the body may become "deaf" to the effect of insulin. This can be caused by a chromium deficiency or the inability of the body to make GTF from chromium.
- Insulin and GTF have a "lock-and-key" fit into the cell membrane to allow glucose into the cells. In the overweight individual, bloating of the cells by excessive fat storage may ruin the lock-and-key fit.

Treatment and Nutrition

If the person has juvenile diabetes, there will probably be a need for daily injections of insulin. Diet must be regulated. Exercise is encouraged.

In the adult diabetic, oral drugs are sometimes given to stimulate the pancreas to secrete more insulin. Weight control and proper diet are important.

Exercise improves the effectiveness of the insulin and therefore improves glucose tolerance in all people. Exercise should be considered almost as important as medication for the diabetic.

Probably a third to a half of all non-insulin-dependent diabetics could have their condition controlled by proper nutrition management. The categories of nutrition involvement include:

Weight maintenance. Often, just losing weight brings the glucose tolerance back to normal. Overfat people are four times more likely to have diabetes.

Diet to stabilize glucose curves. This means small, frequent meals; minimum amounts of refined sugar, caffeine, and alcohol; maximum intake of fiber (whole grains, fresh vegetables and fruit, legumes). Legumes (beans) are the food that provides the most stable blood glucose curves.

Supplementary nutrients. Of these, chromium is probably the most important for stabilizing blood glucose. Most Americans consume between 25 and 33 micrograms of chromium daily, when the minimum acceptable standard is 50 micrograms.[6] In a study using insulin-dependent diabetics, supplements of high-chromium brewer's yeast improved the insulin sensitivity of all six people, thus lowering their insulin needs.[7] In other clinical experiments, high-chromium yeast was given to normal older adults. "Normal" glucose tolerance for older adults might be considered diabetes if it occurred in younger people. Fifty percent of the supplemented older adults had marked improvements in glucose tolerance.[8]

In normal healthy people, chromium from the diet is made into glucose tolerance factor (GTF) in the body. Experts feel that some people cannot make enough of their own GTF from dietary chromium.[9] For these people, GTF from brewer's yeast would become a dietary essential, lest they develop too high (hyperglycemia) or too low (hypoglycemia) blood sugar levels.

There are other vitamin and mineral supplements that could be valuable to the diabetic.[10] Selenium, zinc, vitamin E, and C may improve the lowered immune functions of the diabetic. Selenium, vitamin C, and vitamin E could help lower the major heart disease risk that diabetics face. Vitamins E, C, A, and the mineral selenium may prevent the capillary fragility that causes retinal damage in diabetics. Diabetics are often low in B_6 levels in the blood and also have nerve degeneration and tingling sensations (peripheral neuropathies). These symptoms are often improved with B_6 supplements of up to 50 milligrams per day. Since B_6 is also involved in glucose tolerance, it is not surprising that some studies have shown B_6 to improve the glucose curves of both healthy and diabetic patients.[11]

Diabetics have considerably lower levels of magnesium than normal healthy subjects. This contrast is most blatant in diabetics who have experienced some destruction of the retina. Magnesium loss is high when the diabetic lapses into ketosis, a situation in which the body is trying to primarily burn fats as a fuel, and is doing so rather inefficiently. The by-products of this inefficient fat burning are called ketone bodies. When magnesium is given with insulin during ketosis, the insulin needs are less.[12] Many fatal heart attacks in this country may be due to low magnesium levels. Since diabetics are at higher risk for heart attack, an increase in magnesium intake, makes good sense for them.

Osteoporosis is more common in diabetics than normal subjects, probably due to the excess calcium excretion that accompanies their "limping" kidneys. For this reason, calcium intake should increase for diabetics. Also, since calcium and magnesium compete for the same sites of absorption in the intestines, taking one without the other might create an imbalance.

The diabetic has difficulty converting linoleic acid from the diet into prostaglandins in the body. Gamma-linolenic acid (GLA, often sold as evening primrose oil) provides the ready-to-use material for making prostaglandins. GLA can help lower blood pressure, improve the HDL/LDL ratio, reduce the stickiness of fats in the blood, and may facilitate weight loss.[13] Considering the diabetic's risk for heart disease, GLA may be a valuable supplement.

To date, there is no guaranteed cure for diabetes. In 1921, Banting and Best first produced insulin and the world thought that diabetes was gone forever. Not so. Artificial insulin only prevents the diabetic from dying in the near future of ketosis. Diabetics now have a wide variety of other hurdles to avoid, with death often coming from heart disease due to their abnormal fat metabolism.

Non-insulin-dependent diabetics can improve their situation markedly when they reduce their percent body fat, follow a proper diet, and exercise regularly. Insulin-dependent diabetics must adhere strictly to their program of diet and shots.

27

OSTEOPOROSIS

"A joyful heart is good medicine, but a broken spirit dries up the bones."

PROVERBS 17:22

Osteoporosis is a loss of mineral content or hollowing out of the bones.[1] It affects over 20 million Americans today, at an annual cost of about $3.8 billion. Each year, about 1.3 million bone fractures occur in America as a direct result of osteoporosis. One out of three people age sixty-five and older have some degree of osteoporosis. An English physician recently commented that orthopedic units in English hospitals are so overcrowded with osteoporosis patients that the situation is somewhat reminiscent of the plagues of centuries past. The incidence of hip fractures has doubled in the past 28 years.[2]

Because levels of the female hormone estrogen, which helps keep the bones fortified, decline after menopause, four times more women than men are afflicted. In a recent study of women ages forty-nine to sixty-six, 70 percent consumed less than 800 milligrams daily of calcium and 13 percent consumed less than 400 milligrams.[3] The RDA is 800, and good evidence says that it should be 1,500 for older women.[4] This means that most women are consuming one-half to one-third the calcium they need.

Normal bones break. But osteoporotic bones can shatter like a pane of glass. This makes reassembling these pieces a tricky matter. Such a disabling bone separation can lead to extensive surgery, wheelchairs, crutches, canes, and immobility. One-third of these people die of complications within a year after their bone break.

One of the problems in osteoporosis is detection. Only a few high-powered research techniques such as neutron activation analysis, can detect the osteoporosis early enough to make corrective measures valuable.[5] Conventional X rays cannot detect serious bone demineralization until nearly half of the bone has eroded. At this point the condition may be irreversible. Even if properly treated, it could still be life-threatening.

Another problem is that there are few blatant symptoms. Calcium is critical to proper nerve and muscle functioning. Nature has evolved a complex feedback system that keeps the nerves and muscles (especially the heart) supplied with at least survival levels of calcium. The blood will steal calcium from the bones to keep the heart muscle pumping. Thus, neither X rays nor blood tests will reveal the earlier stages of osteoporosis. A person might have occasional cramps and muscle twitches, but these may go away, be ignored or sedated. Another early warning sign is premature tooth loss, since the jaw is one of the first bones to be eroded when intake of calcium is low. In some people the osteoporosis occurs primarily in the spinal region. As the vertebrae of the spinal column shrink, the nerves radiating from the spine may become compressed. The result is excruciating pain. In the latter stages of osteoporosis, a rounded and humped back is common, with a loss in height of several inches. At this point the condition is very serious.

Major risk factors for osteoporosis include aging (especially postmenopausal women), bearing many children, low calcium intake, low vitamin D intake, sedentary lifestyle, stress, high-protein diets, high-fat diets, high phosphorus intake, and alcoholism.[6]

Other risk factors are smoking, high coffee intake, high aluminum ingestion,[7] use of oral contraceptives, high phytate intake, low fluorine intake, low magnesium intake, alcohol intake.

Program to Prevent or Reverse Osteoporosis

Calcium intake must be 1,200 to 1,500 milligrams per day for postmenopausal women. An interesting study found that older women who used to drink lots of milk had a lower incidence of osteoporosis than women who never were milk drinkers.[8] Apparently, fortifying the bones early in life is a major step toward preventing this disease.

Child bearing and lactation can help prevent osteoporosis, since estrogen flows abundantly in early motherhood. Estrogen prevents bone loss. Yet bearing and nursing many children without sufficient calcium in the diet will result in raiding of calcium bone stores.

Magnesium intake must be 400 to 600 milligrams per day.

Vitamin D intake must be between 400 and 600 I.U. per day. For those who get minimum sun exposure and drink little vitamin-D-fortified milk, supplements may be necessary.

Exercise is mandatory.[9] Astronauts show significant bone loss after only one or two months in space. The skeletal system fortifies itself when stress on the bones (exercise) is regular and sheds this "unnecessary bone mass" when exercise is infrequent.[10] Without activity, the skeleton slims down to a minimum. Exercise has been used successfully to help recalcify osteoporotic bones.[11] Exercise is very effective, free, and side effects are all beneficial.

Control stress. Psychological distress leads to poor absorption of calcium in the intestines and also provokes the loss of bone stores. Hence, the biblical reference at the chapter's beginning is quite true.

Regulate phosphorus intake. This mineral, though essential, can displace calcium to create serious weakening of the bones. Processed foods, meats, colas, and most animal foods are high in phosphorus. Check food labels and watch this.

Minimize or avoid alcohol. Excessive alcohol interferes with nearly every system in the body. Though women are usually the target for osteoporosis, 47 percent of male alcoholics studied had measurable bone loss. Thirty-one percent of the male alcoholics under forty years of age had osteoporosis.[12]

Keep protein intake within 60 to 90 grams per day, depending on body weight. When the body consumes too much protein, it can burn it for fuel or store it as fat. Either of these processes requires the liver and kidneys to convert the protein into something different. This burden causes the kidneys to lose calcium when filtering the blood. Prime rib, roast beef, and other foods high in phosphorus, fat, and protein should not be on the menu often.

Limit fat intake. High-fat diets raise osteoporosis risks by rendering the dietary calcium unavailable for absorption and thus losing it in the stools. Fats can create insoluble soaps out of your dietary calcium and cause it to be lost in the stools.[13]

Follow your physician's advice regarding the use of estrogen therapy and other drugs that can help prevent bone loss after menopause, especially if you began it earlier than normal.

The other risk factors may be insignificant by themselves or catastrophic when they become cumulative. Aluminum displaces bone matter. Fluoride helps solidify bones. Decades of coffee intake and smoking slowly erode bones. Regular fad diets slowly chip away at the body's calcium stores.

The average woman loses about one-fourth of her skeletal mass from age thirty to age seventy. This is not good; it also is not inevitable. Death and aging are not preventable. Osteoporosis probably is.

28

ARTHRITIS

"When in doubt, try nutrition first."
—Professor Roger Williams, University of Texas

Arthritis remains an unsolved mystery. Ten percent of the world's population and 25 percent of Americans have arthritis. More than 20 million Americans suffer to the point of requiring medical care.[1] About 4 million are disabled by the condition. Twice as many women as men are affected. The Arthritis Foundation puts the cost of arthritis in America at $25,000 per minute, or $13 billion per year, in lost wages, lost time at work, medical care, incapacitated people, and lost taxes.

The human side can be felt only when someone you know is crippled by arthritis. Arthritis victims suffer so extensively and conventional medicine offers such limited help that arthritics spend over $400 million annually in worthless cures and remedies for their ailment. In this chapter, we hope to explain the basics of this disease and offer some hope for its victims.

Causes

Arthritis is an inflammation of the joint region.[2] Your body is composed of 206 bones. Any place two movable bones meet, there is a system of tough connective tissue to bond the bones together and a slippery synovial fluid to lubricate the movement. In some people the joint becomes irritated, swelling sets in, and pain and immobility are the results.

The Merck Medical Manual lists dozens of possible causes for arthritis.[3] Some of them are:

- Psychological stress. Guilt, hate, hurt, rejection, and other stressors could provoke it.
- Problems with the body's chemistry, such as gout, diabetes, or scurvy (vitamin C deficiency).
- Infectious organisms, such as bacteria, virus, fungus, and other parasites.

- A fall, shock, or concussion that results in injury to a joint area.
- Allergic reactions in which the body's immune system begins to attack the joints.
- Tumors attacking the joints.

Treatment and Nutrition

There are numerous therapies used, including hot packs, stretching exercises, drugs, injections, and surgery. Some, but not all, cases could be cleared up with a more positive outlook on life. Other people would feel better if they used stretching exercises daily. Find a physician who is flexible, open-minded, and oriented toward treating the condition rather than just the symptoms.

As you can see, arthritis is not an easy disease. It has many causes that result in similar symptoms. As with diabetes, this can confuse people into oversimplifying the disease and its treatments. There are several possible nutritional causes and treatments for arthritis.

Weight control. Obesity places undo stress on the joints. Weight loss will often improve arthritis. Consult the chapter on obesity for more on this subject.

Allergies. Somewhere between 8 and 20 percent of the United States population suffers from some type of allergy. When the body begins its autoimmune response, it attacks its own tissue. If the attack is in the joint region, arthritis can result. See the chapter on food allergies and sensitivities for more on this subject.

Macronutrient intake. Some clinicians have had decent results in changing the normal American diet to a healthier balance. Lowering the fat intake seems to help some people. Lowering the sugar intake can also help. Reducing meat protein and increasing vegetable protein can improve symptoms for some arthritics. Lowering alcohol intake could be valuable. In general, we strongly encourage the arthritic to consume the optimal diet recommended throughout this book. At the very worst, it will help the arthritic feel better and have more energy. And it just may be the cure. There can be near miraculous healings once you begin to optimally nourish your body.

Micronutrient intake. There are very promising possibilities here. Some cases of arthritis can be treated by increasing the intake of one or more of the following nutrients:

niacin (400 mg);
pantothenic acid (100 mg);

riboflavin (50 mg);
vitamin A (10,000 I.U.);
B₆ (50 mg);
folacin (800 micrograms);
vitamin C (1,000 mg);
magnesium (400 mg);
calcium (800 mg as calcium hydrogen phosphate);
high-sulfur proteins (eggs, gelatin, beans).

Leukotrienes are inflammatory agents produced by the body that may cause and support arthritis. There is an entire class of fatty acids called eicosanoids that help prevent the buildup of these "bad guy" leukotrienes. Fish oil is a primary source of a form of this fatty acid (eicosapentanoic acid).[5] In scientific studies done at Harvard University, EPA fish oil has been shown to improve the inflammation and tender joints of arthritis.[6] They also found that there is a safe upper limit to this fish oil consumption. Taking eighteen capsules daily (providing about 3,600 milligrams of EPA) may cause a slight lowering of white blood corpuscles, which could signal lowered disease resistance.[7] As in anything in nutrition and throughout life, it is a question of balance. Extremes are harmful.

Zinc has been shown to improve the clinical management of rheumatoid arthritis.[8] This makes sense in light of zinc's role in inhibiting leukotrienes. Rutin may be a valuable supplement for arthritis.[9]

Antiarthritis Nutrition Program

1. A diet high in complex carbohydrates and fiber and low in fat.

2. At least three ounces of fish consumed at least three times each week (salmon is richest in EPA).

3. A broad spectrum vitamin and mineral supplement that includes 30 milligrams of zinc, 200 milligrams of rutin, 200 micrograms of selenium, plus the other nutrients mentioned above.

4. If no fish is consumed, take ten capsules daily of EPA fish oil.

5. Be aware of possible food allergies. Is there a food that you crave? Or that you eat regularly? Try eliminating that food for at least a week to see if any symptoms clear up. Milk, wheat, and beef are very common allergic foods among Americans.

29

FOOD ALLERGIES AND SENSITIVITIES

"One man's meat is another man's poison."   —LUCRETIUS, 100 A.D.

Some of you may know well the symptoms of hay fever, with its swollen red eyes and runny itchy nose. Others may have swelled up from bee stings. These are allergic reactions. While some experts state that less than 8 percent of the population is afflicted with allergies,[1] others claim that the percentage is much higher.

One person may react to the most minute level of a certain food. Another person may be less sensitive yet eventually react once exposure to the allergen has reached a "critical mass." Some people grow out of their allergies, others may grow into them. A few people will react to a certain substance some of the time but not consistently. Some people may react to an allergen only when there is dust in the air, or an acid food in the stomach, or they are under stress. Some people can be so sensitive to certain substances that their throat will close up and they may die after the least contact with that food. There are thousands of other substances in the air, dirt, food, and surroundings that could also provoke a reaction.

For the purposes of this chapter, an allergy is an internal reaction to a foreign protein. A food sensitivity can be caused by any of the thousands of other substances found in foods.

Allergy Symptoms

The symptoms of allergies range from the classic ones of hay fever—runny nose, itching burning eyes, skin rash, or swollen sinus passages—to swelling, discomfort or irritation anywhere else in the body. Some people may not have the overt symptoms but only the subtle internal ones, or the obvious symptoms may be only a small of the body's reaction to the irritant.

Symptoms in the skin include hives, eczema, fluid seepage, swelling, and itchiness. Internal symptoms may be in the gastrointestinal tract as ulcers, with bloating, flatulence, burning sensations, nausea, indigestion; in the skeletal joints with swelling and arthritislike symptoms; in the pancreas with diabetes as the eventual result of self-destruction of the body's insulin producer; or in the brain with tissue swelling and behavioral changes taking place. Some migraine headaches can be brought on by food allergies.[2]

What Causes an Allergic Response?

In normal digestion, the body takes a large complex protein from food and renders it down to smaller amino acids. The amino acids pass through the intestinal wall and are carried by the blood to tissue that needs these protein building blocks. For most healthy people, 98 percent of protein digestion is handled this way. The remaining 2 percent of the protein is able to slip through the intestinal wall without being properly broken down. For some unhealthy people, much more than 2 percent of the protein may end up intact in the blood stream.[3]

The normal immune system is designed to attack and destroy foreign invaders. In the not-so-healthy individual, the immune bodies will begin attacking the large food proteins that have entered the blood stream. This can lead to a buildup of immune bodies to handle the overwhelming flow of food proteins slipping into the bloodstream. If there is an abundance of immune bodies, they may begin a self-destructive rampage, called the autoimmune response, in which the immune bodies create a sharklike feeding frenzy and may begin indiscriminately destroying surrounding tissue. Attacking joints could create arthritis. Attacking the intestinal lining would cause nausea and indigestion. Attacking the pancreas may end up as diabetes. Attacking the brain may cause swelling and behavioral changes.

Basically, an allergic response is the result of the body's hypersensitive immune system not only overwhelming the invading foreign protein but also attacking its own body tissue.

Why are Allergies so Common Today?

There are several known and a few speculated reasons for the prevalence of allergies.

1. The low incidence of breast-feeding in this country. Mother's milk is the ultimate hypoallergenic food (i.e., very few people react to it). It consists of human proteins, formed by humans for humans. Other milks, including cow and soy, are foreign and may cause a hypersensitive immune system in the young infant. Only 10 to 20 percent of American infants are nursed to six months of age.

2. The early introduction of solid foods.[4] The immature immune system

of a young infant is more likely to react abnormally to a food protein. For decades, people have been introducing foods to their infants as early as one week of life. It is now generally accepted that an infant should not eat food other than mother's milk or formula for the first six months of life.

3. The restrictive dietary selections in America. Noel Vietmeyer, of the National Academy of Sciences, estimates that there are over 20,000 edible species of plants on earth. Only 100 or so are commercially grown around the world.[5] There are hundreds of different potato species, though we rarely see more than three types in our stores. Our ancestors ate many different kinds of fish and animals, yet most Americans eat only beef, chicken, and pork. There are dozens of grains which grow bountifully in North America, yet most Americans restrict themselves to depleted white wheat flour. With some of these proteins passing through the intestinal wall into the bloodstream, the restrictive diet creates a buildup of certain food proteins, which can trigger an autoimmune response. Thus an allergy is born.

4. Many Americans are malnourished. A healthy digestive tract allows only a small portion of proteins through. A healthy immune system attacks only foreign invading organisms. Malnourished people are more likely to exhibit abnormal digestion and hyperactive responses of their immune system.

5. Stress can provoke allergic responses. We are all exposed to more stress than we sometimes care to admit. Catecholamines are the stress hormones that change many chemical and biological parameters in the body. Stress has been positively linked to the immune system in a new science called psychoneuroimmunology.

6. The abundance of pollutants and drugs. Alcohol, tobacco, prescription, over-the-counter, and "recreational" drugs are widely distributed and heavily used in America. We are also exposed to an ever-increasing quantity and variety of pollutants. Though the normally healthy system may not have allergies, the lead-intoxicated system may. Most drugs, including alcohol, have a variety of side effects on the efficiency of the digestive tract.[6] Alcohol can seriously erode the surface of the intestines to interfere with absorption.[7] These changes in digestive and immune functions may provoke an allergic reaction.

Testing for Allergies

There are a variety of assessing methods, none of which is totally satisfactory.

Skin testing. The clinician scratches the patient's back while injecting a potential allergen, such as mold or wheat protein. Swelling may appear as an indicator that the patient might be allergic to that substance. This method does not take into consideration that symptoms may be something other than blatant skin hives. Many physicians now use the back of the arm, since the hyperallergic individual may have a severe reaction once the allergen has been injected. Tourniquets can be applied to the arm more easily than to the back, thus allowing the physician to treat the allergic response. The skin patch test is mildly painful, expensive, and not totally reliable.

Radioallergosorbent test (RAST). A sample of the patient's blood is sent through a complex device and tested for potential allergenic substances. Not all substances can be tested this way. The method is also expensive and not totally reliable.

Basophil histamine release. This method involves test-tube laboratory study of the patient's blood for histamine release. It's very expensive, time consuming, and realistically appropriate only for research.

Cytotoxic testing. Potential allergens are added to the patient's blood in a test tube and the rate of destruction of blood cells is observed. The more blood cells that are destroyed, the greater the person's sensitivity to that food. This method is very controversial, yet many clinicians claim to have good results.

Provocative sublingual testing. A sample of potential allergens is placed under the patient's tongue. The clinician then applies pressure to the patient's arm, which is held parallel to the floor, to test his strength. The theory is that an allergic response will diminish muscle strength and the clinician can easily push down the patient's arm. This method is very controversial and shunned by the core of the medical community. Yet some claim that it is inexpensive, noninvasive, and provides immediate results.

Patient's own response. Though the other methods attempt to elicit some scientifically documented results, they are not reliable in doing so. This is our favorite method: If the food seems to create a response, then don't eat it. It the symptoms go away, then there is some evidence that the food was at fault. As the classic Henny Youngman joke goes: "Doctor, every time I do this it hurts." Doctor's reply: "Then don't do that."

Though it would be nice to have some laboratory readout or X-ray picture that irrefutably identifies the problem, such is not the case with allergies. There are thousands of chemicals in the environment, and thousands of others in our food supply, with thousands of others being found in the human body. The possible combinations among these sets of substances are limitless. The possibility of obtaining reproducible scientific results is slim.

Allergies and Foods

Hypoallergenic foods are those less likely to cause an allergic response in most individuals. These foods include rice, applesauce, pears, carrots, squash, and lamb. They would probably be allowed for even the most allergic person.

Hyperallergenic foods (those more likely to cause an allergic reaction) include eggs (especially the white part), milk, wheat, corn, peanuts, soybeans, chicken, fish, beef, nuts, mollusks, and other shellfish. The mold found in fermented foods such as cheese, dried fruit, yogurt, and wine may create problems for some. Cow's milk contaminated with various antibiotics may cause an allergic reaction in some people. Yellow dye (tartrazine) can provoke a reaction in those sensitive to aspirin. Monosodium glutamate (MSG) can lead to chest pains, labored breathing, and flushing within twenty minutes after ingestion. Spices and chocolate can be laden with insect parts that precipitate a reaction.

Nutritional Treatment

Elimination diet. In this program, the patient is restricted to hypoallergenic foods or perhaps even goes on a three-day fast with only water and vitamin supplements. Once the symptoms have cleared, foods are reintroduced into the diet to see if a symptom is created. If so, that food is removed. After a few days to clear the system, another potential irritant is fed to the patient. After this tedious detective work is completed and the known irritants have been discovered, the patient is sent home with a diet that avoids the allergic foods. In some cases, this can be quite restrictive. People allergic to milk or wheat may have to eliminate many foods that contain these products, such as noodles or bread.

This procedure can be incredibly expensive when conducted under the auspices of a hospital. Save yourself money and find out if certain foods bother you by performing the elimination program at home. Keep a careful record of all foods consumed. Some people crave the food that they are allergic to. The creed of the elimination diet is: If it bothers you, don't eat it.

Rotation diet. For those people who can tolerate small quantities of the allergic food without symptoms, the rotation diet allows a more normal existence. It could be that daily intake of the food causes an allergy, while weekly intake may have no effect at all. These people are placed on a diet that allows the potentially offending food only once a week. This diet prevents any buildup of allergens.

Food Sensitivities

A sensitivity can be caused by any of the thousands of substances found in food. Dr. Ben Feingold, a nationally respected allergist with thirty years of clinical and teaching experience, developed his theory about food sensitivities. In treating a woman for allergies, he removed all processed foods from her diet. Not only did her skin clear up, but her psychiatrist called Dr. Feingold to ask what he had done. The psychiatrist had been working with this woman for years, to no avail, when suddenly she got completely better on Dr. Feingold's diet. There are two values to the Feingold diet: (1) It eliminates all additives. (2) It encourages the intake of healthy fresh produce, which provides nutrients for normal body and brain metabolism.

An additive that has recently been embroiled in controversy is metabisulfite. It is used to prevent the browning that occurs in lettuce, potatoes, and even grapes for wine making. There are between a half million and a million asthmatics in this country who could suffer a fatal encounter with metabisulfite if they ingested it.[8] The FDA has required that restaurants and food processors who use metabisulfite label their products. It has also been suggested that the substance be banned.

Another possible food sensitivity is to candida albicans, a yeast mold found commonly in many foods and in many people. Most people are unaffected by the presence of candida. In a few people, candida can be the cause of physical or mental ailments. Researchers consider candida to be an "opportunistic pathogen,"[9] which means that it becomes a nuisance primarily in people who have some other health malady. Candida is more of a symptom than a cause. Antifungal medication can kill the candida in the patient's body. Yet efforts must be made to find the true physical or emotional problem in the patient. For some people, merely eliminating candida from the body seems to be the total treatment. A high-sugar diet encourages the growth of candida, so this is another reason to minimize sugar intake.

Efforts to treat food sensitivities seem to be very individual and custom tailored. Our recommendations are: Eat foods in as close to their natural state as possible. Eat a wider variety of foods. Avoid drugs, pollutants, and excess alcohol. And if something bothers you, avoid it.

30

SMOKERS

"Tobacco is a dirty weed. I like it. It satisfies no normal need. I like it. It makes you thin. It makes you lean. It takes the hair right off your bean. Its the worst darn stuff I've ever seen. I like it."
—INSCRIPTION ON A CIGARETTE PACK DISPENSER

You are probably aware of some of the monumental risks involved in using tobacco products. You may even have tried to quit smoking. On average, each cigarette takes six minutes off the life of a smoker. Tobacco is considered one of the major preventable risk factors in the world today. A smoker consuming one pack of cigarettes per day has increased his or her risk for the following conditions:[1]

lung cancer (700%)
laryngeal (throat) cancer (500%)
oral cancer (300%)
emphysema (1000%)
esophageal cancer (400%)
bladder cancer (100%)
pancreatic cancer (100%)
kidney cancer (50%)
coronary heart disease (70%)
peptic ulcer (100%)

Pipe and cigar smokers who do not inhale and tobacco chewers all have a much higher risk for mouth cancer.

Smokers bind the vitamin C in their systems, with up to 500 milligrams ruined by a pack of cigarettes. This often leads to elevated fats and cholesterol in the blood, susceptibility to scurvylike gums, premature wrinkling of the skin, and a barrage of other assaults on the health. Supplements of vitamin C can restore serum C levels to normal.[2] Tobacco smoke produces tar to dirty the teeth and lungs, a carcinogenic form of nickel, carbon monoxide to suffocate all body cells, heat to burn the lungs and mouth, nicotine to constrict the blood vessels, and other potent toxins. If you are a smoker, the best course for your health and longevity is to quit. But then, you probably know that. Studies show that smokers are risk takers. They have twice the incidence of driving while drunk and a much lower rate of seat belt use.[3] Barring quitting, cut back. Barring that, we can recommend nutrients that will help reduce the awesome risks you take by continuing to use tobacco.

Our recommended daily supplement program for the smoker is to take a balanced multiple vitamin and mineral supplement, plus 2,000 milligrams of ascorbic acid, 400 I.U. of vitamin E, 200 micrograms of selenium from yeast, 10 milligrams of thiamin HCL, 25,000 I.U. of beta-carotene, and 2 grams of L-cysteine.[4]

Secondhand Smoke

Less than a third of all adults in the United States smoke. Yet only in the past few years have the nonsmoking majority demanded their right to breath clean air. "Passive smoking" (a.k.a. secondhand smoke), in which you inhale someone else's tobacco smoke, is more than an inconvenience; it is a vile threat to health. Some people react violently to this passive smoking with headaches, sinus conditions, asthma, and other problems. Some people just can't stand the smell. Recent studies show that passive smoking may be as deadly as firsthand smoke. It has been found that smokers who live with other smokers have a significantly elevated death rate from breathing their own smoke plus their roommates' exhaled smoke.[5]

Children who are exposed to continuous secondhand smoke in their home elevate their cancer risk by 60 percent. Nonsmoking adults exposed to passive smoking increase their cancer risk by 50 percent. Those non-smokers who are exposed to smoke during both childhood and adulthood more than double their risk for cancer. In passive smoke there is three times as much benzopyrene (a known carcinogen), six times as much toluene (the part of airplane glue that causes brain damage), fifty times as much dimethylnitrosamine (one of the more potent carcinogens known) as the same volume of directly inhaled smoke.[6]

There is great concern now for the developing fetus within the smoking pregnant woman. This unborn infant receiving secondhand smoke has twice the risk for being small at birth and thus experiencing the complications of immature organs and such.[7] This infant also has a significantly higher risk for heart defects and problems of delivery.

Nonsmokers are a majority. They, too, have rights. Ask pleasantly if the person who is smoking nearby will extinguish his cigarette. Most smokers will comply. The helpless nonsmoker, like the developing fetus and young child, deserves protection from secondhand smoke.

Smokeless Tobacco

Chewing tobacco is not inhaled, but it still contains the same carcinogens found in other tobacco products. Dr. Byron Bailey has ample evidence that up to 80 percent of all cancer of the head and neck could be prevented through tobacco avoidance. Beta-carotene (vitamin A) has proved itself to be a staunch adversary of mouth and other types of cancer.[8]

Sugar is used in the tobacco curing procedure. Chewing tobacco is exposed to the teeth for long periods of time. Dental caries are very common in tobacco chewers.

Giving Up Smoking

People who quit smoking often complain of almost immediate and noticeable weight gain. This is easily explained. Nicotine elevates basal metabolism so that the heart and all cells must work harder (and probably die sooner). This higher metabolism inefficiently burns fuel to allow the smoker to eat a bit more than the nonsmoker. Once you quit smoking, you return to your normal healthy rate of metabolism, and you will not be able to eat as many calories.

In addition to the basal metabolism factor, a recent study found that an enzyme involved in fat storage is affected by cigarette smoking.[19]

Don't continue smoking just to keep your weight down. Nicotine elevates set point. Once off tobacco, your body will adjust in about six months. Exercise markedly accelerates this adjustment and keeps the weight off.

Reformed smokers may also have a need for oral satisfaction. For years or even decades, they have had something in their mouths. This habit does not dwindle quickly. There is a chewing gum your doctor can prescribe that appeases the oral need and also provides the body with some nicotine to prevent the sudden effects of "cold turkey" nicotine withdrawal.

The heat from the burning tip of tobacco products will singe the delicate tissue of the mouth and lungs. Once smoking ceases, this tissue begins to heal. Suddenly foods have a taste that the smoker has not experienced for years. Eating can become a passion, as the reformed smoker almost gets drunk on the flavor of various foods. Refer to the chapter on obesity for help with these problems.

The best technique for helping the recently reformed smoker is exercise. Exercise elevates basal metabolism to prevent weight gain and also lowers stress for the jitters of a reformed smoker. Exercise helps clear the lung passages of accumulated tobacco wastes. It helps prevent backsliding into the smoking habit since, once accustomed to exercise, it is nearly impossible to smoke and enjoy one's sport.

Do not be surprised if you feel bad initially after quitting. When you first had a cigarette, it probably made you dizzy and nauseated, yet you persisted until you got used to it. The body can adjust to some rather unhealthy situations. Some people feel better almost immediately after quitting. Others take months or even up to a year to reacclimate their bodies to a normal healthy state. Be patient.

Tobacco is a major risk. If you choose that risk, keep it to yourself and respect the health rights of others, especially unborn infants and children. And remember that you can lower the health risks of tobacco through protective nutrients.

31

MENTAL FUNCTIONS

"Incredible though it may seem, correct nutrition can mean the difference between depression and good cheer, between sanity and insanity, even between law-abiding self-control and criminal behavior."
— DR. MICHAEL LESSER, PSYCHIATRIST

In 1980, the Central Prison of Portugal attempted an experiment allowing an inmate to teach the other prisoners the principles of nutrition. For those interested, a relatively unrefined diet was available. Of the 400 prisoners, 22 tried this unusual prison diet, which followed the seven general rules of nutrition as described in chapter 5. Each of these 22 prisoners now speaks of the difference in behavior and mental outlook due to improved nutrition.[1]

Nutrition can affect the mind in a number of ways:

1. Hypoglycemia. Radical swings in blood glucose are known to influence the brain's performance.

2. Allergies to protein. Reactions may cause the brain to swell and change personality.

3. Vitamin, mineral, or protein deficiencies. There are abundant known deficiencies in this country and many symptoms are manifested in a hobbling mind.

4. Genetics. Some people have a genetically acquired higher need for nutrients, although this is rare.

5. Sensitivity to food additives or substances, which may affect some people's emotions.

6. Substance abuse. Alcohol is the "inspiration" involved in much crime, drunk driving, child and wife abuse, and general depression for the excessive drinker. Drugs distort behavior to cause a once normal person to do something he or she would not otherwise do.

The human mind is very dependent on the diet. The mind is an organ, with nutrient demands like any other area of the body and with the distinct possibility of being interfered with by toxicants.

Oxygen

Although the brain accounts for only about 5 percent of the body weight of an adult, it uses 25 percent of the body's oxygen supply. Roughly 50 percent of young children and menstruating women are at least borderline anemic. Since they don't have sufficient red blood cells to carry oxygen to the body, this often results in fatigue, irritability, and moodiness. In children, this can manifest itself as hyperactivity or other forms of deviant behavior.

Be it moods, thinking, or emotions, all require enough oxygen to the brain, which in turn requires optimal levels of nutrients to build the red blood cells to carry the oxygen to the brain. Iron, copper, folacin, B_{12}, B_6, and protein are the nutrients directly involved in making red blood cells, with all other nutrients indirectly needed.

Glucose

A diesel engine will burn kerosene, jet fuel, or diesels of various grades, but it will run best on diesel fuel. The brain will burn fat, protein, or even the liver by-products of alcohol if necessary, but it operates most efficiently on constant levels of blood glucose. In one medical school, a professor gave each student an injection of insulin to lower blood glucose and let the medical students feel the effects firsthand of hypoglycemia. In this class of healthy, normal, intelligent people, some began sobbing uncontrollably, others developed paranoid symptoms, and some had to be restrained.[2] The brain, lungs, kidneys, and the lens of the eye do not function well without a regular supply of blood glucose.

Dieters who fast or who are on low-carbohydrate diets have felt the effects of a glucose-starved brain. Once the body has depleted its carbohydrate stores of glycogen, it begins burning fats in earnest. The by-products of inefficient fat burning are called ketone bodies. The ketone bodies create a mild stupor as the brain attempts to function amidst these alcohol-like substances.

Children after a candy binge, adults in the throes of a hangover, and hypoglycemics not on a specific nutrition program all have lowered mental functions when their blood glucose levels fall. Diet and exercise can alleviate the symptoms.

Metabolites

Just as an automobile engine requires a spark to burn its fuel, the human body must have enzymes to instigate the "burning" of food. These metabolites include the vitamins thiamin, niacin, riboflavin, biotin, and pantothenic acid. Chromium is required to get the glucose into the cells. If these vitamins and mineral are not present in the right proportion and at the proper time, then the brain cannot properly burn its preferential fuel, glucose. The result is poor mental function.

The Electrolyte "Soup"

Electrolytes are ions that create an electrical charge. Each cell in your body is a tiny battery, with ions of sodium, potassium, chloride, and, to a lesser extent, magnesium and calcium to create this electrical charge.[3] As long as there is the proper electrical charge in each of your cells, you have life in your body. The brain is even more dependent than other body cells for this electrical charge, because the brain transmits nervous impulses through this electrolyte "soup."

Though Americans are rarely deficient in sodium or chloride, potassium is likely to be low in the diet. Calcium and magnesium are not only subordinate ions in this electrolyte soup but they are also involved in the release of the neurochemical transmitters that leap the gap between nerve cells. The body has built-in stabilizing systems to regulate the levels of these ions in the blood. Yet if dietary intake is deficient, the stabilizing systems can only do so much. The ion levels are usually kept within survival minimums that may even appear acceptable on a laboratory blood analysis, but they are often not at levels to provide optimal brain function. There are reserve depots for sodium, chloride, and calcium, but levels of potassium, magnesium, and water are not as closely guarded and hence are more likely to fluctuate, since there is no reservoir.

Neurochemical Transmitters

The human brain is an amazing computer. With about 10 billion separate nerve cells and each nerve cell touching up to 1,000 other nerve cells, the possible number of "switches" between brain cells is almost beyond calculation. These connections are the essence of memory, thought, and behavior. The chemicals that bridge the gap (synapse) between nerve cells are collectively called neurochemical transmitters. Some of these substances excite and some inhibit neighboring cells from "firing." Scientists are only beginning to understand the various types of transmitters and their relationship to the diet.[4] Natural substances in the diet have been shown to relieve pain, induce sleep, alleviate stress, control trembling muscles, and perhaps improve memory and mental acuity.

It has been shown that levels of tryptophan in the brain directly affect the levels of serotonin, that influencing our intellectual and emotional process-es. In a true quirk of biochemistry, the key to getting more tryptophan into the brain is not entirely dependent on having more tryptophan in the blood. A membrane shield selectively allows passage of certain substances into the brain. In order to elevate levels of tryptophan and thus serotonin in the brain, one must have a healthy supply of the amino acid tryptophan and a diet high in complex carbohydrates. The carbohydrates help because they stimulate insulin response, which in turn aids the passage of tryptophan into the brain. Get the recommended 12 percent of your calories from proteins, with the bulk of the diet being provided by complex carbohydrates, to stim-ulate ideal tryptophan into the brain.

Other neurochemical transmitters include dopamine and norepineph-rine, which are both built from the amino acid tyrosine. Gamma amino bu-tyric acid (GABA), is another transmitter, some of which is found in pota-toes. Choline, found in the diet and also made in the body, is converted into acetylcholine in the brain for communication between nerve cells. Choline and lecithin have been used to treat the shakes (tardive dyskinesia) that are created when people are overmedicated for too long.[5] Choline and lecithin also help relieve the stupor of the early stages of Alzheimer's disease.[6]

Humans can stimulate internal production of a morphinelike substance, endorphin, for a "natural high" through exercise, meditation, and probably other means. Some of the research in pain clinics is attempting to get pa-tients to create their own endorphins.

Work done at the Massachusetts Institute of Technology has shown that dietary tyrosine helps improve one's stress tolerance.[7] Tyrosine is used to make norepinephrine, which is a stress hormone and a neurochemical trans-mitter. If too much norepinephrine is used up in stress, less tyrosine is left over for mental functions.

Protein (especially the amino acids tryptophan and tyrosine), complex carbohydrates (especially whole grain cereals, legumes, and vegetables), and various vitamins and minerals are all dietary precursors that will eventually form the hundreds of chemicals to communicate messages between brain cells. All of these chemicals are dependent on raw materials found in the diet.

Interfering Agents in the Brain

Essential nutrients in the diet provide the raw materials for all of the brain's wonderous workings. Other substances, not essential to the body, can jam the proper workings of the brain. Protein allergies are now known to be quite common and possibly involve mental symptoms.[8] A swollen brain can result in significant personality changes in a sensitive person eating a certain protein. Likely foods for allergic responses include fish, nuts, milk, eggs, corn, and wheat. See the chapter on allergies for a more in-depth study of this field.

Lead-laden air is common in large urban areas and is known to retard mental processes, especially in young children. Mercury from silver dental fillings may affect some people's moods and health. Aluminum is found in large levels in the brains of Alzheimer's victims. There are other pollutants likely to affect behavior.

Proper Development

By age five, a child's brain has achieved 90 percent of its adult weight. If the child is not fed right, the brain will never develop to its full potential.[9]

All creatures develop their survival skills as quickly as possible. The survival skill of humans is thought. Thus, the human brain develops early and rapidly. This development is time dependent. If all the right nutrients are not present at the right time, then brain construction is stunted, perhaps permanently. Low zinc in the diet of a pregnant woman may irremedially stunt the brain growth of her developing fetus.[10] Scientists have found direct relationships between brain development and protein, folacin, iodine, iron, lactose, taurine, cholesterol, zinc, gamma linolenic acid, EPA (fish oil), and many other nutrients.

Nutrition is important for all people, all of the time. Yet it is particularly crucial for young people and pregnant women since the nutrients will provide raw materials to properly build a brain. Anything less than ideal nourishment may cause a waste of human potential.

Mind Your Diet

Given the abysmal nutritional intake of many people, we feel that diet could relieve much of the emotional distress in America. The brain must be properly built, then optimally nourished and also shielded from chemicals that may jam its performance. To avoid radical swings in moods, as well as increase mental alertness, eat right to think right.

$$\approx$$

32
SEX

"A man comes to me, suffering from cancer, TB, or many other dangerous diseases, and, in addition, he is impotent. He says, 'Doctor, fix up the impotency and let the cancer go hang.' "
—*"Doctor" John Romulus Brinkley*

Nutrition is most definitely related to sex. The reproductive system is one of the nine systems of the human body. Given all the repercussions that the other systems suffer when the body is malnourished, why should the sexual system be exempt?

Along with the need to eat, drink, sleep, and breathe, sex is one of the stronger biological urges that a healthy adult has. Sexual intercourse has at least three purposes: (1) procreation of the species, (2) emotional bonding, (3) physical release. The mind is the most critical link in the successful and continued enjoyment of sex. You must have an interested and interesting partner. And you must feel good about yourself, your partner, and sex. These two simple rules will go a long way toward alleviating serious sexual dysfunctions. Having paid homage to the psychological aspects of sex, let's talk about the biological aspects. Since your body is built from, repaired by, and fueled by nutrients from your diet, it seems obvious that nutrition would play a key role in the healthy enjoyment of sex.

Male Potency and Libido

Impotency is not uncommon, especially among males aged forty and above. In an interesting study, 440 men in this age group with impotence were given complete medical testing. Ninety-two percent were found to have at least two major risk factors toward heart disease. Eighty percent were found to have occlusions of various blood vessels. These people checked in for their sexual problems yet found out that an overwhelming number had vascular problems.[1] The relationship between vascular health and male potency is critical.

There is a a maze of delicate blood vessels throughout the penis. When the male is excited, chemical messages help close the valves in the penis to trap blood. The penis then begins to expand and become hard. If there is vascular disease, these blood vessels cannot properly trap blood, so that an erection cannot occur. Heart disease is indicative of vascular problems throughout the body. If vessels in the heart region are being obstructed, then it is likely that vessels in the brain or legs or even the penis are also being blocked. Consult the chapter on heart disease in this book to prevent or even reverse the effects of vascular disease, which often stunts a man's sexual pleasure.

Zinc is another critical limiting factor in sex drive and erections. Zinc is found in at least eighty different enzyme systems in the body. It is directly involved in making sperm and the male hormone testosterone. Oysters, an old Oriental aphrodisiac, have roughly ten times the zinc concentration of any other food.[2] If a male were impotent from zinc deficiency and consumed oysters for a few months, there is a good chance that the oysters would be an aphrodisiac of a nutritional nature.

Men on renal dialysis (kidney filtration machines) have a high incidence of impotency. The filtering devices are less efficient than real kidneys in keeping zinc in the blood. On giving zinc supplements to a group of impotent men on renal dialysis, there was a marked increase in potency, sperm count, and sex drive.[3] A sperm discharge requires considerable zinc. So does protecting the skin from infections like acne. An old wives' tale threatened teenage boys with acne if they masturbated. Dr. Carl Pfeiffer has found valid reasons that adolescents who have a high zinc need for growth, a low dietary zinc intake, and considerable zinc losses in ejaculation can end up with acne.[4] Indeed, good studies have shown that zinc often improves acne.[5]

Another nutritional factor that directly affects male potency is alcohol. Alcohol dissolves social inhibitions, which results in increased sex drive. Yet too much alcohol interferes with the normal manufacture of the male hormone responsible for sex drive. Alcohol also creates a serious drain on the body's precious zinc supplies. Alcohol makes the desire for sex greater but may diminish the ability to quench that desire. Many serious drug abusers are either not interested in sex or are impotent or sterile.

Female Fertility

Women are born with all the eggs they will ever need, about 400,000. Malnutrition for a female during her own fetal development can play havoc with her ability to bear healthy infants. This is known as the "grandmother effect." The chapter on pregnancy deals with the nutritional issues of pre-natal nourishment. The infant is totally and irremediably dependent on its mother's diet for proper development.

Not only does the mother's diet influence the development of her unborn child, but it also affects her own system. A well-nourished mother has less likelihood of edema, bloating, toxemia, and the dangerous delivery conditions of pre-eclampsia and eclampsia. Optimal B_6, protein, and magnesium will help prevent this dangerous buildup of fluid in the mother's tissues. In clinical trials, some women who were having difficulty getting pregnant found that B_6 supplements also helped them to conceive.

Male Fertility

A male orgasm releases about 200 million sperm. This mass production, which occurs in the testicles, requires specific contributions from the man's diet. With low quantity or quality of sperm, the chances of impregnating a female are slim.

The American male is not one of the more fertile creatures on earth. Obesity, smoking, stress, alcohol and drug abuse can explain much of this infertility. Smoking creates nutritional deficiencies, introduces toxins, and reduces oxygen flow to all parts of the body. Tobacco smoke contains cadmium, which can displace zinc in the body and cause a zinc deficiency to manifest itself as infertility.[6] The testicles function best away from the body, keeping them a few degrees lower than 98.6º F. Obesity, tight pants, jacuzzis, extensive exercise, and heavy cotton underwear warm the testicles, reducing sperm production.

Nutrients are also important to sperm making. Clumping sperm is improved significantly by taking one gram of vitamin C per day.[7] This clumping effect seriously reduces the chances of fertilizing an egg. Arginine has been used to successfully improve the quality and quantity of sperm for conception.[8]

The prostate gland is a doughnut-shaped organ that encircles the tube (urethra) leading from the bladder to the penis opening. The prostate is responsible for adding fluid to the sperm as it makes its way toward an ejaculation. Many men suffer from an enlarged prostate gland, which tends to pinch the urethra and cause painful urination and dribbling. Though surgery is often used to treat this condition, zinc supplements for two to four months have had great success in reducing the swelling of the prostate.[9] Ask your doctor about this kind of treatment.

Premenstrual Syndrome

The symptoms, severity, and timing of PMS vary. Radical mood swings, tender breasts, fluid retention, painful body, and binge eating (especially on sweets) are the most common symptoms. They can occur at any time in the menstrual cycle but are most likely to occur a week to ten days before menstruation. They often cease just hours after menstruation begins. One out of three women have some degree of PMS.

The best "medicine" for treating PMS is usually composed of nutrients and exercise. Studies show the PMS victim to be seriously low in magnesium and other nutrients.[10] A well-controlled scientific study found that women gained significant relief from their premenstrual symptoms by using a high-potency multiple vitamin/mineral supplement.[11] PMS can worsen with overfatness, sedentary lifestyle, after bearing children, between ages thirty and forty. The following nutritional program will help to minimize PMS.

Take a high quality broad spectrum multiple vitamin and mineral supplement providing all essential nutrients, including:

- 50 milligrams per day of vitamin B_6, which helps in the proper manufacturing of the female hormone estrogen and in regulating fluid balance.[12]
- 500 milligrams of calcium (depending on one's food calcium intake). This aids in normal nerve transmission and muscle contractions and helps to relieve tension and cramps.
- 250 milligrams of magnesium, which aids in normal nerve transmission and muscle relaxation. Can improve disposition and cramps.[13]
- 10,000 international units of vitamin A as beta-carotene.
- 200 I.U. of vitamin E.
- 30 milligrams of zinc.
- Three tablets per day of gamma linoleic acid (evening primrose oil). This may help the body to manufacture the many by-products of the essential fatty acid, including prostaglandins for smooth muscle control.[14] See the chapter on quasi-vitamins for more on this nutrient.

Healthy Breasts

Surgical removal of the breast (mastectomy) has been a common surgical procedure in America for the past twenty years. Some physicians in the past have even advocated removal of the breasts simply as a preventive measure. Granted, without breasts there can be no cancer of the breast. But this line of reasoning defies logic. Medical authorities now speculate that many mastectomies were unnecessary.

Women occasionally develop lumps in their breasts. This condition, cystic mastitis, is not serious unless the lumps become malignant or painful. Oftentimes the lumps just go away. A group of women scheduled for breast surgery due to cystic mastitis were asked to avoid coffee, tea, cola, and chocolate. These foods contain many substances related to caffeine that could provoke breast lumps. Thirteen out of twenty (65 percent) of the women who abstained from these foods for one to six months had complete disappearance of breast nodules, pain, tenderness, and nipple discharge.[15] Of the women who continued caffeine consumption, only one got better without medical intervention. Four hundred I.U. per day of vitamin E has also been shown to be effective in slowly dissolving these benign lumps.[16]

Cancer of the breast has been closely associated with smoking, overfatness, and high-fat diets, and also with a low intake of vitamins C, E, A and the mineral selenium. Selenium has been fairly successful at halting the growth of breast tumors.[17] Ideal nutrition can prevent and sometimes reduce benign lumps and tumors in breasts. But no lump in the breast should be taken lightly; see your doctor about the noninvasive approaches of nutrition before the radical means of surgery need to come into play.

Cervical Abnormalities

Another common surgical procedure in the past twenty years has been removal of the uterus and/or ovaries. Two-thirds of women admitted to the hospital for surgery on their uteruses had one or more blatant nutritional deficiency of vitamins A, C, or folate.[18]

Many cases of abnormal cell growth may have been caused by malnutrition. Since folacin is commonly deficient in the American diet and is directly responsible for rapidly growing cells, it makes good sense that low folacin could lead to abnormal growth of new cells. Optimal nutrition will help insure optimal body functions, including in the uterus and other female organs.

AIDS

AIDS (acquired immune deficiency syndrome) may become the bubonic plague of the late 20th century. It is unique for several reasons.[19]

- AIDS is a very new disease. First discovered in the United States only 7 years ago and in Central Africa in the early 1970s, the AIDS virus may be a genetic mutation.

- At first, it affected primarily male homosexuals and intravenous drug users. However, AIDS now is found in many heterosexuals and recipients of AIDS-infected blood transfusions. On a more global basis, AIDS strikes malnourished people of poor regions; its nickname in Africa is "the slim disease." The highest incidence of AIDS in this country is not in big city regions which would have the greatest concentration of junkies and gays, but Belle Glade, Florida, where many poor people live. The highest incidence of AIDS in the world is in the poverty belts of Haiti and Central Africa.

- The AIDS virus may lie dormant in the host for up to a decade. With such a long time lag, there are probably many people infected with AIDS who are unknowingly spreading the disease.

- There is no cure. There is no vaccine to prevent it.

- Most AIDS victims die within a year, after suffering infections, cancer, and even mental deterioration.

- Approximately $100,000 is spent in health care (usually public funds) for the average AIDS victim. Private health care can not afford an AIDS epidemic.

AIDS is associated with a virus known as human immunodeficiency virus (HIV). The incidence of AIDS has grown exponentially since its discovery. As of February 1987, experts estimated that 1.5 million Americans had been exposed to the AIDS virus through blood-to-blood or sperm-to-blood contact. Of these people, 31,000 have contracted AIDS, of which half have died. By 1991, an estimated 270,000 Americans will have contracted AIDS. On a global basis, AIDS is even more alarming. Over 25 million people in Central Africa have been exposed to the AIDS virus. Some experts predict a population shortage in Central Africa by the end of the century because of the AIDS epidemic.

The AIDS virus cripples the immune system and is particularly destructive to the T lymphocytes. This leaves the AIDS victim open to infections. One of the puzzling aspects of AIDS is that only 30% of the people who are exposed to the virus get the condition, not unlike the way not everyone becomes infected with a flu virus when someone sneezes in a crowded room. The evidence suggests that a well nourished person is much less likely to contract AIDS, even if exposed to the virus.[20]

One interesting theory on the nutrition-AIDS link involves zinc. Gay men often have sex several times a day. Much zinc is required to make sperm. Most Americans are low in their intake of zinc. And zinc is also intimately involved in supporting the immune system. Therefore, one noted physician has proposed that major zinc losses would make a person more vulnerable to the AIDS virus.[21] Another physician who specializes in research on the immune system agrees that those who have a well-nourished immune system (especially with respect to vitamins A and E and zinc) have a much better chance at thwarting the AIDS virus should they be exposed to it.[22]

Although there appear to be no surefire cures for AIDS, large doses of vitamin C (up to 40 grams daily) have been shown to extend the quality and quantity of life for AIDS patients.[23] John Beldekas, Ph.D., formerly of the Boston University School of Medicine, found that AIDS victims showed noticeable relief from their symptoms when placed on a well-balanced vegetarian diet. Vegetarianism may offer a certain amount of prevention against AIDS, as well as relieving symptoms in people who already have AIDS. Much research has shown that positive thinking helps to keep the immune system working ideally.[24] Other non-nutrition approaches to preventing AIDS infection includes the use of condoms during sex, monogamy, and curtailing anonymous blood donations.

Energy, Attitude, and Looks

There are some obvious nutritional relationships to sexual performance. Someone who is always tired or cranky from chronic malnutrition is unlikely to be a fun sex partner. Low energy levels can stem from the anemia of a low red blood cell count, which involves the nutrients iron, B_{12}, folacin, B_6, copper, and protein. Low levels of energy nutrients like niacin, pantothenic acid, biotin, riboflavin, chromium, and thiamin can result in lethargy. Erratic swings in blood glucose could bring about a tempermental or tired person. Fifty million women in the world use oral contraceptives,[25] which can cause deficiencies of numerous nutrients including B_6 and folacin and lead to lethargy and depression.[26]

A good attitude is important to sexual enjoyment and very relevant to nutrition. See the chapter on mental functions to better appreciate the ways nutrients contribute to your moods.

One's appearance can be an important factor in sexual fulfillment. Consult the chapter on obesity for information on how to permanently maintain a lean body. Hair, skin, and nails are manifestations of the body's internal health. Since these tissues are considered sacrificial by the body, their looks will suffer when nutrient intake falls below ideal levels.

For more sex and better sex, for greater potency and fertility, for the healthy outcome of pregnancy, for fewer problems with premenstrual syndrome, for the reduced risk of breast lumps, uterine abnormalities, and prostate swelling, and for greater energy, better attitude, and more attractive looks, keep your nutrient intake tuned to "optimal."

33

THE ATHLETE

"A nutrition chain is only as strong as its weakest link."
—DR. ROGER WILLIAMS, UNIVERSITY OF TEXAS

Of the most susceptible groups within the population—heart attack victims, terminal cancer patients, the listless elderly, and obese individuals—athletes are the most vulnerable to nutrition misinformation. They will try anything. Big money, prestige, careers, years of training, and self-esteem are at stake. When it comes to trimming hundredths of a second off one's time, diet can be the key factor between gold, silver, bronze, and "thanks for coming."

Most Americans are somewhere between marginally and grossly malnourished. Athletes are no exception. Actually, the travel schedule of professional and college athletes often exposes them to a worse-than-normal variety of food. The stress of perform-or-else, along with abundant free time, can drive even the most devoted athlete into regular sessions of junk food eating. Wrestlers, dancers, jockeys and others concerned about their weight are particularly prone to malnutrition.

Energy

For the athlete, the question is how to get enough fuel into the body to prevent weight loss or scavenging of lean tissue. Athletes want their bodies to be burning the optimal fuel during the event. They also need to provide enough energy nutrients to "spark" the fuel.

The body can burn carbohydrate, fat, or protein. Carbohydrates are the preferred fuel. Excellent studies have shown that athletes who consume 60 to 80 percent of their calories from carbohydrates will have more glycogen in their body, and thus more endurance.[1] The average adult body stores about 350 grams of glycogen, providing about 1,400 calories.[2] This will propel someone through about one and a half hours of intense activity. Once the glycogen is gone, the body must adapt to burning fat. In the conversion process, fat-burning enzymes must be built up in the cells. This is a transition phase known as the "wall"; the brain and body is starved of energy, resulting in outrageous fatigue and distress. Some athletes now prefer to start the event in ketosis, already burning fats, in order to avoid confronting the "wall" sometime during the event.

Another approach is to carb load. This involves tricking the body into doubling its normal carbohydrate stores by totally depleting the glycogen supply for several days, then feeding massive "carbs" to this depleted system.

Carb loading follows a specific regimen. Five days before the event, train extensively and vigorously.[3] Drain every ounce of glycogen from your muscle stores. You must avoid restocking the carbohydrates, so eat only protein and fat foods. Four days before the event, train equally hard and eat as you did the day before. This day's training will be difficult, since you now have almost no glycogen for body fuel and will feel very lethargic. Do it anyway to extract the remaining glycogen from the muscles and blood. On the third day before the event, continue eating as above, but do a light workout. You have now finished the depletion phase. Two days before the event, do not train, and begin carb loading. This begins the repletion phase. Select primarily fruits, vegetables, grains and cereals. The day before the event, do the same: no training and high carbohydrate food intake. By the day of the event, you will have supersaturated your muscle tissues with twice the normal glycogen supplies to help prevent encountering the "wall" en route.

For events that go beyond ninety minutes of intense exercise carb loading may be valuable. For other sports it is probably useless. Since it causes extra glycogen and fluids to be stored in the muscles, they can become stiff and less flexible. Diabetics and hypoglycemics should not follow this program, since it creates serious ketosis and abnormal blood glucose levels during the depletion stage.

Another form of maximum energy metabolism is to provide the body with the nutrients to burn the fuel: thiamin, niacin, riboflavin, pantothenic acid, and biotin. Also, chromium is required for glucose to enter the cells.

A Swiss study published in the *Annals of the New York Academy of Sciences* found that trained athletes given 1,000 milligrams of ascorbic acid daily were much better able to burn fats both in muscle and liver cells.[4]

Carnitine, involved in the rate-limiting step (the bottleneck) in burning fats, has been clinically shown to improve athletic performance.[5]

At least tentatively, several other nutrients have been successful in improving muscle functions. Lipoic acid, coenzyme Q, nucleosides of inosine and adenosine, and creatine all have potential for improving athletic performance.[6] Oral zinc supplements increased the stamina of rat muscles.[7]

Since relatively large segments of the population are low in their intake of many of these nutrients, it becomes obvious that better eating habits and supplements would be of value to the athlete. Not only do athletes often eat poorly, but their nutrient requirements are much higher. Thiamin requirements during intense exercise increase fifteenfold.[8] It would be impossible to get this amount of thiamin from food.

The athlete needs copious quantities of calories to maintain ideal body composition during training. Carbohydrates are preferred. Protein is required for tissue repair but can impair energy levels if consumed extensively as fuel. Fat is a concentrated energy source in the diet that can be valuable to the super-active athlete to help avoid weight loss. The percentage of calories in the diet as recommended by the Senate Diet Goals (protein 12 percent, fat 30 percent, and carbohydrates 58 percent) can change to 10:25:65 in the normal athlete and to 8:35:57 in the extremely active athlete.

Caffeine has been shown to increase muscular endurance by 20 percent when 330 milligrams (about three cups of coffee) were given one hour before an event.[9] Caffeine probably helps the athlete via its stimulation of insulin and promotion of extra fats into the bloodstream. Caffeine is also a diuretic, however, and thus can dehydrate the athlete as well as create a need to urinate at inopportune moments.

Ginseng has been a favorite Oriental medicine and tonic for many centuries. Claims of its benefits include enhanced mental, physical, and sexual vigor. Studies in Europe have found that ginsana (a standardized ginseng) improves reactions, coordination,[10] and oxygen-carrying capacity.[11] (Ginseng is more thoroughly discussed in the quasi-vitamins chapter.)

Fluid and Electrolyte Balance

Electrolytes are minerals in the fluid of the body that create low-level electricity, which is essential for the membrane potential in all cells. The body is two-thirds water, with a specific mixture of sodium, potassium, chloride, magnesium, and calcium. Fluid, electrolytes, and some minerals are lost in sweat. The body attempts to keep its temperature within normal range through the evaporative cooling that occurs with perspiration. This loss of precious fluids and minerals retards performance[12] and may even cause death. Every year about five high school athletes die in football practice from dehydration.

Up to ten quarts of water can be lost in one hot day. This could be fatal, unless regular water breaks are taken. The athlete should consume 5 to 10 cups of clear fluids daily, and drink something every ten to twenty minutes during intense, strenuous exercise. The fluid should contain at least some sugar (sucrose, glucose, lactose, fructose, honey) in a 5 percent solution, or about a tablespoon of sugar per quart of fluid.[13] If the day is warm, the fluid should be cool to help lower the core temperature of the body. If the exercise is longer than a half hour, then the addition of electrolytes, especially sodium, potassium, and chloride, may be of benefit. You can make your own electrolyte drink by mixing together the following: one tablespoon of sugar, honey, or sweetener; one-fourth teaspoon of Lite Salt (contains potassium, sodium, chloride, magnesium, and iodide); flavoring; and one quart of clean water.

If the day is hot and muggy, then sweating will not efficiently cool the body and perhaps it would be best to work out in the cool of the morning or evening.

Calcium is important for muscle contraction, while magnesium is crucial for muscle relaxation. Both have their roles as electrolytes and as muscle regulators. One thousand milligrams of calcium daily should prevent muscle fatigue. There is very good evidence that insufficient magnesium levels are responsible for the abundance of sudden heart attacks in this country.[14] Jim Fixx, the well-conditioned guru of runners, died at age fifty-two of a heart muscle spasm (ventricular fibrillation). Although he had also been genetically inclined toward it, a heart attack while running is indicative of magnesium deficiency. It is likely that many athletes experience muscle spasms from low levels of electrolytes, especially magnesium and potassium. Such a muscle spasm occurring in the heart region could be fatal.

Stress Adaptation

In one study, 2,000 milligrams of vitamin C per day were given to a group of people, with another group receiving a placebo. All were then tested for their tolerance of altitude. The vitamin-C-supplemented group had an endurance gain of 26 percent over the placebo group.[15]

South African miners supplemented with 250 milligrams of vitamin C daily were better able to maintain a lower body temperature and lost less body fluids in the stifling heat (about 125° F.) of a deep mine.[16] This and other data show that for athletes exposed to extremes of heat, cold, and altitude, the optimally nourished may be able to tolerate the conditions—and perform—better.

Nutrients to Prevent Accelerated Oxidation

Extremely active people die sooner than others. With all the praise heaped on exercise this may seem a bit surprising. Exercise is, indeed, good for you. Yet exercise accelerates the oxidative "rusting" in the tissues. Supplements can slow down oxidation. Vitamins A, C, E, and the minerals selenium and manganese are all proven antioxidants and would be valuable additions to the active individual's nutrition program.[17, 18]

Nutrition for Bodybuilders

Body builders are interested in maximum lean mass muscle definition in order to look ornately sculptured, so it is crucial for these people to stay on a low-fat diet.

Competitive bodybuilders often pay exorbitant prices for "free amino acids" and other supplements and usually consume far too much protein, thinking that all dietary protein will turn into muscle. Too much protein strains the kidneys and liver, causes loss of calcium from the bones, and lowers energy levels. Even the largest bodybuilders should keep their protein intake near 100 grams per day. Some weight lifters will take large amounts of powdered protein (which is probably unnecessary and may be harmful) yet have no B_6 supplements to process the protein. They could be creating a serious B_6 deficiency from their high protein intake.[19] Long ago it was thought that heat and sweating raised protein needs. A more recent study showed that this is true, but the body quickly adjusts so that within a week or so it is not losing much protein.[20]

Anabolic steroids have been discussed and cursed thoroughly in the scientific literature.[21] There is a safer way to quick muscle development. A 1981 study from the University of Rome found that male volunteers given 1,200 milligrams of l-lysine plus 1,200 milligrams of l-arginine at night on empty stomachs had a remarkable increase in lean mass.[22] Using these supplements, the subjects were able to quickly increase their muscle mass when they followed their normal intense training routine. Carnitine, due to its leading role in fat burning, might help to minimize fat in the skin region.

Steroids have their side effects.[23] Do not believe someone who tells you otherwise. There are already isolated incidences of young and healthy users who have developed liver cancer. Impotence and sterility are also possible side effects.

The Pre-Event Meal

For centuries, the usual pre-event meal consisted of copious quantities of rare meat. If the athlete really believes in this ritual, it may work. But meat and fat should be avoided before a contest. It takes only a few hours for a high-carbohydrate meal to be assimilated; it takes over six hours for a high-protein meal and about twenty-four hours for a high-fat meal to finally pass through the digestive system. Remember, these figures are for normal situations. The stress of a serious competitive event could hardly be considered normal. Therefore, the amount of time required for digestion is even longer.

We recommend that pre-event meals be eaten at least four hours prior to the event and that the meal be high in fluid and carbohydrates. There are many powdered blender drinks that make fine pre-game meals. They are easy on the stomach while providing some energy and fluid. A bloated digestive tract can be a nuisance.

If small amounts of food are taken during competition, they should be soft, high in fluid, high in easily absorbed carbohydrates,[24] and low in fat and spices. Most important, it should be something that the athlete feels comfortable with.

Building Red Blood Cells

Many athletes are anemic, probably because of the abnormally high destruction of red blood cells during intensive exercise.[25] The success of athletic performance depends largely on getting enough oxygen to the muscle tissue. In anaerobic events such as sprints, oxygen transport is not as important since the event lasts only ten or twenty seconds. In an even like the Turkey Climb, a one-mile bike ride up a 20 percent grade in Los Angeles, however, the contestants often end up with blue legs and severe confusion due to a lack of oxygen. Training is a key component of improving oxygen transport to the cells. One recent development for competitive athletes is blood doping, and is certain to create problems in regulating Olympic events. In this method, the athlete trains hard, often at a high elevation to stimulate greater production of red blood cells. A month before the event, a pint of blood is removed from the athlete's body and refrigerated. Just prior to the event, the stored blood (or perhaps some of the red blood cells) is infused into his body, providing an abnormally high number of red blood cells to carry oxygen to the muscles. No one really knows whether there are serious side effects to this technique.

A safer method is through nutrition. Nutrients that are directly involved in building red blood cells include iron, copper, B_{12}, B_6, folacin, and protein.

Recommended Program

1. Eat small frequent meals high in complex carbohydrates. Follow the guidelines in the chapter on the exchange system. While an optimal diet

may seem optional for nonathletes, it is mandatory for serious competitors.

2. Consume large amounts of fluids regularly. Saturate the body with food sources of potassium, magnesium, and calcium before the event. Consume a balanced electrolyte drink during the event. Take 500 milligrams of potassium, 400 milligrams of calcium, and 400 milligrams of magnesium after your workout (with a meal). These electrolyte-minerals will help prevent cramping.

3. Find a vitamin/mineral supplement with nutrient levels in the "supplemental" ranges given in the chapters on vitamins and minerals.

Remember, more is not necessarily better. If you provide your body with an optimal level of nutrients, then your body will reward you with optimal performance.

PART SIX

NUTRITION AND THE GOVERNMENT

AMERICA WAS FOUNDED AS A NATION OF FARMERS. WE HAVE progressed through the manufacturing phase and now into the era of technology and information. Yet it is still our space age farmers who provide the United States with food independence from other nations and something to offset our unfavorable balance of trade. The government tries to keep the food clean, safe, and properly labeled; to provide recommendations for a "decent diet"; to feed those who cannot feed themselves; and to educate those who need nutrition knowledge. This is not always done fully, nor to perfection. But it is a good system upon which to base future improvements. The government's role in the food business of America is extensive. This section is dedicated to unraveling that complex and sometimes insufficient role in the nourishment of Americans.

34

UNITED STATES
RECOMMENDED DAILY
ALLOWANCES

"We the people of the United States . . . promote the general welfare. . . . "
—PREAMBLE TO THE CONSTITUTION OF THE UNITED STATES

In the deep dark moments of World War II, there was considerable food rationing in the United States. The nation's leaders, concerned about the health of the people on these marginal food supplies, asked a panel of scientists to create a guideline for nutrient intake that would probably secure decent health for most adults. This guideline became known as the minimum daily requirement.

After the war and food rationing, the government asked a similar group of scientists at the National Academy of Sciences to develop more than minimum standards. The government wanted nutrient intake levels that would provide a margin of safety for most healthy adults. They created the recommended dietary allowances (RDA), which are amounts of essential nutrients that should keep most people healthy. There are separate RDAs for different ages, men, women, pregnancy, and lactation. The RDAs are updated approximately every five years to include the most current scientific findings. Since not all of the RDAs for each age group could be put on a food label, the Food and Drug Administration was assigned the task of creating one standard of nutrient comparison that would help the consumer understand the nutritional content of a food item. Enter the United States recommended dietary allowance, or USRDA. Based upon many of the higher values of the RDA, the USRDA is the standard used for food label comparison. The World Health Organization (WHO), Food and Agriculture Organization (FAO), and many other developed nations have their own versions of the RDA. Most are quite similar.

Values and Limitations of the RDA

The RDA has value in that it was established by an elite group of scientists; provides the only standard for comparing adequacy of diets; is based upon valid scientific studies; takes into consideration some variance in human needs; and allows a standard for nutrition labelling information.

But the RDA does not allow for optimal levels of health. Although it makes recommendations for all age groups, there is a growing wealth of data that show that the RDA for older, very young, very active, and infirm individuals should be markedly higher. There are nutrients that lie in a gray zone of quasi-nutrients, such as choline, carnitine, and inositol, which are not mentioned in the RDA. Other substances, such as fiber and the essential fatty acid, are recognized as essential nutrients but not mentioned in the RDA. Essential trace elements like chromium and selenium do not have an RDA but rather are given an "acceptable range." Some nutrients, when taken at greater-than-RDA levels, can reduce the damaging effects of pollution. People using tobacco products, drugs of almost any type, or too much alcohol have far higher nutrients needs, also.

There are many problems in creating one nutrient level that millions of people should adhere to. The Food and Nutrition Board of the National Academy of Sciences readily admits that 2.5 percent of the population is not covered by its guidelines due to the numerous fluctuating factors.

The RDA for additional energy needs for a lactating woman is 500 calories. The number of calories needed by a lactating woman is proportional to the volume and calorie density of the milk produced. Both of these factors vary substantially with the size, age, and activity of the infant. How efficiently a woman converts calories in the diet to calories in her milk also varies. From all these variables, the FNB guesstimates that the average woman produces 850 milliliters of milk daily, requiring an additional 750 calories in her diet. The board then goes on to assume that most women gain unwanted fat stores during pregnancy and that a calorie deficiency during lactation will help them to lose this extra weight. Putting together the variables and assumptions, the board decided that 500 extra calories per day will meet the needs of the breast-feeding mother. Although an abundance of scientific data were used to arrive at this number, you can see the obvious shortcomings of reducing millions of unique human situations to one statistical average.

In 1980, the Food and Nutrition Board of the National Academy of Sciences commissioned the Committee on Dietary Allowances to review the RDAs and make recommendations for appropriate changes. Five years and half a million dollars later, that committee, surprisingly, recommended lowering the RDAs for vitamin A (by 25 to 33 percent), C (by 33 to 50 percent), B_6 (by about 10 percent), and iron (by about 16 percent).[1] It did recommend raising the RDAs for calcium by about 25 percent. A wealth of data have shown the protective effect that some of these nutrients exert against certain common ailments like cancer, premenstrual syndrome, and anemia. Deficiencies already exist for these nutrients in much of the American population. Lowering the RDAs may improve the alleged nutritional status of the American people on paper (since fewer people will then be considered deficient) but will only serve to mask and worsen the overall health of this country.

Essentially, the RDA is a target to shoot for. It is the only means we have of comparing a food item or someone's diet to known standards. Those consuming less than the RDA are not guaranteed malnutrition, nor are those consuming the RDA guaranteed good nutritional status. Use the RDA as a guideline, not a law to be inscribed in stone.

35
SENATE DIETARY GOALS

"If a free society cannot help the many who are poor, it cannot save the few who are rich."

—JOHN F. KENNEDY

In 1976, the Senate Select Committee on Nutrition and Human Needs gathered a cadre of prestigious scientists to seek their advice on dietary recommendations for the American people. From dietary surveys performed by the United States Department of Agriculture, they found that we ate too much sugar, salt, fat, refined foods, cholesterol, and not enough complex carbohydrates, fiber, and plant protein.

The first Senate dietary goals did not make any reference to the abundance of calories and alcohol consumed in the U.S., nor did they speak of the benefits of fluoridated water. Yet they performed a significant task in that they told the American people how to lower the risks for degenerative ailments.[1] Among the findings:

Fat. Current daily intake—45 percent of total calories (7 percent polyunsaturated, 19 percent monounsaturated, 16 percent saturated). Recommended daily intake—30 percent of total calories (10 percent polyunsaturated, 10 percent monounsaturated, 10 percent saturated).

Carbohydrates. Current daily intake—46 percent of total calories (18 percent sugar, 28 percent complex and naturally occurring carbohydrates). Recommended daily intake—58 percent of total calories (10 percent sugar, 48 percent complex and naturally occurring carbohydrates).

Protein. Current daily intake—12 percent of total calories. Recommended daily intake—12 percent of total calories (more of it from vegetable protein).

Cholesterol. Current daily intake—600 milligrams. Recommended daily intake—300 milligrams.

Sodium. Current daily intake—6 to 18 grams of salt. Recommended daily intake—5 grams or less of salt.

Fiber. Current daily intake—low. Recommended daily intake—increase substantially.

Calories. Current daily intake—too much (resulting in overweight). Recommended daily intake—balance calorie intake and output.

Dietary Guidelines and Suggested Foods

1. Eat a variety of foods daily. Include these every day: fruits and vegetables; whole grain and enriched breads and cereals; milk and milk products; meats, fish, poultry, eggs; dried peas and beans.

2. Maintain ideal weight. Increase physical activity; reduce calories by eating fewer fatty foods and sweets and less sugar, and by avoiding too much alcohol; lose weight gradually.

3. Avoid too much fat, saturated fat, and cholesterol. Choose low-fat protein sources such as lean meats, fish, poultry, dried peas and beans; use eggs and organ meats in moderation; limit intake of fats on and in foods; trim fats from meats; broil, bake, or boil—don't fry; read food labels for fat content.

4. Eat foods with adequate starch and fiber. Substitute starches for fats and sugars; select whole grain breads and cereals, fruits and vegetables, dried beans and peas, and nuts to increase fiber and starch intake.

5. Avoid too much sugar. Use less syrup and honey; reduce candy, soft drinks, cookies; select fresh fruits or fruits canned in light syrup or their own juices; read food labels (sucrose, glucose, dextrose, maltose, lactose, fructose, syrups, and honey are all sugars).

6. Avoid too much sodium. Reduce salt in cooking; add little or no salt at the table; limit salty items like potato chips, pretzels, salted nuts, popcorn, condiments, cheese, pickled foods, and cured meats; read labels for sodium or salt content, especially in processed and snack foods.

7. If you drink alcohol, do so in moderation. Individuals who drink should limit all alcoholic beverages to one or two drinks per day. Use of alcoholic beverages during pregnancy can result in the birth defects and mental retardation of fetal alcohol syndrome.

36

REGULATION OF THE VITAMIN INDUSTRY

"What do vitamins do for you? Well, I don't know about you, but they built my home, put my kids through college, bought me nice cars. . . ."
—PRESIDENT OF A MAJOR VITAMIN MANUFACTURING FIRM

In 1973, legislation was introduced to make it mandatory to obtain a physician's prescription for any level of nutrients beyond 100 percent of the USRDA. The health food industry responded by soliciting support from its millions of customers across the country. The avalanche of mail that arrived in Washington showed that the people of this country wanted the right of free choice in the nutrition supplement market. Legislators listened and have since abandoned the idea of serious restrictions on the vitamin industry.

There are a few laws that the vitamin industry must heed, however:

• Levels of folacin supplements cannot exceed 400 micrograms per day for adults, and 800 micrograms per day for pregnant women. More than this requires a physician's prescription. Folacin and vitamin B_{12} work closely together in the body. A deficiency of one can often be mistaken for a deficiency of the other. If a person were seriously low in B_{12} and were taking high doses of folacin, the folacin could conceivably mask the symptoms of pernicious anemia (B_{12} deficiency) and lead to permanent nerve damage.

• No claims can be made by a vitamin manufacturer as to health benefits to be derived by taking its products. For instance, a vitamin bottle cannot say, "Cures or prevents heart disease."

• Coated tablets should dissolve in sixty minutes and uncoated tablets in thirty minutes in the stomach of a healthy individual.

• A nutritional product can contain no more than 2 percent impurities (excipients).

• All products must contain what the manufacturer's label states. They must have the same amount of nutrients after a two-year shelf life.

- Due to problems encountered by kidney patients, potassium levels cannot exceed 95 milligrams per day without a prescription.

An attempt was made by the FDA to limit vitamin A levels to 10,000 I.U. per day and vitamin D to 400 I.U. in nutrition supplements. Given the high level of these nutrients found in foods, however, this has been a difficult concept to enforce.

Two-thirds of all households buy vitamin supplements, while one-third of all people take them. But do the people get what they need? In many cases, we don't think so, because of flaws in the governmental regulation of the vitamin industry.

"Bioavailability" refers to how much you absorb of a nutrient. Bioavailability is known to vary considerably among foods.[1] The same probably is true for nutrients from pills. Yet few or no studies are done on this issue when a pill is made. You may be absorbing far less than what the label states, depending on the form of the vitamin or mineral used and the way it was processed. Time release capsules have been found in the feces and large intestines. Time release vitamin C is less efficiently absorbed than regular C.[2] Time release tablets may even accumulate in the stomachs of patients with gastrointestinal problems.[3]

Labels should compare the nutrient content to the USRDA. In an attempt to make their products look more potent, some manufacturers will compare their products to the minimum daily requirements (MDR), which are substantially lower than the USRDA. Other manufacturers will express the units in abnormal ways. For instance, thiamin is usually expressed in milligrams, with 1.5 being the USRDA. A manufacturer may claim 1,200 micrograms of thiamin, an impressive number, but equivalent to only 1.2 milligrams.

Many vitamin formulas seem to have no biochemical rationale. Nutrients that Americans are commonly low in, such as selenium and chromium, are often omitted.

Many nutrients are included in negligible quantities, merely so that the manufacturer can list them on the label. Fifty milligrams of potassium is about 1 percent of an active adult's daily needs, yet it appeals to the consumer who sees this nutrient included.

Many vitamin C products claim to be made with rose hips or acerola cherries, for which the consumer pays nearly triple the price of synthetic C. "Chelated minerals" is another sales pitch. Each of these claims may have some nutritional merit, yet there is no minimum requirement for these substances. A manufacturer can claim chelated minerals or rose hips C and have only 1 percent of these items in the product. Acerola and rose hips C are bulky and expensive. Even a generous manufacturer would give no more than 10 percent of the C in this form. Since there are no federal guidelines for minimum levels, the consumer has no idea of what percentage of the product is chelated or rose hips.

"Natural" and "organic" have no legal meaning. Chemically, they refer to carbon compounds. All vitamins, whether synthetically or naturally derived, are technically organic. All vitamins, natural and synthetic, have the same action in the body. There may be accessory factors found in natural foods that aid in the absorption or action of certain vitamins and minerals, but whether these are found in "natural" vitamins is anybody's guess. Consumers pay more for the "natural" label with no assurance that the product is different or better.

Many people go to health food stores in desperation because of poor health. Once there, they are subjected to the sincere but misleading claims of a sales clerk telling them which nutrients will help what condition. If a registered dietician made the same statements, he or she could be indicted and possibly jailed for practicing medicine without a license. With people's health on the line, there should be certification for "nutritionists," with penalties for fakers.

The 2 percent allowable standard for impurities in vitamins is far higher than the standards set for the drug industry. Since nutrients are being used by trained professionals for therapeutic purposes, vitamin manufacturers should have equally stringent purity codes. The partial nerve paralysis caused by excessive doses of vitamin B_6 does not occur in pharmacological grade B_6. This indicates that the impurities cause the problem, not the vitamin.[4]

Some vitamin manufacturers omit the nutrient that they claim on the label. Drug manufacturers are federally licensed and more likely to be truthful about including all claimed ingredients in their vitamin products, since their licenses are more expensive and inspection by the FDA is more frequent. But for many of the "brand X" vitamin manufacturers, the license is cheap and the inspections are few, if any. These vitamin pills, especially those that seem remarkably cheap, may not contain what it claims. This is illegal. Yet the FDA's manpower is insufficient to police the industry. Also, the FDA feels that the less vitamins present, the less the possibility of harming the consumer. We can only say *caveat emptor*—let the buyer beware. If the vitamin product seems too inexpensive to be possible, think again about buying it.

37

FOOD LABELING

The Food and Drug Administration has the responsibility of overseeing the nutritional comparison of food products, while the United States Department of Agriculture grades and inspects various food items.

All food labels must state:[1]

• The common name of the product (a generic name, such as catsup).
• The name and address of the company responsible for making or distributing the product.
• The net contents by weight, volume, or number of units.
• The ingredients in descending order. Thus the first item listed is the most prevalent in the product.

If any nutritional claims are made about the product, then it must also have:[2]

• Serving or portion size
• Servings per container.
• Calories per serving.
• The amount of protein, fat, carbohydrate in grams per serving.
• The following nutrients as a percentage of the USRDA: protein, vitamin, thiamin, niacin, riboflavin, calcium, iron. If any of these nutrients are found in levels of less than 2 percent of the USRDA, they must have an asterisk (*) and an explanation.

There are several types of claims that are not allowed on food labels:

1. That a food is effective as a treatment for a disease.
2. That the soil on which food is grown may be responsible for deficiencies in quality.
3. That a balanced diet of ordinary foods cannot supply adequate amounts of nutrients (except the iron requirements of infants, children, and pregnant or lactating women).

4. That storage, transportation, processing, or cooking of a food may be responsible for deficiencies in its quality.

5. That a food has particular dietary qualities when such qualities have not been shown to be significant in human nutrition.

6. That a natural vitamin is superior to a synthetic vitamin.

Unfortunately, rules 2, 3, and 4 are not necessarily true statements and therefore do nothing to protect or educate the consumer. Rule 2 is inaccurate since it is known that food grown on selenium-poor soil is significantly lower in selenium than foods grown on selenium-rich soil. Rule 3 is inaccurate since "ordinary food" (i.e., processed) is often nutritionally depleted and cannot maintain ideal health for many people. Rule 4 is also untrue since an abundance of data has proved that the storage, transportation, processing, and cooking of a food can markedly deteriorate its nutrient content.[3]

The Value of Labels

Though there is not much of a plot line to them, labels can make for very interesting reading, especially if you are concerned about health and money. By comparing costs per serving you can determine the best buys. By comparing nutrients present and their percentage of the USRDA you can better select a healthier food item. Food labels can be deceiving, however.

The food manufacturer has conjured up some interesting products to entice the calorie-conscious consumer. A "lo-cal" product may have only a few calories less than the competitive brands and be considerably more expensive. Often a "diet food" contains extra water or has had air whipped into it. The consumer ends up with less product at a higher price. Buy the real food and use less of it, if you need to diet.

The FDA can ask food manufacturers to properly label products, but a request is not as effective as a law. Recently it has been found that bone meal contains significant levels of lead. The FDA requested that bone meal manufacturers put a warning label on their product for children and pregnant and lactating women to be aware of the dangers of lead consumption. Only one of the fifty companies notified by the FDA voluntarily complied with the request.

When a product contains little or none of the food category stated on the label, then it must have "imitation" somewhere on the label. Thus imitation chicken soup or grape juice need not contain any chicken or grapes.

There are about 300 different food items that have an officially sanctioned standard of identity and therefore do not have to put any ingredients on their labels. Thus items (such as catsup, mayonnaise, and butter) are exempt from declaring any ingredients.

Various types of sugar can be split into their specific names so that the food manufacturer does not have to list sugar as the main ingredient. Levulose, glucose, mannose, dextrose, sucrose, and corn syrup, are all different names for one thing: sugar.

Food labels can be the consumer's valuable ally, but only if you read them and read them carefully.

PART SEVEN

PRACTICAL APPLICATIONS OF NUTRITION

THIS SECTION SUMMARIZES THE INFORMATION IN THE EARLI-
er parts of the book and puts it into practical working knowledge for your
everyday life.

The basic elements of an optimal nutrition program should be food as a
foundation and supplemental vitamins as insurance. Chapter 38, on the exchange system, shows you categories of foods, which to eat, when, how
much, and why.

Chapter 39 is critical to applying nutrition principles in the kitchen. The
Pritikin program was effective at lowering fats in the blood, yet the pre-
scribed foods were so austere that they sent all but the most captivated scur-
rying back to their snack cupboard. We teach you how to make nutritious
foods taste delicious.

There are many good foods. But there are a few super foods. Chapter 40
deals with the nutritional talent and versatility of these super foods. Keep
them on your grocery list often.

38

THE EXCHANGE SYSTEM

"Nothing in education is so astonishing as the amount of ignorance it accumulates in the form of inert fact."

—HENRY ADAMS

What good is abundant nutrition knowledge unless one can select the right foods to eat? The essence of optimal nutrition begins with food. You may not remember much of the thousands of details of this book when you put it down, but you should remember this chapter.

In the 1940s, scientists knew enough about nutrition to be able to make some recommendations about what to eat; they formulated the seven food groups. Educators trying to teach nutrition found this system too complicated. So, in 1956, the USRDA consolidated the seven food groups into the four food groups:

fruits and vegetables
breads and cereals
meats
dairy

This system answered the call to simplify and is still used today by many health educators. Yet the four food groups method has some major flaws. Half of the groups are high in fat and cholesterol. It provides fewer plant selections. It classifies fruits and vegetables together as though they contribute similar nutrients, which they don't. It has a vague method of portion control. "One serving" could be interpreted as anything from a half cup to two cups. Since overweight is so common in this country, portion control should be emphasized. There is no allowance for fats and condiments. Butter on bread or the absorbed oil in a piece of fried chicken isn't counted. Fatty meat counts the same as lean fish. It shouldn't. The meats group leaves few options for vegetarians. And studies found that even when satisfying the "basic four" requirements, a person could be deficient in numerous nutrients.[1]

The exchange system, formulated by the American Diabetic and Dietetic associations, improves drastically on the old method. We now have the following groups:

protein/meat (high, medium, and low fat)
vegetables
fruits
breads and cereals
dairy
fats
free (mostly fluid and fiber foods or condiments)

"Exchange" merely means that, within each group, one selection may be exchanged for another and still provide similar calories, protein, carbohydrate, and fat. A small tortilla is equal in these respects to a piece of bread or half a bagel.

Each group has a reason for being in your daily diet. If you tried to rely on nutritional powders and pills for your nutrient intake, you would be taking handfuls of pills and still probably develop some deficiency or imbalance. Foods are the essence of optimal nutrition, while supplements are of secondary importance.

This system has been finely tuned and time tested so that it is sanctioned by all major health agencies in the United States, including the American Dietetic Association, the United States Department of Public Health, the American Diabetic Association, and the American Medical Association. The exchange system is an ideal compromise: It provides the accuracy not found in the four food groups and the simplicity not found in looking each food up in the USDA's *Nutrient Analysis Guide*.

"Leader nutrients" refers to the nutrients contributed uniquely by each of the six groups in the exchange system of meal planning. The leader nutrients for each group are:

Protein/meat: protein, B_{12}, zinc, iron, B_6, niacin, carnitine, phosphorus, choline, myoinositol.

Fruit: vitamin A, C, simple carbohydrates (especially fructose), fluid, fiber, bioflavonoids, potassium.

Vegetables: vitamin A, K, C, folacin, potassium, fluid, fiber, chlorophyll, cruciferous vegetables, naturally occurring complex and simple carbohydrates.

Dairy: protein, calcium, lactose, vitamin A, D, niacin, riboflavin, biotin, gastroinositol, fluid, lactobacillus bacteria.

Breads and cereals: chromium, silicon, vitamin E, thiamin, niacin, magnesium, iron, complex carbohydrates, fiber (all primarily from whole grain products).

Fats: high in calories, vitamin E, linoleic acid, linolenic acid, choline.

What follows is a list of representative members of each group. Be aware of the need for honesty with yourself. One small apple equals one fruit exchange, which is roughly 40 calories. There are gorgeous apples that are nearly softball size. These would be four or five fruit exchanges, or 160 to 200 calories. Similarly, one slice of bread is a bread exchange. Yet home-made bread can be cut in any thickness, and store-bought bread varies in its weight and fiber content. Therefore, a sandwich made on a submarine bun would provide perhaps four bread exchanges.

Vegetables: ½ cup

asparagus	green pepper	onions
bean sprouts	greens	rhubarb
beets	beet	rutabaga
broccoli	chard	sauerkraut
Brussels sprouts	collards	squash, summer
cabbage	dandelion	string beans
carrots	kale	tomato juice
cauliflower	mustard	tomatoes
celery	spinach	turnips
cucumber	turnip	veg. juice
dandelion	mushrooms	zucchini
eggplant	okra	

Fruits: ½ to 1 cup measure. The sweeter the fruit, the greater the natural sugar content, and the less you get for one exchange. The dried or juiced equivalent, such as 2 apricots yield 4 dried apricot halves or 12 grapes yield ¼ cup of grape juice, all have the same calories but occupy less volume.

apple, small	grapes, 12	pineapple, ½ c.
apple juice, ⅓ c.	mango, ½	pineapple juice ⅓ c.
applesauce, ½ c.	nectarine, 1	plums, 2
apricots, 2	orange, 1	prune juice, ¼ c.
banana, ½ small	orange juice, ½ c.	prunes, 2
cherries, 10	papaya, ⅓	raisins, 2 tbl
dates, 2	peach, 1 med.	tangerine, 1
grapefruit, ½	pear, 1 small	watermelon, 1 c.
grape juice, ¼ c.	persimmon, 1	

Fats: 1 teaspoon of pure fat (like oil) or one tablespoon of high-fat food (like bacon or nuts).

avocado, ⅛	margarine, butter, oil,	nuts, large, 6
bacon, 1 strip	lard, bacon fat,	nuts, small, 20
heavy cream, cream cheese, salad dressing, 1 tbl.	mayonnaise, 1 tsp.	olives, 5 small

Breads and cereals: Approximately 1 ounce of grain product or its equivalent in starchy vegetables. Those higher in air, like puffed cereal and popcorn, are allowed more volume though they still end up the same in weight and calories. Note that beans, peas, peanut butter, and lentils can qualify for either this group or the protein group if one is a vegetarian.

crackers	beans, peas, lentils, ½ c.	mashed potato, ½ c.
arrowroot, 3	bran flakes, ½ c.	parsnips, ⅔ c.
graham, 2	bread, 1 slice	pasta cooked, ½ c.
squares	cooked cereal, ½ c.	peas, ½ c.
matzoh, 2	corn, ⅓ c.	popcorn, 3 c.
oyster, 20	corn on cob, 1 small	potato, 1 small
pretzels, 25 small	cornmeal, 2 tbl.	puffed cereal, 1 c.
rye wafer, 3	English muffin, ½	rice or barley, ½ c.
saltines, 6	flour, 2½ tbl.	squash, ½ c.
soda, 4	grits, ½ c.	tortilla, 1 6-inch
bagel, ½	hamburger bun, ½	wheat germ ¼ c.
baked beans, ¼ c.	lima beans, ½ c.	yam, ¼ c.

Protein/meats: About 1 ounce of each of these foods. Note that the higher the fat content, the more calories must be allowed for it. Some of these selections are higher in starch (beans, peas, lentils) and must also be considered a bread exchange. Some are higher in fat, like peanut butter, and must include two fat exchanges in addition to the protein exchange.

Low fat

lean beef, lamb,	clams, oyster, scallops,	beans, peas, lentils
pork, poultry, veal	shrimp, 5	(plus 1 bread),
fish, 1 oz.	lobster, salmon, tuna,	½ c.
farmer's cheese, 1 oz.	cottage cheese, ¼ c.	crab, ¼ c.

Medium fat

organ meats, 1 oz.	peanut butter	parmesan cheese,
mozzarella, 1 oz.	(plus 2 fats), 2 tbl.	3 tbl.
canadian bacon,	pork, veal, fish,	egg, 1
1 oz.	beef, lamb, 1 oz.	

High fat

capon	frankfurters	salami
cheeses	goose	sausage
cold cuts	hamburger	spare ribs
duck	lamb breast	steak

Milk and dairy: 1 cup (8 fluid ounces) measure. Note that nonfat milk is the standard here. If low-fat milk is selected, it counts as a milk exchange plus a fat. Whole milk is considered a milk exchange plus two fat exchanges.

| skim, nonfat, or buttermilk, nonfat yogurt, 1 c. | low-fat milk or yogurt (plus 1 fat), 1 c. | whole milk or yogurt (plus 2 fats), 1 c. |

Free: These foods are sufficiently high in fluids or fiber or noncaloric substances that they contribute negligible calories to the diet in normal portions.

artifical sweeteners	parsley	vanilla
chicory	radishes	vinegar
coffee	spices	water
endive	tea	watercress
lettuce		

TABLE 23: Guide to Exchange System (Grams)

	Protein	Fat	Carbohydrates	Calories
milk (nonfat)	8	-	12	80
vegetables	2	-	5	25
fruit	-	-	10	10
breads	2	-	15	70
meat/protein				
low fat	7	3	-	55
medium fat	7	5½	-	77
high fat	7	8	-	100
fats	-	5	-	45

To get some practice, let's analyze a sample (but not recommended) meal using this exchange system of meal planning.

Salad bar: ½ cup broccoli, ¼ cup carrots, ¼ cup bean sprouts (total of 1 cup of vegetables, which is 2 vegetable exchanges at 25 calories each; total: 50 calories), 2 tablespoons of creamy Italian dressing (2 fat exchanges at 45 calories each equals 90 calories total).

Soup: ½ cup black bean (low-fat protein exchange of 55 calories, plus a bread exchange of 70 calories; total: 125 calories), salt, spices, onions (insignificant calories).

TABLE 24: **Sample Exchange Patterns**

| | Calories/Day | | | |
	1,000	1,200	1,900	2,400
milk (nonfat)	2	2	3	4
vegetables	4	4	7	7
fruit	3	4	7	10
breads	3	5	8	11
meat/protein				
low fat	5	5	5	5
medium fat	(1 protein + ½ fat exchange)			
high fat	(1 protein + 1 fat exchange)			
fats	3	3	8	10

Bread: small loaf of sour dough (equals four bread exchanges at 70 calories each; total: 280 calories).

Condiments on bread: 5 pats of butter (5 fat exchanges at 45 calories each; total: 225 calories), 2 tablespoons of jelly (jelly is primarily sugar and thus qualifies as empty calories; 90 calories in this case).

Starch: 1 cup white rice (2 bread exchanges at 70 calories each; total: 140 calories) with seasonings (free), cooked in 2 teaspoons of butter (2 fat exchanges at 45 calories each; total: 90 calories).

Entree: 10 ounces of prime rib (10 high-fat protein exchanges at 100 calories each; total: 1,000 calories).

Beverage: 2 large cocktails (at 300 empty calories each; total: 600 calories).

In sum, here is how the calories break down:

	Sample Meal	Ideal
total calories	2,690	800
percent calories from:		
carbohydrate	17	58
fat	32	30
protein	16	12
alcohol	22	less than 5
empty food	26	less than 5

Now let's try a more recommended meal. Use the same salad bar but deduct the Italian dressing and use vinegar (free group). The soup was quite acceptable. Make the bread selection two pieces of whole wheat with only two pats of butter and no jelly. Use steamed brown rice instead of white rice cooked in butter. Have six ounces of halibut (low-fat meat exchange) rather than ten ounces of prime rib. Sip one glass of dry white wine (90 calories) instead of the cocktails. This would still be considered a pleasant and tasty meal.

Note that the exchange system encourages low-fat and nonfat foods. Whole milk qualifies as a milk exchange plus two fat exchanges. Four ounces of hamburger qualifies as four low-fat protein exchanges plus four fat exchanges. The ideal pattern leans heavily toward grains, fruits, and vegetables in order to comply with the Senate Diet Goals.

With a little practice, you can use this exchange system to create your own balanced, optimal diet of the right foods in the correct portions.

39

MAKING IT NUTRITIOUS AND DELICIOUS

"The most nourishing meal in the world is useless unless it is eaten."
—QUILLIN AND REYNOLDS

Thousands of guests have been through the La Costa Spa in the last twenty years and most have commented on how delicious the food was. The food served in the spa dining room is low in salt, fat, cholesterol, and calories, while being high in fiber and many essential nutrients. We offer no refined or processed foods and even use sugar substitutes sparingly.

Eating should be a pleasure. It should also be a nourishing experience for your body. The two can coexist. One doesn't need to feel depriced eating basically natural food. If a sweetener is necessary, a little unfiltered honey is better than sugar, and apple or fruit concentrate is even better then honey. Fish can be broiled or poached in wine and garlic instead of butter.

There is no all or none in nutrition. The Senate Diet Goals recommended that we (the average "healthy" person) cut our sugar and cholesterol consumption in half, eat only one-third of our current salt intake, and cut fat consumption by about 30 percent. These are all very realistic and attainable goals, and they don't mean you can never add salt to anything again.

Most of us taste only the condiments used to flavor the food, never the food itself. In the case of bland white bread and canned vegetables, there is good reason to hide the flavor and better reasons not to eat them. The wild, grainy flavor of whole wheat bread and the subtle tastes in fresh vegetables can stand on their own.

If you have trouble changing your tastes, we recommend a slow "withdrawal" period. Your taste buds will adapt and become more sensitive to the fabulous flavors of foods. Slowly withdraw salt, fat, and sugar condiments from your diet, and slowly begin trying the suggestions in this chapter. Try to eat natural foods as much as possible, limiting refined or processed foods. You will feel better and enjoy your food more.

Substitutions

Here are tips that will dramatically improve the nutrient quality of your meals when preparing food in the kitchen.

Instead of this	Try this
sour cream	low-fat yogurt, whipped 1% fat cottage cheese
salt	Lite salt, vinegar, lemon juice, spices, salt substitutes like Mrs. Dash or Spike
sugar	fructose, honey, dried fruit, molasses, concentrated fruit juice, sugar substitutes
chocolate	carob with chocolate (3 to 1 ratio)
cream in coffee	whole or low-fat milk
deep fry	broil, bake, steam, microwave
high-fat beef	pressure-cooked chuck, flank, sirloin
regular hamburger	ground turkey (same price, lower in fat)
instant mashed potatoes	pressure-cooked (10 minutes) with skins on, then beaten
whipped cream	whipped evaporated skim milk
bacon	Canadian bacon (thin cut lean ham)
oil-packed tuna	water-packed tuna
cream cheese	low-fat, high-protein variation
regular cheese	low-fat cheese

There are dozens of excellent cookbooks, some of which are listed at the end of this chapter. We have included a mere sprinkling of our favorite recipes. At least one of these foods is bound to spring a leak in your saliva glands.

People with serious health problems are often put on very restrictive diets for salt, fat, sugar, cholesterol, and other food substances. This chapter is for the healthy active person who wants to stay that way. The ailing person under a physician's care should follow his or her particular dietary prescription.

Enjoy!

FIG PUDDING

Not only is this a delicious dessert, but figs are unmatched for soluble dietary fiber.

   2 tablespoons apple juice concentrate

   1 egg, separated

   ¼ cup chopped dried figs

¼ Granny Smith apple, peeled and sliced

zest of lemon

¼ teaspoon vanilla extract

¼ cup golden raisins

¼ cup buckwheat grouts

½ cup soft wholewheat bread crumbs

¼ cup whole wheat flour

½ teaspoon baking powder

¼ teaspoon baking soda

¼ teaspoon cinnamon

½ teaspoon nutmeg

¼ teaspoon ground cloves

Separate eggs, setting whites aside. Beat yolks until creamy, mix in apple juice concentrate. In blender, chop figs and apples with apple juice to make a jam-like paste. Combine with lemon zest, vanilla, raisins, grouts, breadcrumbs, and the yolk mixture. Sift the flour with the baking powder, soda, cinnamon, nutmeg, and cloves. Beat egg whites until stiff. Combine wet ingredients with dry, then gently fold in egg whites. Bake in custard cups in water bath at 350° F. Turn out of custard cup onto plate.

LA COSTA SPA GRANOLA

This is another tasty item that is a nourishing meal and a fabulous snack for all active people. The kids will be clamoring for this one.

2 cups rolled oats

⅓ cup steel cut oats

⅓ cup rye flakes

½ cup apple juice

⅓ cup millet

¼ cup nonfat dry milk powder

1 tablespoon vanilla

1½ tablespoons cinnamon

¼ teaspoon ground cloves

½ teaspoon nutmeg

¼ cup apple juice concentrate

2 tablespoons raisins

1 tablespoon unsweetened coconut, toasted

¼ cup dried apricots, chopped

1 vanilla bean

Place oats and rye flakes in bowl, add apple juice and mix gently with fork. Add millet, powdered milk, vanilla, seasonings and apple juice concentrate; mix gently with fork and place on teflon baking sheet (or use nonstick vegetable spray to prevent sticking). Bake at 325⁰ F. for 30 minutes or until granola is golden brown. Cool and add raisins, toasted coconut and apricots. Store in tightly sealed jar with vanilla bean. Serving size is ¼ cup.

Note: Pour apple juice concentrate over this and make into bars. Bake at 350⁰ F. 20-25 minutes until crispy.

FRUIT SMOOTHIE

Use the blender often with such nourishing ingredients as fresh fruit, yogurt, wheat germ, and lecithin. Make a chocolate shake with yogurt, banana, and carob. Make delicious creamed soups out of leftovers. Make your own frozen desserts by blending fresh fruit and pouring it into ice cube trays with wooden sticks inserted. Here's one of our blender favorites.

1 tablespoon honey (optional)

2 cups nonfat yogurt

2 ripe medium-size bananas, or 1 cup cantaloupe or other fruit, or 2 cups orange juice

6 ice cubes

Purée in blender until smooth.

YOGURT CHEESE

Cream cheese is a very high fat dairy product yet is useful in many tasty meals. You can make your own version with almost identical flavor yet with much less fat and calories and even more protein.

Place 2 cups yogurt in double cheesecloth (or a clean nylon that has been washed in hot water) and let hang over a bowl for 24 hours. Remove hardened yogurt cheese ball and refrigerate. Use in place of cream cheese. Excellent for frostings and dips.

BANANA WALDORF

This is excellent by itself, or over a salad, or served in carved-out cantaloupe halves.

2 cups diced banana
1½ cups diced apple
1 cup diced celery
½ cup chopped walnuts
½ cup raisins (optional)
½ cup yogurt
1 tablespoon lemon juice

Use well-chilled fruit. Combine all ingredients. Mix well and serve on lettuce leaves or alfalfa sprouts. Yields 7 small servings.

OVEN FRENCH FRIES

No reason for feelings of deprivation. The healthy potato can still be enjoyed as a fat-free french fry.

1 baking potato
1 egg white, unbeaten
onion and garlic powder or parmesan cheese

Preheat oven 425° F. Cut potato into strips. Dip strips into unbeaten egg whites. Place on nontick pan sprayed with vegetable spray and sprinkle with onion and garlic powder or parmesan cheese. Bake for 25 minutes.

FAST VEGGIE SOUP

Leftover foods, especially vegetables, can be blended into a fantastic soup. Hot fluids, like soup, when served 20 minutes before mealtime have been shown to substantially reduce appetite and the possibility of overeating.

2 cups milk
1 cup cooked vegetables
1 tablespoon miso
1 teaspoon soy sauce (optional)

Put all ingredients in blender. Cover and purée till smooth. Pour into a saucepan and cook over low heat till hot. Makes 2-3 servings.

ONION SOUP

Here is another sumptuous appetizer to increase your dining pleasure and subtract from total calories consumed, not to mention the potent benefits of onion.

2 medium onions, sliced

1 bay leaf

1 cup defatted chicken stock

1 teaspoon basil

½ teaspoon black pepper

1 cup defatted beef stock

1 ounce sherry

Preheat a large skillet over medium heat. Spray skillet with a nonstick vegetable spray. Sauté onions in skillet slowly, until lightly browned. Add seasonings as you are sautéing onions. Then add chicken stock, consommé, and sherry. Simmer for 1 hour. Serve hot.

EASIEST CHICKEN DINNER

The deep-fried chicken found in fast-food places has twice the calories of a normal piece of chicken. This meal is delicious, quick, cheap, and good for you.

4-6 pieces of chicken

dijon mustard or egg whites (optional)

4 baking potatoes

Wash chicken and place in oven-proof pan with enough room so pieces aren't crowded. (For extra flavor, try dipping the chicken in egg white or spread with dijon mustard before baking.) Scrub potatoes and poke with a knife several times. Place chicken and potatoes in oven and cook at 375° F. for 45 to 50 minutes. Serve with fresh fruit or sliced tomatoes.

FISH

We have talked throughout this book about the near miraculous health benefits of regular fish intake. Fish can be baked, broiled, or barbecued to maintain its low levels of fat and calories. This recipe adds unique flavors and textures that will convert even the confirmed fish hater in your family.

4 4-ounce Dover sole fillets, folded into thirds or rolled.

1 cup defatted chicken broth

1 ounce dry white wine

1 shallot, chopped fine

3-4 drops fresh lemon juice

julienne 1 tablespoon each of: leeks, carrots and celery hearts

Pour the white wine into a hot shallow skillet. Remove the skillet from the fire and allow the alcohol to evaporate. Add the chicken broth, shallots and, when hot, the rolls of sole. Sprinkle the fresh julienned vegetables on top. Cover and simmer gently for a few minutes or until the sole becomes milky and firm. Do not overcook. Using a spatula, remove the fish to a hot plate and store in a warm place until the sauce has been reduced to a few tablespoons. Spoon the sauce over the fish. Top each fillet with julienned vegetables and serve at once.

BEAN TACO

    4 corn tortillas, or taco shells
    12 ounces pinto beans, cooked
    ½ medium onion
    2 cloves garlic, minced
    1 bell pepper
    1 tablespoon chopped cilantro
    ½ green chili, chopped
    ½ medium tomato, chopped
    ½ teaspoon cumin
    ¼ teaspoon chili powder
    1 bay leaf

GARNISH:

2 cups lettuce, chopped
1 tomato, diced
1 scallion, diced
2 radishes, sliced
2 ounce shredded, low-fat cheddar cheese

Sauté onion, bell pepper, garlic, green chili and seasonings. Mix in the tomatoes. Crisp the tortilla shells in the oven at 350° F. for about 10 minutes. Place one fourth of the bean mixture on each tortilla shell and top with garnish ingredients. Place the completed taco under the broiler for 30 seconds to melt the cheese. Serve with homemade salsa (see page 00).

BROWN RICE AND APPLES

Even your staunchest health food antagonists will have to admit to liking this one.

1 cup brown rice

2 cooking apples, cored and chopped

¼ cup apple juice concentrate

½ cup chopped walnuts or almonds

½ cup diced celery

Cook rice according to the package directions. In 10-inch nonstick skillet sprayed with vegetable spray, add apples, apple juice concentrate, and celery. Cook and stir until apples are tender but hold their shape, about 5-8 minutes. Stir in hot cooked rice and nuts. Makes 6 servings.

BULGUR PILAF

Bulgur is whole wheat that has been coarsely ground, then partially steam cooked and dried. It has nearly all the nutrients of whole wheat and offers a distinct flavor and texture that makes it a favorite in the Middle East and Eastern Europe.

2 tablespoons defatted chicken broth

½ cup celery chopped

1 medium onion chopped

1 cup raw burgur

¼ teaspoon dill weed

¼ teaspoon oregano

½ teaspoon salt (optional)

¼ teaspoon pepper

2 cups water with 1 to 2 tablespoons miso mixed in

1 tablespoon parsley chopped

Add vegetables and bulgur to heated nonstick skillet. Stir constantly until vegetables are tender and bulgur is golden. Add seasonings and water. Bring to boil. Stir. Reduce heat and simmer 15 minutes.

VARIATIONS

Add chopped green pepper, chopped nuts, sliced mushrooms, grated carrots or sliced olives.

RICE AND LENTILS

Combining grains (rice) with legumes (lentils) provides a complete protein of similar quality to steak, yet much less expensively. Make a large batch of this and keep it in the refrigerator. Just warm it up in the microwave or oven for a delightful meal in itself or as a starch component of a meal.

1 cup brown rice

½ cup lentils

2 teaspoons soy sauce

¼ cup chopped fresh parsley (optional)

1 tablespoon miso (optional)

Cook rice and lentils according to their directions. Mix the two together. Stir in rest of the ingredients. To cook the brown rice faster, put in a pressure cooker with ½ cup less water and cook for 20 minutes.

GARBANZO BEAN SPREAD

All varieties of beans are very nourishing, cheap, easy to store, and can be quite appetizing. The Greeks use a similar recipe in their famous hummus.

2 cups cooked garbanzo beans (drained)

2 tablespoons tahini (sesame seed paste)

1½ tablespoons soy sauce

¾ teaspoons vitamin C powder

5 tablespoons olive oil

2 teaspoons lemon juice

¼ teaspoon dill weed

¼ teaspoon onion powder

¼ teaspoon garlic

½ tablespoon mustard (not the dried type)

1 teaspoon salt

1 tablespoon vinegar

Mix all ingredients in a blender or food processor until well blended. Use as a spread for crackers or on warmed tortillas with grated cheese and alfalfa sprouts.

HOMEMADE SALSA

This has become a ubiquitous condiment for us. Use it on anything from fish to eggs. It turns many Mexican-American dishes into gringo favorites. With its high nutrient density, plus the therapeutic value of red pepper (capsicum), you need not hide this food from anyone.

2 green onions, chopped

4 large tomatoes, chopped

½ onion, chopped

1 clove garlic, chopped

1 chili pepper

1 jalapeno pepper (chopped fine)

¼ cup cilantro, chopped

¼ cup unsalted tomato juice

2 drops tabasco (optional)

1 teaspoon Lite salt (optional)

Blend ingredients to the consistency you like. Use generously and often.

Use powdered vitamin C for tartness in recipes. It also preserves foods and markedly increases your C intake, and can be found at most vitamin stores. Use garlic, red pepper, onion, and ginger often.

There are potential hazards in consuming too much aluminum. Nearly all commercial baking powders use aluminum as an anticaking additive. You can easily and cheaply make a healthier version of baking powder by mixing: 1 tablespoon baking soda, 2 tablespoons cream of tarter, and 2 tablespoons arrowroot.

Cookbooks That Offer Nutritious and Delicious Recipes

Hoshijo, K., *Kathy Cooks Naturally*, San Francisco: Harbor Publishing, 1981. Send to P.O. Box 6853, Ventura, CA 93006.

Moyer, A., *Better Food for Public Places*, Emmaus, PA: Rodale Press, 1977.

James, J., and Goulder, L., *The Dell Color Coded Low Fat Living Guide*, New York: Dell, 1980.

Margie, Levy, and Hunt, *Living Better—Recipes for a Healthy Heart*, Radnor, PA: HLS Press, Chilton Book Co., 1981.

Morash, M., *The Victory Garden Cookbook*, New York: Knopf, 1982.

Hewitt, J., *New York Times Natural Foods Cookbook*, New York: Avon, 1972.

Robertson, L. et. al., *Laurel's Kitchen: A Handbook for Vegetarian Cookery and Nutrition*, Petaluma, CA: Nilgiri Press, 1978.

Lappe, F., *Diet for a Small Planet*, New York: Ballantine, 1975

Gerras, C., ed., *Rodale's Naturally Great Foods Cookbook*, Emmaus, PA: Rodale Press, 1977.

40
Super Foods

"Eat to live and not live to eat."
—BENJAMIN FRANKLIN

There are many good foods. But there are a few that are super foods. These super foods are nutritious, relatively inexpensive, easy to prepare and store, widely available, and tasty. Many of them have incredible life-giving properties.

Soybeans

Soybeans are truly a super food. Varieties of soybeans can be grown from the subarctic regions of central Canada to the tropics of Bolivia. Soybeans, as legumes, have nitrogen-fixing bacteria nodules on their roots which allow the plant to take nitrogen from the air to form protein. This not only produces nourishing foods but also replenishes the soil. Soybeans have an excellent shelf life, lasting at least a year when stored in a cool dry place in a sealed container. Of all the legumes, soy is the highest in oil, primarily polyunsaturated fatty acids, with a generous portion of lecithin. Both polyunsaturated fats and lecithin have the ability to help lower fats in the blood.

Many products can be made from the humble soybean. The whole cooked bean can be fermented with a special bacteria to form tempeh, a staple food in Indonesia; it has a flavor and texture not unlike the white meat of chicken. The whole bean may also be sprouted and blanched, adding a nutty-grainy flavor to an entrée or salad. Soy flour, both regular and defatted, can be used in bread and other baked goods.

Texturized vegetable protein (TVP) made from soy, with a small amount of additives, can be made to look, taste, and feel like beef, chicken, and other animal tissue. And soy is cheap.

Puréed whole cooked soybeans yield soy milk (the fluid portion) and okara (the remaining solids). Okara can be lightly toasted to provide a nutritious addition to homemade granola, cookies, and casseroles. The soy milk can be chilled and consumed as is, or curdled with calcium or magnesium salts to form a curds-and-whey mixture. The curds are compressed to create tofu, which is tasty in burritos, Oriental meals, and casseroles. Tofu can be frozen and then plunged into boiling water to develop a meatlike texture. Add some soy sauce and you have an excellent meat substitute for everything from spaghetti to chili. The fluid left over from making tofu can be used for any number of things, from soup base to fertilizer to insect repellent to soap (because of the lecithin content). The soy milk can be cooked and layers of coagulated soy milk scooped off the top and dried. This dried bean curd (yuba) can be soaked in soy sauce and fried like bacon or used like seaweed or tortillas to wrap around other foods.

Soy has impressive nutrition credentials. About 45 percent of the dried bean is protein. Soy has a decent-quality protein that can be further enhanced by matching with grains. Experts claim that using soy protein to replace some animal protein in the diet would lower heart disease risk.[1] Soy is a rich source of magnesium. When tofu is made with calcium salts it becomes an incredibly dense source of calcium. Soybeans are also a rich source of vitamin B_6. Tempeh and miso are excellent sources of B_{12} for the vegetarian. Soy is the richest source of lecithin and therefore choline as well. Soy is high in potassium and low in sodium and phosphorus, all worth boasting about. Beans provide excellent fiber and promote regular bowel movements,[2] and are the best of all foods at stabilizing blood glucose levels,[3] essential to diabetics, hypoglycemics, and alcoholics and important to everyone else.

There is evidence that people with diets high in soybeans are less susceptible to cancer. This may be due to soybeans' high vitamin and mineral content, or their low fat, or high fiber. Or perhaps there is an unknown factor in soy that exerts potent anticancer properties.

Fish

The domestic animal trade has been accused of using chemicals to rear beef, chicken, and pork; yet fish in the ocean still live in a relatively pristine environment. Fish caught near the industrially polluted areas of Japan in the 1970s were tainted, as is the PCB-laden fish of the Great Lakes. Yet most other fish is relatively pollution free.

Most fish, except sardines and shellfish, are very low in cholesterol. Whole cooked fish, like canned salmon, are high in calcium. Fish from the ocean are high in iodine. Seafood is one of the few reliable sources of selenium. For centuries, cod liver oil saved thousands of children from the ravages of rickets, since fish liver is one of the few rich dietary sources of vitamin D. High in niacin, B_6, pantothenic acid, choline, iron and other essential nutrients, fish seem to form their own cornucopia.

The best is yet to come. Discussed thoroughly in the chapter on quasi-vitamins, fish oil is practically a panacea. Found in fish oil are fatty acids called eicosanoids, including eicosapentanoic acid (EPA) and docosahexanoic acid (DHA). EPA has been shown to be so effective at improving circulation and preventing circulatory disorders, that some reputable scientists suggest an RDA be established for fish oil.[4] Studies have found that people who included as little as 2 ounces of fish in their diet per week had half the incidence of heart disease as those who did not eat any fish.[5]

There are only two principal sources of DHA: fish and mother's milk. DHA has been shown to be important in the development of the central nervous system of the young infant and is important if not essential for the proper growth of the human brain. Infant formulas have negligible levels of DHA. Grandma's old adage that "fish is brain food" is true because fish is high in: (1) DHA, which is involved in brain development; (2) choline, which aids in making a vital brain chemical, acetylcholine; (3) tryptophan and B_6, which are involved in making another essential chemical of thought, serotonin.

Because of its polyunsaturated fats, fish tends to go rancid quickly if not properly stored. For this reason, many people have a poor impression of the taste of fish. Fresh or properly frozen fish has no "fishy" flavor. Fresh fish should have a translucent or pinkish tint to it. When it develops a gray or wax-paper-like pallor, it is too old to enjoy at the dinner table.

Some fish, like the shellfish lobster and abalone, can be very expensive and do not have as many health benefits as scaled fish. Most fish is in the same price range as beef. Since fish has less fat trimmings and no large bones, it is a relatively good bargain.

For variety, fish even outdoes soybeans. There are literally hundreds of types of edible and nourishing fish. Given the hundreds of ways they can be prepared, there should be no boredom when including fish regularly on your menu.

Garlic

Some Eastern Europeans have children wear cloves of garlic around their necks to protect them from colds and infections. Now garlic has been scientifically proved to be a potent force against bacteria and fungus in the human body.

Garlic is cheap and easy to grow in most climates. It was initially used as a flavor enhancer and is still prized by the world's finest chefs as a primary condiment.

The health benefits of garlic have staggered even the most skittish of medical scientists.[6] In addition to its antibacterial and antifungal properties,[7, 8] it apparently slows the growth of tumors.[9] It has been proved to lower fats and cholesterol in the blood[10] while simultaneously raising the HDLs that protect against heart disease,[11] and reducing the "stickiness" of blood cells.[12] It is effective at lowering blood pressure. It also increases physical endurance in laboratory animals.[13] It even keeps insects away,[14] and helps to stabilize high blood sugar levels.

Americans have habitually used fat, salt, and sugar to season food; using any of the allium family, including onions, shallots, and especially garlic, can reduce the intake of dubious condiments and introduce a new subtle flavoring agent with near miracle health benefits. (It is questionable whether powdered garlic or deodorized garlic tablets have the same therapeutic value as whole fresh garlic cloves.)[15] For a longer and healthier life, include garlic often in your cooking.

Ginger

Found commonly in many Oriental dishes, ginger is a root food that provides flavor and aroma. It also has been scientifically found to be more effective at quelling motion sickness than the most commonly used drug, Dramamine.[16] In addition to this unusual property, ginger has been shown to dramatically reduce cholesterol levels in the blood.[17]

Peppers

Green chili peppers are one of nature's richest sources of vitamin C. Green, red, and yellow chilies are grown throughout the United States and provide color, taste, and nourishment for otherwise bland foods. The most impressive members of this group are red hot peppers. These have been scientifically proved to reduce the blood clotting that can cause vessel blockage. A group of researchers found that Thai people have less blood clotting in their vessels due to their regular consumption of red hot peppers containing capsicum.[18] Since diseases of the vascular network are the primary killers in developed nations, we would all profit in adding some red hot peppers to the diet on a regular basis. Also, we do mean red peppers, not black. Black pepper may be carcinogenic and is not recommended. Although red peppers have been historically restricted for ulcer patients, new studies tell us that peppers do not impair the ulcer healing process.[19] But do not eat so many red peppers that stomach discomfort sets in.

Peppers are easy to grow in any size garden, cheap to buy at the store, and proved to be very valuable to one's health. Onions, garlic, ginger, and red pepper not only lack the detrimental effects of typical American condiments but also are potent life extenders.

Sprouts

Sometime in the course of human evolution, we lost the ability to make our own vitamin C, which most other creatures on earth can still do. (There is evidence that some humans do make their own vitamin C.[20]) Most humans have to scramble to find a regular and dependable source of vitamin C in any climate and throughout the year. Sprouts are the answer. Any seed of an edible plant that is capable of germinating can be used. When kept in a sealed container in a cool dry place, unsprouted seeds have a shelf life of at least a year. Remember that transportation and storage time lead to a lower vitamin C content in even the most dependable sources.

Sprouting improves the bioavailability of the seed's protein content, increases vitamin levels,[21] eliminates the digestion-interfering agents called phytates, eliminates much of the naturally occurring toxins,[22] and adds considerable water and fiber to the diet.[23] Wheat sprouts were shown to have potent anticancer abilities.[24]

Sprouts are easy to grow, require no sun or soil, are inexpensive, and provide truly fresh produce for anyone, anywhere, any time. While many people spend exorbitant sums on such nutrient-poor produce as lettuce, they could be growing their own produce, sprouts, in their own kitchen. Children will often eat sprouts, even though they may not like other vegetables, just because they get to participate in the growing of this unique vegetable.

Nearly any seed will work, but those tested in research include peas (Dwarf Gray, early Alaska, Laxton progress, Mammoth melting, Thomas Laxton, Wando) and beans (Executive bunch, Top Crop bunch, Burpee stringless, Great Northern, pinto, Tennessee green pod, red kidney, red valentine, sulfur, white navy, soybean, and mung bean). Alfalfa seeds work well, too.

To sprout seeds, you will need a glass jar (quart size or more), a screen for the top, and a rubber band to hold the screen in place. You can use clean plastic screening or even nylon hosiery. Place one or two tablespoons of seeds in the glass container and secure the screen on top. Keep in mind that seeds will increase in volume about tenfold before they are ready to eat. Allow enough room for expansion. Fill the container half-full with water and let stand overnight to get the seeds started. Next morning drain and rinse. It is best to leave your sprout garden in a dimly lit area. Rinse and drain two or three times each day for the next four or five days. Let the jar stand inverted at an angle after rinsing. This allows the seeds to drain thoroughly and avoids fermentation by providing a regular flow of air into the container.

Larger seeds, like peas and beans, should not be allowed to grow longer than a half inch. Soybean sprouts should be steamed for ten minutes before eating. Smaller seeds like alfalfa can grow up to an inch in length with no bitter flavor. For extra vitamin A, let your alfalfa sprouts sit in a sunny window for an hour or two to develop beta-carotene.

Wheat, Oats, Barley, and Rice

There are many grains that could be highlighted here. Quinoa and amaranth are very nutritious grains common to western South America. Millet, corn, barley, and sorghum are found throughout the world. Yet wheat, oats, barley, and rice are special.[25] They are easy to grow, nutritious, and good for the soil. Corn depletes the soil and encourages erosion. Rice and oats have among the highest-quality protein of all the grains. Wheat has been adapted to every region from subarctic Canada to the southwest desert. Wheat is the cereal grain of choice in most of the developed nations of the world, primarily because of its unique ability to make strands from its gluten protein. These gluten strands give bread its characteristic texture.

Oats and rice are equally impressive in their nutritional value. Oats grow well even in poor soil. They are high in iron, thiamin, riboflavin, fiber, complex carbohydrates, chromium, molybdenum, and other nutrients. The protein quality of oats is so high that it is the preferred grain for horses, oxen, and other beasts of burden.

Rice is an excellent source of protein, thiamin, niacin, fiber, complex carbohydrates, manganese, silicon, and chromium. A new rice flour has been developed that has 25 percent protein, compared with the normal 8 percent.[26] Once again, beware of the grand theft that occurs in the nutritional quality of these whole grains when they are processed into refined products, such as converted or "instant" rice.

Whole grains are rich in polyunsaturated fats, have almost no saturated fats, no cholesterol, are low in sodium, high in potassium, and good sources of vitamin E. If oats, wheat, and rice were included in the diet more often, we would see a marked reduction in the incidence of obesity, heart disease,[27] diabetes,[28] and various other nutritionally related conditions.[29]

Related to these grains, which are the "fruit" of the grass, are the benefits of the grass plant itself. Wheat grass and barley grass are high in chlorophyll, which may account for their talents as anticancer and antiradiation agents.[30] In order to derive these benefits, sprinkle wheat or barley grains on top of the soil in a planter and keep the seeds damp. Within a week or so you will have a two- to three-inch-high "lawn" of grass that can be clipped into a salad bowl so that the plant can continue to produce more grass. Some health food stores offer pure juice from wheat or barley grass, but the price is understandably high.

Wheat and rice germ are particularly nourishing foods. They are high in vitamins E, B_6, and protein.

Cruciferous Vegetables

Vegetables from the cabbage family help protect the intestinal tract against cancer.[31] Broccoli, Brussels sprouts, cabbage, and cauliflower could reduce the incidence of cancer of the gastrointestinal tract by as much as 50 percent if consumed regularly. They also protect against the effects of radiation.[32] At a meeting of the American Cancer Society in Illinois in September of 1983, new research was reported that something in Brussels sprouts could inhibit the development of certain cancers in laboratory animals.[33]

Fermented Foods

Since mankind first saw food rot, we have attempted to control food-altering microbes. Eight thousand years ago, in Mesopotamia, grains were fermented to produce alcohol. Five thousand years ago, the Egyptians discovered how to use yeast to ferment grains and thus make bread. Milk was fermented into yogurt, kefir, and cheese. Coincidentally, the ideal temperature for the fermentation of milk into yogurt is about daytime desert temperature, 115° F. Desert nomads found that fermentation would allow them to better use their milk products.[34]

Yogurt has been apocryphally associated with a long lifespan. We are not sure about this claim, but yogurt and kefir are good for you. Yogurt lowers cholesterol levels in the blood.[35] Yogurt is also valuable in maintaining a benevolent culture of bacteria in the intestines, which helps digestion, production of nutrients (such as vitamin K and biotin), absorption of minerals, and may ward off marginal cases of food poisoning. Yogurt is also well tolerated by people with lactose intolerance, apparently because the bacteria fermenting the yogurt continue to help digest the lactose in the intestines.[36] The bacteria in yogurt (lactobacillus) is also discussed in the chapter on quasi-vitamins.

There are numerous other fermented foods that are not as common on Western tables. Miso, tempeh, and soy sauce are fermented soy products. Studies have found these fermented versions have a lower phytate content,[37] greater availability of protein,[38] lower trypsin-inhibitor content, massive increase in vitamin B_{12} and iron, and improvements in texture and flavor.[39]

Bananas

Most tropical fruit arrives in a battered and discolored condition at the urban grocery store. Bananas are one of the few that can be shipped to market nearly anywhere in the world and provide tasty, nourishing, inexpensive, good-looking fruit. Bananas are very high in vitamin B_6, naturally occurring carbohydrates, and pectin. Bananas are a good source of potassium, magnesium, and vitamin C. When used in a blender, they give a thick maltlike texture to any drink. Peel a banana and put it in a sealed plastic container in the freezer, and you will have a delicious, nourishing frozen desert in a few hours. Bananas are usually affordable throughout the year. For nutrition, cost, taste, versatility, and availability, keep bananas on your grocery list regularly.

Citrus Fruits

Limes were shown in 1749 to cure scurvy. Citrus fruits are one of the few sources of rutin, a bioflavonoid known to prevent capillary fragility. Rutin is found on the white part of the rind. In addition to their vitamin C content, citrus fruits are a favorite for their sweet-tasting and energy-charging fructose. They are also high in fiber, calcium, and potassium, yet low in fat and calories. Citrus fruit makes an ideal snack. Oranges, limes, lemons, tangerines, tangelos, and grapefruit are the best-known members of this group. Ripe fruit will keep reasonably well for a month if stored in a cool, dry, dark place.

Dark-Green Leafy Vegetables

Green plants provide an abundance of vitamin A in the form of beta-carotene, which has been well documented to be an anticancer factor. Vitamin A is in short supply in many diets around the world, and the victims of this shortage suffer everything from frequent infections to permanent blindness. Chlorophyll is a potent anticancer agent.[40] Dark-green leafy vegetables are a primary source of folacin, a B vitamin commonly low in the American diet.

Many dark-green leafy vegetables, such as parsley and spinach, also contribute substantial vitamin C and some calcium. Parsley, considering its nutritive value and low cost, is probably one of the better buys on the produce shelf. Kale, turnip greens, beet greens, and dandelion greens are others in this category of cheap, tasty, and nutritious foods.

Liver

Liver is high in cholesterol, which would make it a restricted food for people with a heart disease risk. Liver is the detoxifying organ of the body. If an animal were exposed to an abundance of pollution and toxins, the liver may be one of the more questionable parts of that animal to eat. Yet most domestic animals live in a healthier and cleaner environment than most people. In our opinion, the benefits of liver far outweigh the risks.

Liver is the richest source of vitamin A, riboflavin, niacin, B_6, B_{12}, folacin, biotin, pantothenic acid, choline, and iron. It is one of the richest sources of potassium, sulfur, magnesium, zinc, copper, chromium, molybdenum, and protein. It is less expensive than the cheapest hamburger and has no fat or bone waste. Pork liver is not only the richest source of iron known, but has a texture similar to steak. Soak the pork liver in milk for two hours in the refrigerator. Then rinse and fry in a little butter with onions and garlic.

Apples

Apples grow well throughout most of the temperate zones of the United States. The skin is a rich source of pectin, which is considered the best of the fibers at keeping blood fats low and purging the gastrointestinal tract. Apples are a valuable detergent food: they clean your teeth while you eat. Apples store reasonably well and appeal to most people's taste buds. An apple a day may indeed keep the doctor away. Our endorsement does not extend to apple juices or drinks, however, because much of the beneficial nutrients have been processed out of them.

Home Garden

Children who dislike produce will often eat vegetables that they helped to grow. You can teach them and feed them with a garden project.[41] In growing your own produce, you can minimize the use of lethal chemicals. A garden guarantees the freshest, most nourishing vegetables available. Considering the time and money that some people spend on a lawn, the same effort could yield a bountiful harvest of nourishing fruits and vegetables worth over a thousand dollars annually.

Community gardens are cropping up around this country where bare land is scarce. The nutritive value and flavor of garden-fresh vegetables make gardens worth the effort.

AFTERWORD

THIS BOOK HAS BEEN DEDICATED TO THE ISSUE OF MALNU-
trition in America, a major factor in the poor health of this country. Malnutrition on a global basis is a very different picture. Americans suffer from an
excess of calories, fat, salt, sugar, cholesterol, food additives, alcohol, and
caffeine, and have deficiencies in some vitamins, minerals, complex carbohydrates, and fiber. But the world's poor suffer from many more deficiencies, including such essentials as protein, calories, iodine, vitamin A, and
iron. There are more than 400 million iodine-deficient people in Asia
alone.[1] Iodine deficiency can lead to permanent retardation in children. In
southeast Asia, it is considered unmanly to eat vegetables; over a quarter of a
million children in that area of the world go blind from vitamin A deficiency
every year.[2] Riboflavin deficiency causes up to thirty million cases of cataracts a year in India alone.[3]

A half billion people in the world are severely malnourished;[4] more than
half of them suffer from protein/calorie malnutrition—they can't get
enough food to eat, let alone the right nutrients—and more than half of
these are preschool-age children. More people die of starvation every three
days (fifteen to twenty million people yearly) than died in the bombing of
Hiroshima.[5] The lowered disease resistance that comes with malnutrition
contributes to more deaths. More than one billion people drink contaminated water, which claims twenty-five million lives each year.

Yet the world produces enough food to provide two pounds of grain a
day for every person on earth—3,000 kilocalories per person, more than
enough to fulfill the average need of 2,300 kilocalories a day. In other
words, we already have the capacity to feed everyone, but we aren't doing
it.

There are many issues involved in world hunger: water scarcity, transportation limitations, inefficiency, ignorance, greed, political corruption,
and not using available technology. Swelling populations worsen the problem, although hungry people have large families because so few live to ma-
turity, parents need help with the chores, and children are the "social security" of most cultures. (Once the Social Security system was implemented
in America, the birth rate dropped dramatically.)

The issue of world hunger is a large, complex, often overwhelming one,
but there are solutions. Produce more food. Encourage family planning.
Better use the resources we have. Genetic engineering can produce

drought-resistant plants tailored to certain climates and nutritional needs. The United States has enough food rotting in storage from government subsidy buyouts to feed a good percentage of the starving masses.

The spectre of world hunger looms over all nations, even ours. We can help these people and, in doing so, help ourselves.

NOTES

Part One

1. Menzel, P. , *Medical Costs, Moral Choices* (New Haven: Yale University, 1985).
2. Garrett, M., *Los Angeles Times*, Apr. 7, 1985, part 1, p. 25.
3. Wagner, M., *Lancet*, Nov. 27, 1982, p. 1207.
4. Klock, H., *Personnel*, vol. 62 (July 1985), p. 13.
5. U.S. Bureau of the Census, *Statistical Abstract of the United States: 1985*, 105th ed., Washington, D.C., 1984.
6. AMA Council on Scientific Affairs, *Journal of the American Medical Association*, vol. 249 (Feb. 11, 1983), p. 784.
7. Louis Harris Organization, Mount Sinai Hospital Medical Center health-care report 1, *Time*, Chicago regional edition, Jan. 17, 1977.

Chapter 1: Why Nutrition is Important to Everyone

1. Bortz, W., *Journal of the American Medical Association*, vol. 248 (Sept. 10, 1982), p. 1203.
2. Crews, E. et. al., *American Journal of Physiology*, vol. 216, no. 2 (Feb. 1969), p. 359.
3. Blair, S., et. al., *Journal of the American Medical Association*, vol. 252 (July 27, 1984), p. 487.
4. Galbo, H. et. al., *Journal of Applied Physiology*, vol. 40 (June 1976), p. 855.
5. Weltman, A. et. al., *American Journal of Clinical Nutrition*, vol. 33 (May 1980), p. 1002.
6. Lohmann, D. et. al., *Metabolism*, vol. 27, no. 5 (May 1978), p. 521.
7. Wechsler, H. et. al., *New England Journal of Medicine*, vol. 308 (Jan. 13, 1983), p. 97.
8. Snyder, S., *Scientific American*, vol. 236, no. 3 (Mar. 1977), p. 44.
9. Welin, L. et. al., *Lancet*, Apr. 20, 1985, p. 915.

Chapter 2: Malnutrition in the Land of Plenty

1. Pastides, H., *Yale Journal of Biology and Medicine*, vol. 54 (1981), p. 265.
2. Reed, P. , *Nutrition: An Applied Science* (St. Paul, MN: West Publishing Company, 1980).
3. National Research Council, *Diet, Nutrition, and Cancer* (Washington, D.C.: National Academy Press, 1982).
4. Clark, L., *Federation Proceedings*, vol. 44 (June 1985), p. 2584.
5. Anderson, R. et. al., *American Journal of Clinical Nutrition*, vol. 41 (June 1985), p. 1177.
6. Leibovitz, B., *Carnitine* (New York: Dell, 1984), p. 85.
7. Colman, N., *Nutrition Reviews*, vol. 40, no. 8 (Aug. 1982), p. 225.
8. Smithells, R., *Pediatrics*, vol. 69 (Apr. 1982), p. 498.
9. Butterworth, C. et. al., *American Journal of Clinical Nutrition*, vol. 35 (Jan. 1982), p. 73.

10. Walsh, J. et. al., *Annals of Nutrition and Metabolism*, vol. 25 (1981), p. 178.
11. Kathman, J. et. al., *Nutrition Research*, vol. 4 (1985), p. 245.
12. Kritchevsky, D., *Federation Proceedings*, vol. 41 (Sept. 1982), p. 2813.
13. Guhrie, H. et. al., *Journal of Nutrition Education*, vol. 13 (1981), p. 46.
14. Ziporyn, T., *Journal of the American Medical Association*, vol. 253 (Apr. 5, 1985), p. 1846.
15. Chen, L. et. al., *Drug-Nutrient Interactions*, vol. 3, no. 2 (1985), p. 73.
16. U.S. Bureau of the Census, *Statistical Abstract of the United States: 1985*, 105th ed., Washington, D.C., 1984.
17. Atwood, J. et. al., *Archives of Internal Medicine*, vol. 145 (July 1985), p. 1185.
18. Roe, D., *Journal of the American Dietetic Association*, vol. 85 (Feb. 1985), p. 174.
19. Roehm, J. et. al., *Archives of Internal Medicine*, vol. 128 (1971), p. 88.
20. Myers, C. et. al., *Annals of the New York Academy of Sciences*, vol. 393 (1982), p. 419.
21. Whanger, P. , *Selenium in Biology and Medicine*, ed. J. Spallholz et. al., (Westport: AVI Publishing, 1981), p. 230.
22. *Nutrition Reviews*, vol. 42 (1984), p. 260.
23. Ip, C. et. al., *Carcinogenesis*, vol. 2 (1981), p. 435.
24. Tewfik, H. et. al., *International Journal for Vitamin and Nutrition Research*, supp.23 (1982), p. 265.
25. Rabinowitz, M. et. al., *Lancet*, Jan. 18, 1983, p. 63.
26. Mirvish, S. et. al., *Journal of the National Cancer Institute*, vol. 55 (1975), p. 633.
27. Nomura, A. et. al., *Cancer Research*, vol. 45 (May 1985), p. 2369.
28. O'Dea, K., *Diabetes*, vol. 33 (June 1984), p. 596.
29. Schroeder, H., *American Journal of Clinical Nutrition*, vol. 24 (May 1971), p. 562.
30. Mitchell, H. et. al., *Nutrition in Health and Disease*, 16th ed. (Philadelphia: J.B. Lippincott, 1976), p. 18.
31. Welsh, S. et. al., *Food Technology*, Jan. 1982, p. 70.
32. See note 29 above.
33. Colgan, M., *Your Personal Vitamin Profile* (New York: Quill, 1982), p. 32.
34. McEndree, L. et. al., *Nutrition Reports International*, vol. 27 (Jan. 1983), p. 199.
35. AMA Council on Foods and Nutrition, ed., *Nutrients in Processed Foods* (Acton, Mass: Publishing Science Group, 1974).
36. Shils, M., *Federation Proceedings*, vol. 43 (Apr. 1984), p. 1412.

Chapter 3: Why All the Confusion?

1. Consensus Development Conference on Osteoporosis, *Journal of the American Medical Association*, vol. 252 (Aug. 10, 1984), p. 799.
2. Mazess, R. et. al., *American Journal of Clinical Nutrition*, vol. 42 (Sept.1985), p. 568.
3. Guthrie, H., *Introductory Nutrition*, 5th ed. (St. Louis: Mosby Company, 1983), p. 269.
4. Hendler, S., *The Complete Guide to Anti-Aging Nutrients* (New York: Simon & Schuster, 1985).
5. Herbert, V., in *Present Knowledge in Nutrition*, 4th ed. (Washington, D.C.: Nutrition Foundation, 1976), p. 201.
6. Williams, R., *Nutrition Against Disease* (New York: Pitman, 1971).
7. Alvarez-Dardet, C. et. al., *New England Journal of Medicine*, vol. 312 (June 6, 1985), p. 1521.
8. Rimland, B. et. al., *American Journal of Psychiatry*, vol. 135 (1978), p. 472.
9. London, R. et. al., *Obstetrics and Gynecology*, vol. 65 (Jan. 1985), p. 104.
10. Hittner, H. et. al., *New England Journal of Medicine*, vol. 305 (Dec. 3, 1981), p. 1365.
11. Laurence, K. et. al., *British Medical Journal*, vol. 282 (May 9, 1981), p. 1509.
12. *Lancet*, June 9, 1984, p. 1308.
13. Goodwin, J. et. al., *Journal of the American Medical Association*, vol. 251 (May 11, 1984), p. 2387.
14. Leibovitz, B., *Carnitine* (New York: Dell, 1984), p. 21.

15. Borum, P., *Annual Review of Nutrition*, vol. 3 (1983), p. 233.
16. Kwee, H. et. al., *Journal of Nuclear Medicine*, vol. 26 (July 1985), p. 790.
17. Mertz, W., in *Present Knowledge in Nutrition*, 4th ed. (Washington, D.C.: Nutrition Foundation, 1976), p. 373.
18. Salmenpera, L., *American Journal of Clinical Nutrition*, vol. 40 (Nov. 1984), p. 150.
19. Yung, S. et. al., *Journal of Pharmaceutical Sciences*, vol. 71 (Mar. 1982), p. 282.
20. Oliver, M., *Lancet*, May 11, 1985, p. 1087.

Chapter 4: Assessing Your Nutritional Status

1. Barrett, S., *Journal of the American Medical Association*, vol. 254 (Aug. 23, 1985), p. 1041.
2. Deeming, S. et. al., *American Journal of Clinical Nutrition*, vol. 31 (July 1978), p. 1175.
3. Golden, M. et. al., *Lancet*, Dec. 11, 1982, p. 1338.
4. Laker, M., *Lancet*, July 31, 1982, p. 260.
5. Morris, J. et. al., *Biological Trace Element Research*, vol. 5 (1983), p. 529.
6. Hallfrisch, J. et. al., *Nutrition Research*, vol. 2 (1982), p. 263.

Chapter 5: The Seven General Rules of Nutrition

1. Saab, R. et. al., *Journal of Food Science*, vol. 46 (1981), p. 662.
2. Thompson, H. et. al., *Carcinogenesis*, vol. 5 (1984), p. 849.
3. Randall, E. et. al., *Journal of the American Dietetic Association*, vol. 85 (July 1985), p. 830.
4. Leveille, G. et. al., *Nutrition Today*, Nov. 1974, p. 4
5. Fabry, P. et. al., *American Journal of Clinical Nutrition*, vol. 23 (Aug. 1970), p. 1059.

Chapter 6: Carbohydrates

1. *Mosaic*, May 1975, p. 13.
2. Consolazio, C. et. al., *American Journal of Clinical Nutrition*, vol. 25 (Jan. 1972), p. 85.
3. Worthington, B. et. al., *Journal of the American Dietetic Association*, vol. 64 (Jan. 1974), p. 47.
4. Bolton, R., *Ethnology*, vol. 12 (July 1973), p. 227.
5. Jenkins, D. et. al., *American Journal of Clinical Nutrition*, vol. 34 (Mar. 1981), p. 362.
6. Young, C. et. al., *Journal of the American Dietetic Association*, vol. 59 (Nov. 1971), p. 473.
7. Long, P. et. al., *Nutrition: An Inquiry into the Issues* (Englewood Cliffs, N.J.: Prentice-Hall, 1983), p. 59.
8. Haverberg, L. et. al., *American Journal of Clinical Nutrition*, vol. 33 (1980), p. 17.
9. *Consumer Reports*, Mar. 1978, p. 136.
10. Sreebny, L., *Community Dentistry and Oral Epidemiology*, vol. 10 (Feb. 1982), p. 1.
11. Sheiham, A., *Lancet*, Feb. 5, 1983, p. 282.
12. Goodhart, R. et. al., *Modern Nutrition in Health and Disease* (Philadelpha: Lea & Febiger, 1973), p. 635.
13. Welborn, T. et. al., *Diabetes Care*, vol. 2 (1979), p. 154.
14. Story, J., *Federation Proceedings*, vol. 41 (Sept. 1982), p. 2797.
15. Offenbacher, E. et. al., *Diabetes*, vol. 29, no. 11 (Nov. 1980), p. 919.
16. Elias, A. et. al., *General Pharmacology*, vol. 15, no. 6 (1984), p. 535.
17. Lester, M. et. al., *Nutrition and Behavior*, vol. 1 (1982), p. 3.
18. Hallfrisch, J. et. al., *Journal of Nutrition*, vol. 109 (Nov. 1979), p. 1909.
19. Wurtman, R., *Lancet*, Nov. 1985, p. 1060.
20. Morgan, K. et. al., *Journal of the American Dietetic Association*, vol. 85 (Mar. 1985), p. 352.
21. See note 9 above.

22. Kessler, I. et. al., *Journal of the American Medical Association*, vol. 240 (July 28, 1978), p. 349.
23. Sheiham, A., *Lancet*, Feb. 5, 1983, p. 282.
24. Koivisto, V., et.al, *Journal of Applied Physiology*, vol. 51, no. 4 (Oct. 1981), p. 783.

Chapter 7: Fiber

1. Pavlovic, M. et. al., *Diabetologia Croatica*, vol. 13 (Nov. 1, 1984), p. 199.
2. Kirby, G. et. al., *American Journal of Clinical Nutrition*, vol. 34 (1981), p. 824.
3. Van Der Aar, P. et. al., *Journal of Nutrition*, vol. 113 (Mar. 1983), p. 653.
4. *Mosaic*, May 1975, p. 13.
5. Van Ness, M. et. al., *American Family Physician*, vol. 31, no. 4 (Apr. 1985), p. 198.
6. Steggerda, F., *Annals of the New York Academy of Sciences*, vol. 150 (1960), p. 57.
7. Murphy, E. et. al., *American Journal of Digestive Diseases*, vol. 17 (1972), p. 639.
8. Yatzidis, H., *British Medical Journal*, vol. 4 (1972), p. 51. Hall, R. et. al., *American Journal of Gastroenterology*, vol. 75 (1981), p. 192.
9. Wilmshurst, P. et. al., *British Journal of Nutrition*, vol. 44 (1980), p. 811.
10. Anderson, J. et. al., *Obesity and Bariatric Medicine*, vol. 9 (1980), p. 109.
11. Evans, E. et. al., *Nutrition and Metabolism*, vol. 18 (1975), p. 199.
12. Hillman, L. et. al., *American Journal of Clinical Nutrition*, vol. 42 (Aug. 1985), p. 207.
13. Vahouny, G., *Federation Proceedings*, vol. 41 (Sept. 1982), p. 2801.
14. Anderson, J., *Annals of Internal Medicine*, vol. 98, no. 2 (1983), p. 842.
15. Anderson, J., *Medical Times*, vol. 108, no. 5 (May 1980), p. 41.
16. Watanabe, K. et. al., *Journal of the National Cancer Institute*, vol. 63 (1979), p. 141.
17. National Research Council, *Diet, Nutrition, and Cancer* (Washington, D.C.: National Academy Press, 1982).
18. Graf, E. et. al., *Cancer*, vol. 56 (Aug. 15, 1985), p. 717.
19. Ershoff, B., *American Journal of Clinical Nutrition*, vol. 27 (1974), p. 1395.
20. Holt, S. et. al., *Lancet*, Mar. 24, 1979, p. 636.
21. Burkitt, D. et. al., eds., *Refined Carbohydrate Foods and Disease* (London: Academic Press, 1975).
22. Andersson, H. et. al., *Human Nutrition: Applied Nutrition*, vol. 39A (Apr. 1985), p. 101.
23. Bass, L., *American Journal of Nursing* (Feb. 1977), p. 254.
24. Brender, J. et. al., *American Journal of Public Health*, vol. 75 (Apr. 1985), p. 399.
25. Kromhout, D. et. al., *Lancet*, Sept. 4, 1982, p. 518.

Chapter 8: Protein

1. Weitzman, M. et. al., *Immunology*, vol. 128 (1982), p. 2770.
2. Hellebostad, M. et. al., *Acta Paediatrica Scandinavica*, vol. 74 (1985), p. 191.
3. McEndree, L. et. al., *Nutrition Reports International*, vol. 27 (Jan. 1983), p. 199.
4. Carroll, K., *Federation Proceedings*, vol. 41 (Sept. 1982), p. 2792.
5. Rouse, I. et. al., *Lancet*, Jan. 1, 1983, p. 5.
6. *The Nutrition Report*, vol. 3, no. 6 (June 1985), p. 43.
7. Taber, L. et. al., *Journal of the American Dietetic Association*, vol. 76 (Jan. 1980), p. 21.
8. Nader, C. et. al., *Nutrition Reports International*, vol. 23, no. 1 (Jan. 1981), p. 113.
9. Ellis, F. et. al., *American Journal of Clinical Nutrition*, vol. 25 (1972), p. 555.
10. Pixley, F. et. al., *British Medical Journal*, vol. 291 (July 6, 1975), p. 11.
11. Howie, B. et. al., *American Journal of Clinical Nutrition*, vol. 42 (July 1985), p. 127.
12. Snowdon, D. et. al., *American Journal of Public Health*, vol. 75 (May 1985), p. 507.
13. Gersovitz, M. et. al., *American Journal of Clinical Nutrition*, vol. 35 (Jan. 1982), p. 6.
14. Sherman, A. et. al., *Journal of Nutrition*, vol. 115 (May 1985), p. 607.

Chapter 9: Fat

1. Danforth, E., *American Journal of Clinical Nutrition*, vol. 41 (May 1985), p. 1132.
2. National Research Council, *Diet, Nutrition, and Cancer* (Washington, D.C.: National Academy Press, 1982), chapter 1, p. 5.
3. Mills, D. et. al., *Proceedings of the Society for Experimental Biology and Medicine*, vol.176 (1984), p. 32.
4. Thomassen, M. et. al., *British Journal of Nutrition*, vol. 51 (May 1984), p. 315.
5. Sgoutas, D. et. al., *American Journal of Clinical Nutrition*, vol. 23 (Aug. 1970), p. 1111.
6. Kritchevsky, D., *Federation Proceedings*, vol. 41 (Sept. 1982), p. 2813.
7. Smith, E., *Lancet*, Mar. 8, 1980, p. 534.
8. See note 6 above.
9. National Research Council, *Diet, Nutrition and Cancer*, chapter 5, p. 5.
10. Mattson, H. et. al., *American Journal of Clinical Nutrition*, vol. 25 (June 1972), p. 589.
11. Saba, P. et. al., *Current Therapeutic Research*, vol. 24, no. 3 (Aug. 1978), p. 299.
12. Mickelsen, O. et. al., *Journal of Nutrition*, vol. 57 (1955), p. 541.
13. See note 2 above.
14. Snowdon, D., *Journal of the American Medical Association*, vol. 254 (July 19, 1985), p. 356.

Chapter 10: Water

1. Kott, E. et. al., *European Neurology*, vol. 24 (1985), p. 221.
2. Consumer Guide, *Family Medical and Health Guide* (Skokie, Ill: Publications International, 1984).
3. Brody, J., *Jane Brody's Nutrition Book* (New York: W.W. Norton, 1981).
4. Colgan, M., *Your Personal Vitamin Profile* (New York: Quill, 1982).
5. Magnuson, E. et. al., *Time*, October 14, 1985, p. 76.
6. *The San Diego Union*, Dec. 18, 1980, p. A-12.
7. Marier, J., *Reviews of Cancer and Biology*, vol. 37 (1978), p. 115.

Chapter 11: Vitamins

1. Zile, M. et. al., *Proceedings of the Society for Experimental Biology and Medicine*, vol. 172 (1983), p. 139.
2. Gunby, P. , *Journal of the American Medical Association*, vol. 247 (Apr. 2, 1982), p. 1799.
3. Solomons, N. et. al., *American Journal of Clinical Nutrition*, vol. 33 (Sept. 1980), p. 2031.
4. *Nutrition and the M.D.*, vol. 8 (1982), p. 1.
5. Morley, J. et. al., *American Journal of Clinical Nutrition*, vol. 34, (Aug. 1981), p. 1489.
6. Sommer, A. et. al., *American Journal of Ophthalmology*, vol. 93, no. 1 (Jan. 1982), p. 84.
7. Hodges, R. et. al., *American Journal of Clinical Nutrition*, vol. 31 (May 1978), p. 876.
8. *Lancet*, July 3, 1982, p. 28.
9. Mathews-Roth, M. et. al., *Archives of Dermatology*, vol. 113 (Sept. 1977), p. 1229.
10. Ames, S., *American Journal of Clinical Nutrition*, vol. 22 (July 1969), p. 934.
11. Bieri, J. et. al., *American Journal of Clinical Nutrition*, vol. 34 (Feb. 1981), p. 289.
12. Ram, M. et. al., *American Journal of Obstetrics and Gynecology*, vol. 135, no. 4 (Oct. 15, 1979), p. 470.
13. Peto, R. et. al., *Nature*, vol. 290 (Mar. 19, 1981), p. 201.
14. Wechsler, H., *Archives of Dermatology*, vol. 115, no. 1 (Jan. 1979), p. 73.
15. Hustead, V. et. al., *Journal of Pediatrics*, vol. 105 (1984), p. 610.
16. Solon, F. et. al., *Journal of the American Dietetic Association*, vol. 74 (Feb. 1979), p. 112.

17. Chernov, M. et. al., *American Journal of Surgery*, vol. 122 (1971), p. 674.
18. Smith, F. et. al., *New England Journal of Medicine*, vol. 294 (1976), p. 805.
19. Farrington, K. et. al., *British Medical Journal*, vol. 282 (June 20, 1981), p. 1999.
20. *CRC Critical Reviews in Toxicology*, vol. 9 (1979), p. 351.
21. Baxi, S. et. al., *Western Journal of Medicine*, vol. 137, no. 5 (Nov. 1982), p. 429.
22. Selhorst, J. et. al., *Journal of the American Medical Association*, vol. 252 (Dec. 28, 1984), p. 3365.
23. Farris, W. et. al., *Journal of the American Medical Association*, vol. 247 (Mar. 5, 1982), p. 1317.
24. Ragavan, V. et. al., *American Journal of the Medical Sciences*, vol. 283 (May 1982), p. 161.
25. Kemmann, E. et. al., *Journal of the American Medical Association*, vol. 249 (Feb. 18, 1983), p. 929.
26. Ziporyn, T., *Journal of the American Medical Association*, vol. 250 (Oct. 21, 1983), p. 1951.
27. Peng, S et al., *Arterial Wall*, vol. 4 (1978), p. 229.
28. Jibani, M. et. al., *British Medical Journal*, vol. 290 (Mar. 9, 1985), p. 748.
29. Leach, A. et. al., *Aviation, Space, and Environmental Medicine*, vol. 47, no. 6 (Jun 1976), p. 630.
30. Clemens, T. et. al., *Lancet*, Jan. 9, 1982, p. 74.
31. Greer, F. et. al., *Journal of Pediatrics*, vol. 98 (May 1981), p. 696.
32. Lawson, D., *Journal of Human Nutrition*, vol. 35, no. 1 (Feb. 1981), p. 61.
33. Cockburn, F. et. al., *British Medical Journal*, July 5, 1980, p. 11.
34. Offermann, G. et. al., *Epilepsia*, vol. 20, no. 1 (Feb. 1979), p. 3.
35. *Science News*, June 4, 1983, p. 367.
36. Maclennan, W. et. al., *British Medical Journal*, vol. 2 (Oct. 1, 1977), p. 859.
37. O'Hare, A. et. al., *Archives of Disease in Childhood*, vol. 59 (1984), p. 766.
38. Elidrissy, A. et. al., *Calcified Tissue International*, vol. 36 (1984), p. 266.
39. Scott, J. et. al., *American Journal of Medicine*, vol. 63 (Sept. 1977), p. 488.
40. FitzGerald, G. et. al., *Annals of the New York Academy of Sciences*, vol. 393 (1982), p. 209.
41. Ip., C. et. al., *American Association of Cancer Research*, vol. 24 (Mar. 1983), p. 96.
42. Wartanowicz, M. et. al., *Annals of Nutrition and Metabolism*, vol. 28 (1984), p. 186.
43. Muller, D. et. al., *Lancet*, Jan. 29, 1983, p. 225.
44. Robison, W. et. al., *Investigative Ophthalmology and Visual Science*, vol. 18, no. 7 (July 1979), p. 683.
45. Burton, G. et. al., *Lancet*, Aug. 7, 1982, p. 327.
46. Hornsby, p. , *Journal of Cellular Physiology*, vol. 112, no. 2 (Aug. 1982), p. 207.
47. Ayres, S. et. al., *Cutis*, vol. 21, no. 3 (Mar. 1978), p. 321.
48. Wald, N. et. al., *British Journal of Cancer*, vol. 49 (1984), p. 321.
49. Weder, B. et. al., *Neurology*, vol. 34 (Dec. 1984), p. 1561.
50. Kligman, A., *Archives of Dermatology*, vol. 118 (May 1982), p. 289.
51. Tsai, A. et. al., *American Journal of Clinical Nutrition*, vol. 31 (1978), p. 831.
52. *Nutrition and the M.D.*, vol. 8 (Mar. 1982), p. 1.
53. Corigan, J. et. al., *American Journal of Clinical Nutrition*, vol. 34 (Sept. 1981), p. 1701.
54. Saperstein, H. et. al., *Archives of Dermatology*, vol. 120 (July 1984), p. 906.
55. See note 11 above.
56. Hittner, H. et. al., *New England Journal of Medicine*, vol. 305 (Dec. 3, 1981), p. 1365.
57. Castillo, R. et. al., *Journal of Pediatrics*, vol. 99 (Oct. 1981), p. 583.
58. Sokol, R. et. al., *American Journal of Clinical Nutrition*, vol. 41 (Jan. 1985), p. 66.
59. Machlin, L. et. al., *Journal of Nutrition*, vol. 110 (1980), p. 1958.
60. Shearer, M. et. al., *Lancet*, Aug. 28, 1972, p. 460
61. Cummings, M., *American Journal of Clinical Nutrition*, vol. 34 (Feb. 1981), p. 297.
62. Turley, S., *Atherosclerosis*, vol. 24 (1976), p. 1.
63. Rao, B. et. al., *American Journal of Clinical Nutrition*, vol. 31 (Jan. 1978), p. 169.

64. Beetens, J. et. al., *Archives Internationales De Pharmacodynamie Et De Therapie*, vol. 259 (1982), p. 300.
65. Ginter, E. et. al., *Journal of Nutrition*, vol. 99 (1969), p. 261.
66. Reuler, J. et. al., *Journal of the American Medical Association*, vol. 253 (Feb. 8, 1985), p. 805.
67. Goodwin, J. et. al., *Journal of the American Medical Association*, vol. 249 (June 3, 1983), p. 2917.
68. Wassertheil-Smoller, S. et. al., *American Journal of Epidemiology*, vol. 114, no. 5 (Nov. 1981), p. 714.
69. Finley, E. et. al., *American Journal of Clinical Nutrition*, vol. 37, no. 4 (1983), p. 553.
70. Dannenberg, J., *Journal of the American Dental Association*, vol. 105 (Aug. 1982), p. 172.
71. Briggs, M. et. al., *Lancet*, 1973, p. 201.
72. Pru, C. et. al., *Nephron*, vol. 39, no. 2 (Feb. 1985), p. 112.
73. Shilotri, S. et. al., *American Journal of Clinical Nutrition*, vol. 30 (July 1977), p. 1077.
74. Rhead, W. et. al., *Nutrition Reviews*, vol. 29 (1971), p. 262.
75. See note 74 above, p. 260.
76. Sarji, K. et. al., *Thrombosis Research*, vol. 15, no. 516 (1979), p. 639.
77. Fazio, V. et. al., *American Journal of Clinical Nutrition*, vol. 34 (Nov. 1981), p. 2394.
78. Hornig, D. et. al., *International Journal for Vitamin and Nutrition Research*, vol. 50, no. 3 (1980), p. 309.
79. Pelletier, O., *Nutrition Today*, Autumn 1970, p. 12.
80. Jones, E. et. al., *IRCS Medical Science*, vol. 12 (1984), p. 320.
81. Elmer, G., *Nurse Practitioner*, Nov. 1981, p. 40.
82. Brand, J. et. al., *Lancet*, Oct. 16, 1982, p. 873.
83. Garry, P. et. al., *American Journal of Clinical Nutrition*, vol. 36 (Aug. 1982), p. 332.
84. Salmenpera, L., *American Journal of Clinical Nutrition*, vol. 40 (Nov. 1984), p. 150.
85. Addis, G. et. al., *Medical Laboratory Sciences*, vol. 42 (1985), p. 90.
86. See note 66 above.
87. Hoyt, C. et. al., *Medical Journal of Australia*, vol. 1 (Jan. 15, 1977), p. 65.
88. Harrill, I. et. al., *American Journal of Clinical Nutrition*, vol. 30 (Mar. 1977), p. 431.
89. Henshaw, J.L. et. al., *Journal of the American Dietetic Association*, vol. 57 (Nov. 1970), p. 436.
90. Heller, S. et. al., *American Journal of Clinical Nutrition*, vol. 27 (Nov. 1974), p. 1221.
91. *Medical Tribune*, May 12, 1982.
92. Prchal, J. et. al., *Lancet*, Jan. 7, 1978, p. 12.
93. Tremblay, A. et. al., *Nutrition Research*, vol. 4 (1984), p. 201.
94. Belko, A. et. al., *American Journal of Clinical Nutrition*, vol. 37 (Apr. 1983), p. 509.
95. Elmer, G., *Nurse Practitioner*, Sept. 1981, p. 40.
96. Vir, S. et. al., *International Journal for Vitamin and Nutrition Research*, vol. 47, no. 4 (1977), p. 336.
97. Ajayi, O. et. al., *American Journal of Clinical Nutrition*, vol. 39 (May 1984), p. 787.
98. Kane, J. et. al., *New England Journal of Medicine*, vol. 304 (Jan. 29, 1981), p. 251.
99. Krehl, W., *Federation Proceedings*, vol. 40 (Apr. 1981), p. 1527.
100. Alhadeff, L. et. al., *Nutrition Reviews*, vol. 42 (Feb. 1984), p. 33.
101. Lee, C. et. al., *Annals of Clinical and Laboratory Science*, vol. 14 (1984), p. 151.
102. *Lancet*, Apr. 10, 1976, p. 788.
103. Adams, p. et. al., *Lancet*, Aug. 31, 1974, p. 516.
104. Root, E. et. al., *American Journal of Clinical Nutrition*, vol. 37 (Apr. 1983), p. 540.
105. Schaumberg, H. et. al., *New England Journal of Medicine*, vol. 309 (1983), p. 445.
106. Rudman, D. et. al., *New England Journal of Medicine*, vol. 309 (Aug. 25, 1983), p. 488.
107. Adams, P. et. al., *Lancet*, Apr. 28, 1973, p. 7809.
108. Haspels, A. et. al., *Maturitas*, vol. 1, no. 1 (June 1978), p. 15.
109. Singleton, N. et. al., *Journal of Nutrition for the Elderly*, vol. 1, no. 1 (Spring 1980).

110. Kleiner, M. et. al., *American Journal of Clinical Nutrition*, vol. 33 (July 1980), p. 1612.
111. Wighton, M. et. al., *Medical Journal of Australia*, vol. 2 (July 14, 1979), p. 1.
112. Roach, E. et. al., *American Family Physician*, vol. 25 (Jan. 1982), p. 111.
113. Elmer, G., *Nurse Practitioner*, Nov. 1981, p. 40.
114. Chanarin, I. et. al., *Lancet*, Sept. 6, 1980, p. 505.
115. Dong, A., *Annals of Nutrition and Metabolism*, vol. 26 (1982), p. 209.
116. Golden, R., *American Journal of Psychiatry*, vol. 140, no. 2 (Feb. 1983), p. 218.
117. Shojania, A., *Canadian Medical Association Journal*, vol. 126 (Feb. 1, 1982), p. 244.
118. Rodbro, p. , *Acta Medica Scandinavica*, vol. 188 (1970), p. 457.
119. Tchernia, G. et. al., *Developmental Pharmacology and Therapeutics*, vol. 4, suppl.1 (1982), p. 58.
120. Orr, J. et. al., *American Journal of Obstetrics and Gynecology*, vol. 151 (Mar. 1, 1985), p. 632.
121. Rhoads, G. et. al., *American Journal of Epidemiology*, vol. 120 (Dec. 1984), p. 803.
122. Mukherjee, M. et. al., *American Journal of Clinical Nutrition*, vol. 40 (Sept. 1984), p. 496.
123. Deacon, R. et. al., *Scandinavian Journal of Haematology*, vol. 28, no. 4 (Apr. 1982), p. 289.
124. Enk, C. et. al., *Scandinavian Journal of Haematology*, vol. 25, no. 1 (July 1980), p. 63.
125. Barlow, G. et. al., *Clinica Chimica Acta*, vol. 29 (1970), p. 355.
126. Butterworth, C. et. al., *American Journal of Clinical Nutrition*, vol. 35 (Jan. 1982), p. 73.
127. Alhadeff, L. et. al., *Nutrition Reviews*, vol. 42 (Feb. 1984), p. 33.
128. Tanaka, K., *New England Journal of Medicine*, vol. 304 (Apr. 2, 1981), p. 839.
129. Packman, S. et. al., *Lancet*, June 26, 1982, p. 1435.
130. Bonjour, J., *International Journal for Vitamin and Nutrition Research*, vol. 47 (Feb. 16, 1977), p. 111.
131. Barton-Wright, E. et. al., *Lancet*, Oct. 26, 1963, p. 862.

Chapter 12: Minerals

1. Ackley, S. et. al., *American Journal of Clinical Nutrition*, vol. 38 (1983), p. 457.
2. Marie, P. et. al., *New England Journal of Medicine*, vol. 307 (Sept. 2, 1982), p. 584.
3. Schwartz, R. et. al., *American Journal of Clinical Nutrition*, vol. 26 (May 1973), p. 519.
4. Stewart, A. et. al., *New England Journal of Medicine*, vol. 306 (May 13, 1982), p. 1136.
5. Avioli, L., *Federation Proceedings*, vol. 40 (July 1981), p. 2418.
6. Sowers, M. et. al., *American Journal of Clinical Nutrition*, vol. 42 (July 1985), p. 135.
7. Roberts, H., *New England Journal of Medicine*, vol. 304 (Feb. 12, 1981), p. 423.
8. Kromhout, D. et. al., *American Journal of Clinical Nutrition*, vol. 41 (June 1985), p. 1299.
9. Henningsen, N. et. al., *Lancet*, Jan. 15, 1983, p. 133.
10. Kopyt, N. et. al., *New England Journal of Medicine*, vol. 313 (Aug. 29, 1985), p. 582.
11. AMA Council on Scientific Affairs, *Journal of the American Medical Association*, vol.249 (Feb. 11, 1983), p. 784.
12. Ibid.
13. Dyckner, T. et. al., *British Medical Journal*, vol. 1 (1978), p. 822.
14. Johnasson, G. et. al., *Journal of the American College of Nutrition*, vol. 1 (1982), p. 179.
15. Marier, J., *Revue Canadienne De Biologie Experimentale*, vol. 37 (1978), p. 115.
16. Cohen L. et. al., *Journal of the American Medical Association*, vol. 249 (May 27, 1983), p. 2808.
17. See note 15 above.
18. Gordon, E. et. al., *Journal of Pediatrics*, vol. 99 (Sept. 1981), p. 341.
19. Mahajan, S. et. al., *Annals of Internal Medicine*, vol. 97 (Sept. 1982), p. 357.
20. Hunt, I. et. al., *American Journal of Clinical Nutrition*, vol. 40 (Sept. 1984), p. 508.

21. Meadows, N. et. al., *Lancet*, Nov. 21, 1981, p. 1135.
22. Cherry, F. et. al., *American Journal of Clinical Nutrition*, vol. 34 (Nov. 1981), p. 2367.
23. Atik, O., *Journal of the American Geriatrics Society*, vol. 31 (1983), p. 790.
24. Richardson, J. et. al., *Journal of Sports Medicine*, vol. 19 (1979), p. 133.
25. Klevay, L., *American Journal of Clinical Nutrition*, vol. 28 (1975), p. 764.
26. Bakan, R., *Lancet*, Oct. 13, 1984, p. 874.
27. Helliwell, M. et. al., *Annals of the Rheumatic Diseases*, vol. 43 (1984), p. 386.
28. Crouse, S. et. al., *Journal of the American Medical Association*, vol. 252 (1984), p. 785.
29. Hopper, p. et. al., *Journal of the American Medical Association*, vol. 244 (1980), p. 1960.
30. Fischer, P. et. al., *American Journal of Clinical Nutrition*, vol. 40 (Oct. 1984), p. 743.
31. Harland, B. et. al., *Journal of Food Science*, vol. 50 (May 1985), p. 832.
32. Mukherjee, M. et. al., *American Journal of Clinical Nutrition*, vol. 40 (Sept. 1984), p. 496.
33. Anderson, R. et. al., *Biological Trace Element Research*, vol. 6 (1984), p. 327.
34. Sandstrom, L. et. al., *Journal of Nutrition*, vol. 114 (Dec. 1984), p. 411.
35. *Lancet*, May 4, 1985, p. 1041.
36. Moore, M. et. al., *Journal of Pediatrics*, vol. 105 (Oct. 1984), p. 600.
37. Jain, V. et. al., *Nutrition Research*, vol. 4 (1984), p. 537.
38. Collipp, p. et. al., *Annals of Nutrition and Metabolism*, vol. 26 (1982), p. 287.
39. See note 33 above.
40. Krebs, N. et. al., *American Journal of Diseases of Children*, vol. 138 (Mar. 1984), p. 270.
41. *Nutrition Reviews*, vol. 43 (May 1985), p. 158.
42. Garrison, R. et. al., *The Nutrition Desk Reference* (New Canaan: Keats, 1985), p. 66.
43. Leibel, R., *Journal of the American Dietetic Association*, vol. 71 (Oct. 1977), p. 398.
44. Walter, T. et. al., *Journal of Pediatrics*, vol. 102 (Apr. 1983), p. 519.
45. *Advances in Experimental Medicine and Biology*, vol. 91 (1978), p. 229.
46. See note 43 above.
47. Walford, R., *Maximum Lifespan* (New York: W.W. Norton, 1983).
48. Beutler, E., *Modern Nutrition in Health and Disease* (Philadelphia: Lea and Febiger, 1980), p. 324.
49. Sullivan, J., *Lancet*, June 13, 1981, p. 1293.
50. Baumann, M. et. al., *New England Journal of Medicine*, vol. 307 (Dec. 2, 1982), p. 1459.
51. Guthrie, H., *Introductory Nutrition* (St. Louis: C.V. Mosby, 1983), p. 179.
52. Rao, B. et. al., *American Journal of Clinical Nutrition*, vol. 31 (Jan. 1978), p. 169.
53. Breskin, M. et. al., *American Journal of Clinical Nutrition*, vol. 38 (Dec. 1983), p. 943.
54. Morck, T. et. al., *American Journal of Clinical Nutrition*, vol. 37 (Mar. 1983), p. 416.
55. Rossander, L. et. al., *American Journal of Clinical Nutrition*, vol. 32 (Dec. 1979), p.2484.
56. Gershoff, S. et. al., *American Journal of Clinical Nutrition*, vol. 30 (Feb. 1977), p. 226.
57. Schrumpf, A. et. al., *Acta Medica Scandinavica*, vol. 186 (1969), p. 561.
58. Prohaska, J. et. al., *Science*, vol. 213 (July 31, 1981), p. 559.
59. Walker, W. et. al., *Agents and Actions*, vol. 6, no. 4 (1976), p. 454.
60. Hooper, P. , *Journal of the American Medical Association*, vol. 244 (Oct. 1980), p. 1960.
61. Mertz, W. et. al., *Federation Proceedings*, vol. 41 (Sept. 1982), p. 2807.
62. Tilson, M., *Archives of Surgery*, vol. 117 (Sept. 1982), p. 1212.
63. Soskel, N. et. al., *American Review of Respiratory Disease*, vol. 126 (1982), p. 316.
64. *WHO Technical Report Series*, no. 462 (Geneva, 1971).
65. See note 30 above.
66. Snook, J. et. al., *American Journal of Clinical Nutrition*, vol. 37 (Apr. 1983), p. 532.

67. Shils, M., *Federation Proceedings,* vol. 43 (Apr. 1984), p. 1412.
68. Yan-You, W. et. al., *Lancet,* Sept. 7, 1985, p. 518.
69. Bruhn, J. et. al., *Journal of Food Protection,* vol. 48 (May 1985), p. 397.
70. See note 61 above.
71. Mossop, R., *Central African Journal of Medicine,* vol. 29 (1983), p. 80.
72. Mertz, W., in *Chromium in Nutrition and Metabolism,* ed. D. Shapcott et. al. (Amsterdam: Elsevier, 1979), p. 1.
73. Schroeder, H., *Journal of Nutrition,* vol. 88 (1966), p. 439.
74. Saner, G., *Chromium in Nutrition and Disease* (New York: Alan R. Liss, 1980), p. 129.
75. Anderson, R. et. al., *American Journal of Clinical Nutrition,* vol. 41 (June 1985), p. 1177.
76. See note 33 above.
77. Elwood, J. et. al., *Journal of the American College of Nutrition,* vol. 1 (1982), p. 263.
78. McIntosh, E., *American Journal of Public Health,* vol. 72 (Dec. 1982), p. 1412.
79. See note 33 above.
80. See note 67 above.
81. Levander, O. et. al., *American Journal of Clinical Nutrition,* vol. 34 (Dec. 1981), p. 2662.
82. Masukawa, T. et. al., *Biochemical Pharmacology,* vol. 33, no. 16 (1984), p. 2635.
83. Spallholze, J., *Advances in Experimental Medicine and Biology,* vol. 135 (1981), p. 43.
84. Whanger, P. , in *Selenium in Biology and Medicine,* ed. J. Spallholz et. al., (Westport: AVI Publishing, 1981).
85. Spallholz, J. et. al., *Proceedings of the Society for Experimental Biology and Medicine,* vol. 143 (1973), p. 685.
86. Lawson, T. et. al., *Chemico-Biological Interactions,* vol. 45 (1983), p. 95.
87. Milner, J. et. al., *Cancer Research,* vol. 41 (1981), p. 1652.
88. Myers, C. et. al., *Annals of the New York Academy of Sciences,* vol. 393 (1982), p. 419.
89. Masukawa, T. et. al., *Experientia,* vol. 39 (1983), p. 405.
90. Doni, M. et. al., *Haemostasis,* vol. 13 (1983), p. 248.
91. Shamberger, R. et. al., *Trace Substances and Environmental Health,* vol. 9 (1975), p. 15.
92. Clark, L., *Federation Proceedings,* vol. 44 (June 1985), p. 2584.
93. Orndahl, G. et. al., *Acta Medica Scandinavica,* vol. 211 (1982), p. 493.
94. Perry, H., Jr. et. al., *Federation Proceedings,* vol. 33 (1974), p. 357.
95. Palmer, I. et. al., *Journal of the American Dietetic Association,* vol. 82 (May 1983), p. 511.
96. Spallholz, J., Report to the *Third International Symposium on Selenium in Biology and Medicine,* Beijing, China, June 1984.
97. Caillie-Bertrand, M. et. al., *Acta Paediatrica Scandinavica,* vol. 71 (1982), p. 203.
98. Palmer, I. et. al., *Journal of Food Science,* vol. 47 (1982), p. 1595.
99. Gallagher, M. et. al., *Nutrition Research,* vol. 4 (1984), p. 577.
100. Committee on Nutritional Misinformation, Food and Nutrition Board, *Nutrition Reviews,* vol. 34 (1976), p. 347.
101. Abumrad, N. et. al., *American Journal of Clinical Nutrition,* vol. 34 (Nov. 1981), p. 2551.
102. Burrell, R. et. al., *Journal of the National Cancer Institute,* vol. 36, no. 2 (Feb. 1966), p. 201.
103. Mertz, W., *Science,* vol. 213 (Sept. 18, 1981), p. 1332.
104. *Nutrition Reviews,* vol. 43 (June 1985), p. 187.
105. Michael, H. et. al., *British Medical Bulletin,* vol. 37 (1981), p. 31.
106. Thompson, H. et. al., *Carcinogenesis,* vol. 5 (1984), p. 849.
107. Perry, M., *Journal of the American Dietetic Association,* vol. 62, 1973, p. 631.
108. Rabinowitz, M. et. al., *Lancet,* Jan. 1, 1983, p. 63.

Chapter 13: Quasi-Vitamins

1. Kuksis, A. et. al. in *Present Knowledge in Nutrition* (Washington, D.C.: Nutrition Foundation, 1984), p. 383.
2. Ibid, chapter 27, passim.
3. Kapp, J. et. al., *Journal of Neurosurgery*, vol. 32 (Apr. 1970), p. 468.
4. Bartus, R. et. al., *Science*, vol. 209 (1980), p. 301.
5. Cohen, C. et. al., *American Journal of Psychiatry*, vol. 137, no. 2 (Feb. 1980), p. 242.
6. Simons, L.A. et. al., *Australian and New Zealand Journal of Medicine*, vol. 7 (1977), p. 262.
7. Saba, P. et. al., *Current Therapeutic Research*, vol. 24, no. 3 (Aug.1978), p. 299.
8. Signoret, J. et. al., *Lancet*, (Oct. 14, 1978), p. 837.
9. Toouli, J. et. al., *Lancet* (Dec.6, 1975), p. 1124.
10. Gelenberg, A. et. al., *American Journal of Psychiatry*, vol. 136, no. 6 (June 1979), p. 772.
11. Wood, J. et. al., *Federation Proceedings*, vol. 41, (Dec. 1982), p. 3015.
12. Kuksis, A. et. al., *Nutrition Reviews*, vol. 36 (1978), p. 233.
13. Guthrie, H., *Introductory Nutrition*, (St. Louis: C.V. Mosby, 1983).
14. Simmons, D. et. al., *Science*, vol. 217 (Aug. 1982), p. 848.
15. Bremer, J., *Physiological Reviews*, vol. 63, no. 4 (Oct.1983), p. 1420.
16. Leibovitz, B., *Carnitine* (New York: Dell, 1984).
17. Folts, J. et. al., *American Journal of Cardiology*, vol. 41 (1978), p. 1209.
18. Lacour, B. et. al., *Lancet*, (Oct. 11, 1980), p. 763.
19. Thomsen, J. et. al., *American Journal of Cardiology*, vol. 43 (1979), p. 300.
20. Garzya, G. et. al., *International Journal of Tissue Reactions*, vol. 11 (1980), p. 175.
21. Suzuki, Y. et. al., *Japanese Heart Journal*, vol. 23 (1982), p. 349.
22. Schiavoni, G. et. al., *Clinical Therapeutics*, vol. 96 (1981), p. 263.
23. Rudman, D. et. al. in *Carnitine Biosynthesis, Metabolism, and Functions*, ed. R. Frenkel et. al. (New York: Academic Press, 1980), p. 307.
24. Kohengkull, S. et. al., *Fertility and Sterility*, vol. 23 (1977), p. 1333.
25. Kosolcharoen, p. et. al., *Current Therapeutic Research*, vol. 30 (1981), p. 753.
26. McCarty, M., *Medical Hypotheses*, vol. 8 (1982), p. 269.
27. McCarty, M., *Medical Hypotheses*, vol. 13 (1984), p. 139.
28. Hahn, P. , *Federation Proceedings*, vol. 44 (Apr. 1985), p. 2369.
29. Hendler, S., *The Complete Guide to Anti-aging Nutrients*, (New York: Simon & Schuster, 1985).
30. Lorenz, R. et. al., *Circulation*, vol. 67, no. 3 (Mar. 1983), p. 504.
31. Fischer, S. et. al., *Nature*, vol. 307 (Jan. 12, 1984), p. 165.
32. Kromhout, D et. al., *New England Journal of Medicine*, vol. 312 (May 9, 1985), p. 1205.
33. Dyerberg, J., *Philosophical Translations of the Royal Society of London*, vol. B294 (1981), p. 373.
34. Rudin, D., *Biological Psychiatry*, vol. 16 (1981), p. 837.
35. Phillipson, B. et. al., *New England Journal of Medicine*, vol. 312 (May 9, 1985), p. 1210.
36. Kremer, J., *Lancet* (January 26, 1985), p. 184.
37. Prickett, J. et. al., *Immunology*, vol. 46 (1982), p. 819.
38. Strasser, T. et. al., *Proceedings of the National Academy of Sciences*, vol. 82 (Mar.1985), p. 1540.
39. Prickett, J. et. al., *Journal of Clinical Investigation*, vol. 68 (Aug. 1981), p. 556.
40. Culp, B. et. al., *Prostaglandins*, vol. 20, no. 6 (Dec.1980), p. 102.
41. Black, K. et. al., *Stroke*, vol. 15, no. 1 (1984), p. 65.
42. Phillipson, B. et. al., *New England Journal of Medicine*, vol. 312 (May 9, 1985), p. 1210.
43. Karmali, R. et. al., *Journal of the National Cancer Institute*, vol. 73, no. 2 (Aug. 1984), p. 457.

44. Lee, T. et. al., *New England Journal of Medicine*, vol. 312 (May 9, 1985), p. 1217.
45. *Nutrition Reviews*, vol. 42 (May 1984), p. 189.
46. Singer, P. et. al., *Prostaglandins, Leukotrienes, and Medicine*, vol. 15 (1984), p. 159.
47. Harris, W. et. al., *American Journal of Clinical Nutrition*, vol. 40 (Oct. 1984), p. 780.
48. Horrobin, D., *Yearbook of Nutritional Medicine* (New Canaan: Keats, 1985), p. 23.
49. Wright, S. et. al., *Lancet*, Nov. 20, 1982, p. 1120.
50. Mills, D. et. al., *Proceedings of the Society for Experimental Biology and Medicine*, vol. 176 (1984), p. 32.
51. Van der Merwe, C., *South African Medical Journal*, vol. 65 (May 5, 1984), p. 712.
52. Makila, U., *American Journal of Obstetrics and Gynecology*, vol. 148 (1984), p. 772. Lewis, P. , *British Journal of Hospital Medicine*, Oct. 1982, p. 393.
53. Horrobin, D., *Journal of Reproductive Medicine*, vol. 28 (1983), p. 465.
54. Horrobin, D. et. al., *Lipids*, vol. 18 (1983), p. 558.
55. Glen, I. et. al., paper presented at the International Conference on Pharmacological Treatments for Alcoholism, Institute of Psychiatry, University of London, England, Mar. 29, 1983.
56. Horrobin, D., *Lipids*.
57. Dippenaar, N. et. al., *South African Medical Journal*, vol. 62 (Oct. 1982), p. 505.
58. Ziff, M., *Arthritis and Rheumatism*, vol. 26, no. 4 (Apr. 1982), p. 457.
59. Havsteen, B., *Biochemical Pharmacology*, vol. 32, no. 7 (1983), p. 1141.
60. Hendler, S., *Anti-Aging Nutrients*, p. 267.
61. Marshall, M., *Fortschritte der Medizin*, vol. 102, no. 29-30 (Aug. 16, 1984), p. 772.
62. Shub, T. et. al., *Antibiotiki*, vol. 26 (1981), p. 268.
63. Sasajima, M. et. al., *Folia Pharmacologica Japonica*, vol. 74 (1978), p. 897.
64. Becker, Y. et. al., *Connective Tissue Research*, vol. 8, no. 77 (1981).
65. Paintz, M. et. al., *Pharmazie*, vol. 34 (1979), p. 839.
66. Kinoshito, J., *Journal of the American Medical Association*, vol. 246 (1981), p. 257.
67. Bennett, J. et. al., *Drug Research*, vol. 31 (1981), p. 433.
68. Miller, D. et. al., *Proceedings of the National Academy of Sciences*, vol. 78 (1981), p. 3605.
69. Molnar, J. et. al., *Neoplasma*, vol. 28 (1981), p. 11.
70. Huang, M. et. al., *Journal of Biological Chemistry*, vol. 256 (1981), p. 10897.
71. *Dorland's Medical Dictionary* (Philadelphia: W.B. Saunders, 1974), p. 1371.
72. Guthrie, H., *Introductory Nutrition*, p. 336.
73. Bliznakov, E., *Mechanisms of Ageing and Development*, vol. 7 (1978), p. 189.
74. Cortes, E. et. al., *Cardiac Treatment Reports*, vol. 62 (1978), p. 887.
75. *Resident and Staff Physician*, vol. 29, no. 8 (1983), p. 102.
76. Wilkinson, E. et. al., *Research Communications in Chemical Pathology and Pharmacology*, vol. 12 (1975), p. 111.
77. Yamagami, T. et. al., *Research Communications in Chemical Pathology and Pharmacology*, vol. 14 (1976), p. 721.
78. Angelucci, L. et. al., *Nature*, vol. 181 (1958), p. 911.
79. McCarty, M., *Medical Hypotheses*, vol. 7 (1981), p. 515.
80. Klein, C., *Munchener Medizinische Wochenschrift*, vol. 117 (1975), p. 957.
81. McCarty, M., *Medical Hypotheses*.
82. Ibid.
83. Kintzel, H. et. al., *Acta Pediatrica Scandinavica*, vol. 60 (1971), p. 1.
84. Sullivan, W., *Australian and New Zealand Journal of Medicine*, vol. 3 (1973), p. 417.
85. Kelley, W. et. al., *Metabolism*, vol. 19 (1970), p. 1023.
86. Mertz, W., in *Present Knowledge in Nutrition*, p. 373.
87. Rabinowitz, M. et. al., *Diabetes Care*, vol. 6, no. 4 (July 1983), p. 319.
88. Elwood, J. et. al., *Journal of the American College of Nutrition*, vol. 1 (1982), p. 263.
89. McCarty, M., *Medical Hypotheses*, vol. 14 (1984), p. 307.
90. Sinai, Y et. al., *Infection and Immunology*, vol. 9, no. 5 (May 1974), p. 781.
91. Hayes, KC, *Nutrition Reviews*, vol. 43 (Mar. 1985), p. 65.
92. Hendler, S., *Anti-Aging Nutrients*, p. 210.

93. Barbeau, A. et. al., *Life Sciences*, vol. 17, no. 5 (Sept. 1, 1975), p. 669.
94. Huxtable, R. et. al., *Progress in Clinical Biological Research*, vol. 125 (1983), p. 5.
95. Pasantes-Morales, H. et. al., *Journal of Neuroscience Research*, vol. 11 (1984), p. 303.
96. Takagi, K. et. al., *Japanese Journal of Pharmacology*, vol. 22 (1972), p. 245.
97. Brekhman, I. et. al., *Drug Research*, vol. 25 (1975), p. 539.
98. Ibid.
99. Quiroga, H., *Orientacion Medica*, vol. 31, no. 1281 (1982), p. 201.
100. Dorling., E. et. al., *Notabene Medici*, vol. 10, no. 5 (1980), p. 241.
101. Forgo, I. et. al., *Medizinische Welt*, vol. 32, no. 19 (1981), p. 751.
102. Idem, *Notabene Medici*, vol. 12, no. 9 (1982), p. 721.
103. Tanaka, O. et. al., *Fortschritte Der Chemie Organischer Naturstoffe*, vol. 46 (1984), p. 1.
104. Gilliland, S. et. al., *Applied and Environmental Microbiology*, vol. 49, no. 2 (Feb. 1985), p. 377.
105. *Nutrition Reviews*, vol. 42 (Nov. 1984).
106. McDonough, F. et. al., *American Journal of Clinical Nutrition*, vol. 42 (Aug. 1985), p. 345.
107. Ngumbi, P., et. al., *East African Medical Journal*, vol. 61, no. 5 (May 1984), p. 372.
108. Gregori, G. et. al., *Acta Bio-Medica De L Ateneo Parmense*, vol. 56, no. 1 (1985), p. 23.
109. *New York*, Mar. 13, 1978.
110. Chitnis, M.P. et. al., *Journal of Cancer Research and Clinical Oncology*, vol. 109, no. 3 (1985), p. 208.
111. Riemschneider, R. et. al., *Fortschritte der Medizin*, vol. 102, no. 12 (Mar. 29, 1984), p. 339.
112. Rastopchin, I.P., *Zhurnal Nevropatologii I Psikhiatrii Imeni S.S. Korsakova*, vol. 84, no. 7 (1984), p. 1020.
113. Nagorna-Stasiak, B. et. al., *Polskie Archiwum Weterynaryjne*, vol. 23, no. 4 (1983), p. 63.
114. Grabner, C. et. al., *Journal of Infectious Diseases*, vol. 143, no. 1 (Jan. 1981), p. 101.
115. Nakazawa, K. et. al., *Journal of International Medical Research*, vol. 6, no. 3 (1978), p. 217.
116. Zidenberg-Cherr, S. et. al., *American Journal of Clinical Nutrition*, vol. 37, no. 1 (Jan. 1983), p. 5.

Chapter 14: Alcohol

1. U.S. Bureau of the Census, *Statistical Abstract of the United States: 1985*, 105th ed., Washington, D.C., 1984.
2. Hoyumpa, A. et. al., *American Journal of Clinical Nutrition*, vol. 31 (June 1978), p. 938.
3. Thomson, A. et. al., *Journal of Laboratory and Clinical Medicine* (July 1970), p. 34.
4. Halsted,C. et. al., *New England Journal of Medicine*, vol. 285 (Sept. 23, 1971), p. 703.
5. Baker, H. et. al., *American Journal of Clinical Nutrition*, vol. 28 (1975), p. 1377.
6. Barbariak, J. et. al., *Journal of the American Dietetic Association*, vol. 72 (May 1978), p. 493.
7. Reuler, J. et. al., *New England Journal of Medicine*, vol. 312 (Apr. 18, 1985), p. 1035.
8. Pollack, E. et. al., *New England Journal of Medicine*, vol. 310 (Mar. 8, 1984), p. 617.
9. Gruchow, H. et. al., *American Journal of Clinical Nutrition*, vol. 42 (Aug. 1985), p. 289.
10. Lieber, C., *Journal of the American Medical Association*, vol. 233 (1975), p. 1077.
11. Eisenstein, A., *Journal of the American Dietetic Association*, vol. 81 (1982), p. 247.
12. Hippchen, L., *Ecologic-Biochemical Approaches to Treatment of Delinquents and Criminals* (New York: Van Nostrand Reinhold, 1978), chapter 2.
13. Groves, P. et. al., *Biological Psychology* (Dubuque: Wm. C. Brown Co., 1982), p. 151.
14. Russell, R., *American Journal of Clinical Nutrition*, vol. 33 (1980), p. 2741.

15. Hamilton, E. et.al., *Nutrition: Concepts and Controversies* (St.Paul: West Publishing, 1985), p. 475.
16. Weiner, L. et. al., *Clinical Nutrition*, vol. 4 (Feb. 1985), p. 10.
17. *Lancet*, Mar. 26, 1983, p. 682.
18. Willett, W. et. al., *New England Journal of Medicine*, vol. 303 (Nov. 13, 1980), p. 1159.
19. Camargo, C. et. al., *Journal of the American Medical Association*, vol. 253 (May 17, 1985), p. 2854.
20. Blackwelder, W. et. al., *American Journal of Medicine*, vol. 68 (Feb. 1980), p. 164.
21. Read, M. et. al., *Journal of the American Dietetic Association*, vol. 82 (Apr. 1983), p. 401.
22. Graham, T. et. al., *Aviation, Space and Environmental Medicine*, Aug. 1980, p. 793.
23. Graham, T., *Canadian Journal of Applied Sport Sciences*, vol. 6, no. 1 (1981), p. 27.
24. Kromhout, D. et. al., *American Journal of Clinical Nutrition*, vol. 41 (June 1985), p.1299.
25. *Nutrition Reviews*, vol. 24, no. 8 (Aug. 1966), p. 239.
26. Lindenbaum et. al., *New England Journal of Medicine*, vol. 281 (Aug. 14, 1969), p. 335.
27. Schnitzler, C. et. al., *South African Medical Journal*, vol. 66, no. 19 (Nov. 10, 1984), p. 730.
28. Brody, J., *Jane Brody's Nutrition Book* (New York: W.W. Norton, 1981), chapter 14.
29. *San Diego Union*, July 27, 1985, p. 3.
30. Agarwal, D. et. al., *Alcoholism: Clinical and Experimental Research*, vol. 5 (1981), p. 12.
31. Williams, R., *Nutrition Against Disease* (New York: Pitman, 1971), chapter 11.
32. Bland, J. et. al., *1984-85 Yearbook of Nutritional Medicine* (New Canaan: Keats, 1985), p. 31.
33. See note 28 above.
34. Kastenbaum, R., *Journal of Nutrition for the Elderly*, vol. 4 (Spring 1985), p. 15.
35. Williams, R., *The Prevention of Alcoholism Through Nutrition* (New York: Bantam Books, 1981).
36. Sprince, H. et. al., *Agents and Actions*, vol. 4, no. 2 (1974), p. 125.

Chapter 15: Caffeine

1. Brody, J., *Jane Brody's Nutrition Book* (New York: W.W. Norton, 1981), chapter 12.
2. Williams, P. et. al., *Journal of the American Medical Association*, vol. 253 (Mar. 8, 1985), p. 1407.
3. Lecos, C., *FDA Consumer*, Oct. 1980, p. 6.
4. Brody, J., *Nutrition*, p. 241.
5. Linn, S. et. al., *New England Journal of Medicine*, vol. 306 (1982), p. 141.
6. Ibid.
7. Morrison, A. et. al., *Journal of the National Cancer Institute*, vol. 68 (Jan. 1982), p. 91.
8. Minton, J. et. al., *Nutrition Action*, vol. 135, no. 1 (1979), p. 157.
9. Lam, L., *Cancer Research*, vol. 42 (Apr. 1982), p. 1193.
10. Gershbein, L. et. al., *Research Communications in Chemical Pathology and Pharmacology*, vol. 28, no. 3 (June 1980), p. 457.
11. Costill, D. et. al., *Medicine and Science in Sports*, vol. 10, no. 3 (1978), p. 155.

Chapter 16: Food Additives

1. Levine, A. et. al., *New England Journal of Medicine*, vol. 312 (Mar. 7, 1985), p. 628.
2. Long, P. et. al., *Nutrition: An Inquiry into the Issues* (Englewood Cliffs, NJ: Prentice-Hall, 1983), p. 389.
3. Winter, R., *The Consumer's Dictionary of Food Additives* (New York: Crown, 1978).

4. Harman, L., *Age*, vol. 3 (1980), p. 100.
5. Maeura, B. et. al., *American Association of Cancer Research Abstracts*, 1983, p. 87.
6. Petersen, J., *British Journal of Dermatology*, vol. 94 (1976), p. 233.
7. Taylor, R., *Food Additives* (New York: John Wiley, 1980).
8. Tomita, I. et. al., *IARC Scientific Publications*, vol. 57 (1984), p. 33.
9. Koepke, J. et. al., *Annals of Allergy*, vol. 54, no. 3 (Mar. 1985), p. 213.
10. Lucas, J., *Our Polluted Food* (New York: John Wiley, 1974).

Chapter 17: Naturally Occurring Toxins in Food

1. Sapeika, N., in *Toxic Constituents of Animal Foodstuffs*, ed. I. Liener (New York: Academic Press, 1974), p. 1.
2. Chung, S. et. al., *Journal of Food Science*, vol. 46 (1981), p. 272.
3. Bain, R., *British Medical Journal*, vol. 290 (June 1, 1985), p. 1624.
4. Olson, R. et. al., in *Present Knowledge in Nutrition*, 5th ed. (Washington, D.C.: Nutrition Foundation, 1984), chapter 55.
5. *Medical Tribune* (May 18, 1985), p. 8.
6. Robinson, C. et. al., *Fundamentals of Normal Nutrition*, 3rd ed. (New York: Macmillan, 1978), p. 173.
7. Caster, W. et. al., *International Journal for Vitamin and Nutrition Research*, vol. 54 (1984), p. 371.
8. National Research Council, *Diet, Nutrition, and Cancer* (Washington, D.C.: National Academy Press, 1982), chapter 13.
9. Lucas, J., *Our Polluted Food* (New York: John Wiley, 1974).
10. Levick, R., *New England Journal of Medicine*, vol. 304 (Jan. 15, 1981), p. 172.
11. Hendler, S., *The Complete Guide to Anti-aging Nutrients* (New York: Simon & Schuster, 1985).
12. *Los Angeles Times*, part 5, Aug. 11, 1985, p. 3.
13. See note 9 above.
14. *San Diego Union*, July 13, 1983, p. B-3.
15. Sawhney, B. et. al., *Journal of Food Protection*, vol. 48 (May 1985), p. 442.
16. Schauss, A., *Diet, Crime and Delinquency* (Berkeley: Parker House, 1981), p. 32.
17. National Institute for the Foodservice Industry, *Applied Foodservice Sanitation*, 2nd ed. (Lexington, MA: D.C. Heath, 1978).
18. Hobbs, B., *Food Poisoning and Food Hygiene*, 2nd ed. (London: Edward Arnold, 1968).
19. MacDonald, K. et. al., *Journal of the American Medical Association*, vol. 253 (Mar. 1, 1985), p. 1275.
20. Bodey, G. et. al., *Candidiasis* (New York: Raven Press, 1985).
21. Winner, H. et. al., *Symposium on Candida Infections* (Edinburgh: E & S Livingstone, 1966).

Chapter 18: Pregnancy

1. Guthrie, H., *Introductory Nutrition*, 5th ed. (St. Louis: C.V. Mosby, 1983), chapter 16.
2. Henry, H. et. al., *Journal of the American Dietetic Association*, vol. 85 (Feb. 1985), p. 182.
   Belizan, J. et. al., *Journal of the American Medical Association*, vol. 249 (Mar. 4, 1983), p. 1165.
3. Hunt, I. et. al., *American Journal of Clinical Nutrition*, vol. 40 (Sept. 1984), p. 508.
4. Meadows, N. et. al., *Lancet*, Nov. 21, 1981, p. 1135.
5. Fortmann, S., *American Journal of Clinical Nutrition*, vol. 34 (Oct. 1981), p. 2030.
6. Sandstead, H., *Nutrition Reviews*, vol. 43 (May 1985), p. 129.
7. Cefalo, R., *Medical News*, Apr. 28, 1980, p. 14.

8. Worthington-Roberts, B., *Contemporary Developments in Nutrition* (St. Louis: C.V. Mosby, 1980), chapter 16.
9. Winick, M., *Malnutrition and Brain Development* (New York: Oxford University Press, 1976), pp. 38-40.
10. Baker, H. et. al., *American Journal of Clinical Nutrition*, vol. 28 (Jan. 1975), p. 59.
11. Mukherjee, M. et. al., *American Journal of Clinical Nutrition*, vol. 40 (Sept. 1984), p. 496.
12. Blot, I. et. al., *Bynecologic and Obstetric Investigation*, vol. 12, no. 6 (Aug. 1981), p. 297.
13. Hollingsworth, D., *Diabetes Care*, vol. 4, no. 6 (Nov. 1981), p. 647.
14. Sulik, K. et. al., *Science*, vol. 214 (1981), p. 936.
15. Jenkins, S. *British Journal of Nutrition*, vol. 43 (1980), p. 95.
16. Sexton, M. et. al., *Journal of the American Medical Association*, vol. 251 (Feb 17, 1984), p. 911.
17. Ericson, A. et. al., *American Journal of Obstetrics and Gynecology*, vol. 135 (1979), p. 348.
18. Linn, S. et. al., *New England Journal of Medicine*, vol. 306 (Jan. 21, 1982), p. 141.
19. Guthrie, *Introductory Nutrition*, p. 416.
20. Winick, M., *Modern Medicine*, Oct. 15, 1977, p. 108.
21. Dostalova, L. et. al., *Developmental Pharmacology and Therapeutics*, vol. 4, suppl. 1 (1982), p. 45.
22. See note 3 above.

Chapter 19: Infancy

1. Schneider, M. et. al., in *Contemporary Developments in Nutrition* (St. Louis: C. V. Mosby, 1980), chapter 17.
2. Styslinger, L. et. al., *American Journal of Clinical Nutrition*, vol. 41 (Jan. 1985), p. 21.
3. Krebs, N. et. al., *American Journal of Clinical Nutrition*, vol. 41 (Mar. 1985), p. 560.
4. Moser, P. et. al., *Journal of the American Dietetic Association*, vol. 84 (Jan. 1984), p. 42.
5. Huang, L. et. al., *Nutrition Research*, vol. 4 (1984), p. 977.
6. Hamilton, E. et. al., *Nutrition: Concepts and Controversies*, 3rd ed. (St. Paul: West, 1982).
7. *Nutrition Reviews*, vol. 41 (Mar. 1983), p. 80.
8. Chandra, R., *Acta Paediatrica Scandinavica*, vol. 68 (1979), p. 691.
9. Nelson, G. et. al., *Journal of the American Medical Association*, vol. 253 (Apr. 5, 1985), p. 1880.
10. Freundlich, M. et. al., *Lancet*, Sept. 7, 1985, p. 527.
11. National Research Council, *Recommended Dietary Allowances*, 9th ed. (Washington, D. C.: National Academy of Sciences, 1980), p. 27.
12. Anderson, D. et. al., *Journal of the American Dietetic Association*, vol. 85 (June 1985), p. 715.
13. Sims, A., *American Dietetic Association*, vol. 73 (Aug. 1978), p. 139.
14. Cockburn, F. et. al., *British Medical Journal*, (July 5, 1980), p. 11.
15. Acosta, P. et. al., *American Journal of Clinical Nutrition*, vol. 27 (Dec. 1974), p. 1359.
16. Wallenburg, H. et. al., *Journal of Perinatal Medicine*, vol. 12 (1984), p. 7.
17. Oski, F. et. al., *Pediatric*, vol. 71 (June 1983), p. 877.
18. Idem, *Pediatric Clinics of North America*, vol. 32 (Apr. 1985), p. 493.
19. Schearer, M. et. al., *Lancet*, Aug. 28, 1982, p. 460.
20. Curtis, J. et. a., *Canadian Medical Association Journal*, vol. 128 (Jan. 15, 1983), p. 150.
21. Barness, L., *Nutritional Support of Medical Practice*, ed. H. Schneider et. al. (Hagerstown, Md.: Harper & Row, 1977), p. 455.
22. Orzalesi, M., *Acta Paediatrica Scandinavica*, suppl. 299 (1982), p. 77.
23. Bell, E. et. al., *Pediatrics*, vol. 63, no. 6 (1979), p. 830.

Chapter 20: Childhood

1. Waxman, M. et. al., *Journal of Pediatrics*, vol. 96, no. 2 (Feb. 1980), p. 187.
2. Rogers, C. et. al., *Home Economics Research Journal*, vol. 8, no. 3 (Jan. 1980), p. 173.
3. Goldsmith, R., *Nutrition and Learning* (Bloomington, IN: Phi Delta Kappa Educational Foundation, 1980).
4. Collipp, P. et. al., *Annals of Nutrition and Metabolism*, vol. 26 (1982), p. 287.
5. Choudhry, M. et. al., *Indian Journal of Nutrition and Dietetics*, vol. 21 (Jan. 1984), p. 1.
6. Kadam, S. et. al., *Indian Journal of Nutrition and Dietetics*, vol. 21 (Feb. 1984), p. 69.
7. *Science*, vol. 160 (1968), p. 322.
8. Kohrs, M. et al., *American Journal of Clinical Nutrition*, vol. 32 (1979) p. 1206.
9. Rao, B., *British Medical Bulletin*, vol. 37 (1981), p. 25.
10. Krebs, N. et. al., *American Journal of Diseases of Children*, vol. 138 (Mar. 1984), p. 270.
11. Deringer, S., *Journal of School Health*, vol. 43, no. 8 (Oct. 1973), p. 528.
12. Ashbrook, S. et. al., *Journal of Nutrition Education*, vol. 17 (Mar. 1985), p. 5.
13. Egger, J. et. al., *Lancet*, Mar. 9, 1985, p. 540.
14. Hamilton, E. et. al., *Nutrition: Concepts and Controversies*, 3rd ed. (St. Paul: West, 1985), p. 440.
15. United States Senate Select Committee on Nutrition and Human Needs, *Nutrition and Mental Health* (Berkeley: Parker House, 1980), p. 70.

Chapter 21: Adolescense

1. Driskell, J. et. al., *Journal of the American Dietetic Association*, vol. 85 (Jan. 1985), p. 46.
2. Kathman, J. et. al., *Nutrition Research*, vol. 4 (1984), p. 245.
3. Wynn, V., *Lancet*, Mar. 8, 1975, p. 561.
4. Winston, F., *American Journal of Psychiatry*, vol. 130, no. 11 (Nov. 1973), p. 1217.
5. Larsson-Cohn, U., *American Journal of Obstetrics and Gynecology*, vol. 121 (Jan. 1, 1975), p. 84.
6. *American Dietetic Association*, vol. 68 (May 1976), p. 419.
7. Kligman, A. et. al., *International Journal of Dermatology*, vol. 20, no. 4 (May 1981), p. 278.
8. Verma, K. et. al., *Acta Dermato-Venereologica*, vol. 60 (1980), p. 337.
9. "A Report from Congressman Bill Lowery," compiled by the Library of Congress, Nov. 1985.
10. Deisher, R. et. al., *Pediatrics*, vol. 44 (July 1969), p. 131.
11. Martinez, F. et. al., *Journal of Neurology*, vol. 48, no. 3 (Dec. 1980), p. 315.
12. Alvarez-Dardet, C., et. al., *New England Journal of Medicine*, vol. 312 (June 6, 1985), p. 1521.
13. Guthrie, H., *Introductory Nutrition*, 5th ed. (St. Louis: C. V. Mosby, 1983), p. 487.
14. Gold, E., *Journal of the American Dietetic Association*, vol. 55 (1969), p. 27.

Chapter 22: Older Adulthood

1. Guthrie, H., *Introductory Nutrition*, 5th ed. (St. Louis: C. V. Mosby, 1983), p. 504.
2. Stini, W., *Federation Proceedings*, vol. 40 (Sept. 1981), p. 2588.
3. Recker, R., *New England Journal of Medicine*, vol. 313 (July 11, 1985), p. 70.
4. Ross Laboratories, *Aging and Nutrition* (Ft. Wayne, IN.: Ross Laboratories, 1979).
5. Hendler, S., *The Complete Guide to Anti-Aging Nutrients* (New York: Simon & Schuster, 1985), p. 23.
6. Bortz, W., *Journal of the American Medical Association*, vol. 248 (Sept. 10, 1982), p. 1203.

7. Munro, H., *British Medical Bulletin*, vol. 37 (1981), p. 83.
8. Seals, D. et. al., *Journal of the American Medical Association*, vol. 252 (Aug. 3, 1984), p. 645.
9. Roe, A., *Geriatric Nutrition* (Englewood Cliffs, N.J.: Prentice-Hall, 1983), p. 38.
10. Brown, P. et. al., *American Dietetic Association*, vol. 71 (July 1977), p. 41.
11. Dychtwald, K. et. al., eds., *Millennium: Glimpses into the 21st Century*, (Los Angeles: J. P. Tarcher, 1981).
12. Fisher, S. et. al., *American Journal of Clinical Nutrition*, vol. 31 (1978), p. 667.
13. Baker, H. et. al., *Journal of the American Ceriatrics Society*, vol. 26, no. 5 (1978), p. 218.
14. Geissler, C. et. al., *American Journal of Clinical Nutrition*, vol. 39 (Mar. 1984), p. 478.
15. Kohrs, M. et. al., *American Journal of Clinical Nutrition*, vol. 31 (1978), p. 2186.
16. Masoro, E., in *Nutrition and Aging*, ed. M. Winick (New York: John Wiley, 1975).
17. Neldner, K., *Geriatrics*, Feb. 1984, p. 69.
18. Pangborn, R. et. al., *Food Technology*, Aug. 1975, p. 75.
19. Robinson, C., *Fundamentals of Normal Nutrition*, 3rd ed. (New York: Macmillan, 1978), p. 328.
20. Weinberg, J., *Journal of the American Dietetic Association*, vol. 60 (1972), p. 293.
21. McCann, M. et. al., *New Physician*, Apr. 1978, p. 41.
22. Todhunter, E. et. al., *Geriatrics*, June 1978, p. 49.
23. Schorah, C. et. al., *Lancet*, Feb. 24, 1979, p. 403.
24. Lawson, M. et. al., *British Medical Journal*, vol. 2 (Aug. 4, 1979), p. 303.
25. Kastenbaum, R., *Journal of Nutrition for the Elderly*, vol. 4 (Spring 1985), p. 15.
26. Gelenberg, J. et. al., *American Journal of Psychiatry*, vol. 136, no. 6 (June 1979), p. 772.
27. Lacour, B. et. al., *Lancet*, Oct. 11, 1980, p. 763.
28. Mahajan, S. et. al., *Annals of Internal Medicine*, vol. 97 (Sept. 1982), p. 357.
29. Tanaka, O. et. al., *Fortschritte Der Chemie Organischer Naturstoffe*, vol. 46 (1984), p. 1.
30. Timmreck, T., *Geriatrics*, Oct. 1977, p. 137.

Chapter 23: Obesity

1. Bennion, L. et. al., *Journal of Clinical Investigation*, vol. 56 (Oct. 1975), p. 996.
2. Bialkowska, M. et. al., *Materia Medica Polona*, vol. 3, no. 32 (1977), p. 244.
3. Tullis, F. et. al., in *Nutritional Support of Medical Practice*, ed. H. Schneider et. al. (Hagerstown, Md: Harper & Row, 1977), p. 392.
4. Swaminathan, R. et. al., *American Journal of Clinical Nutrition*, vol.42 (Aug. 1985), p. 177.
5. Hallfrisch, J. et. al., *Nutrition Research*, vol.2 (1982), p. 263.
6. Prentice, A. et. al., *Lancet*, June 22, 1985, p. 1419.
7. Garrow, J. et. al., *Lancet*, Mar. 2, 1985, p. 670.
8. Chalmers, J., *Lancet*, Feb. 2, 1985, p. 287.
9. Surgeon General, *Healthy People* (Washington, D.C.: U.S. Department of Health, Education, and Welfare, 1979).
10. Ferguson, J., in *Lipoplasty*, ed. G. Hetter (Boston: Little, Brown, 1984), chapter 7.
11. See note 8 above.
12. Kark, A., *American Journal of Clinical Nutrition*, vol. 33 (Feb. 1980), p. 420.
13. *Journal of the American Medical Association*, vol. 224 (June 4, 1973), p. 1415.
14. Lee, C. et. al., *American Journal of Clinical Nutrition*, vol. 34 (May 1981), p. 819.
15. Leveille, G. et. al., *Nutrition Today*, Nov/Dec. 1974, p. 4.
16. Clausen, J. et. al., *Journal of the American Dietetic Association*, vol. 77 (Sept. 1980), p. 249.
17. Danforth, E., *American Journal of Clinical Nutrition*, vol. 41 (May 1985), p. 1132.

18. Mickelsen, O. et. al., *Journal of Nutrition*, vol. 57 (1955), p. 541.
19. Acheson, K. et. al., *American Journal of Physiology*, vol. 246 (1984), p. 62.
20. Taber, L. et. al., *Journal of the American Dietetic Association*, vol. 76 (Jan. 1980), p. 21.
21. Bjorntorp, P., *Clinics in Endocrinology and Metabolism*, vol. 5, no. 2 (July 1976), p. 431. Allen, D. et. al., *Medical Journal of Australia*, vol. 2 (Sept. 24, 1977), p. 434.
22. Babirak, S. et. al., *Journal of Nutrition*, vol.104 (1974), p. 452.
23. Braitman, L. et. al., *Journal of Chronic Diseases*, vol. 38 (1985), p. 727.
24. *Journal of Nutrition Education*, vol. 7, no. 2 (Apr. 1975), p. 65. Stuart, R. et. al., *Journal of the American Dietetic Association*, vol. 75 (Sept. 1979), p. 258.
25. Drabman, R. et. al., *Journal of Nutrition Education*, vol. 9, no. 2 (Apr. 1977), p. 80.

Chapter 24: Heart Disease

1. U.S. Bureau of the Census, *Statistical Abstract of the United States: 1985*, 105th ed., Washington, D.C., 1984.
2. Braunwald, E., *New England Journal of Medicine*, vol. 309 (Nov. 10, 1983), p. 1181.
3. Levy, R., *American Journal of Cardiology*, vol. 54 (Aug. 27, 1984), p. 70.
4. Kushi, L. et. al., *New England Journal of Medicine*, vol. 312 (Mar. 28, 1985), p. 811.
5. Kaplan, N., *Annals of Internal Medicine*, vol. 102 (Mar. 1985), p. 359.
6. Duva, J. et. al., *Mount Sinai Journal of Medicine*, vol. 46, no. 4 (July 1979), p. 416.
7. Paffenbarger, R. et. al., *Journal of the American Medical Association*, vol. 252 (July 27, 1984), p. 491.
8. Noppa, H. et. al., *American Journal of Epidemiology*, vol. 3, no. 6 (1980), p. 682.
9. Bertino, M. et. al., American Journal of Clinical Nutrition, vol. 36 (Dec. 1982), p. 1134.
10. Newman, H. et. al., *Clinical Chemistry*, vol. 24 (1978), p. 541.
11. Mertz, W., *Federation Proceedings*, vol. 41, no. 11 (Sept. 1982), p. 2807.
12. Salonen, J. et. al., *Lancet*, July 24, 1982, p. 175.
13. Kromhout, D. et. al., *New England Journal of Medicine*, vol. 312 (May 9, 1985), p. 1205.
14. Johnson, N. et. al., *American Journal of Clinical Nutrition*, vol. 42 (July 1985), p. 12.
15. See note 11 above.
16. Hubbard, J. et. al., *New England Journal of Medicine*, vol. 313 (July 4, 1985), p. 52.

Chapter 25: Cancer

1. Willett, W. et. al., *New England Journal of Medicine*, vol. 310 (Mar. 8, 1984), p. 633. Also Mar. 15, 1984, p. 697.
2. Ibid.
3. U.S. Bureau of the Census, *Statistical Abstract of the United States: 1985*, 105th ed., Washington, D.C., 1984
4. See note 1 above.
5. *Los Angeles Times*, Feb. 10, 1985, part 1, p. 6.
6. Beral, V. et. al., *Lancet*, Aug. 7, 1982, p. 290.
7. Lawrence, W., *Cancer*, vol. 43, no. 5 (May suppl., 1979), p. 2020.
8. See note 1 above.
9. Maugh, T., *Science*, vol. 217 (July 2, 1982), p. 36.
10. *Lancet*, May 29, 1982, p. 1223.
11. National Research Council, *Diet, Nutrition, and Cancer* (Washington, D.C.: National Academy Press, 1982).
12. Ibid.
13. Salonen, J. et. al., *American Journal of Epidemiology*, vol. 120 (1984), p. 342.
14. Shamberger, R., in *Proceedings of the Symposium on Selenium-Tellurium in the Environment* (Pittsburgh: Industrial Health Foundation, 1976), p. 253.

15. Hendler, S., *The Complete Guide to Anti-Aging Nutrients* (New York: Simon & Schuster, 1985), p. 168.
16. Carroll, K., *Cancer Research*, vol. 35 (1975), p. 3374.
17. See note 1 above.
18. Edes, T. et. al., *Proceedings of the Society for Experimental Biology and Medicine*, vol. 162, no. 1 (1979), p. 71.
19. Van Rensburg, S., *Journal of the National Cancer Institute*, vol. 67 (Aug. 1981), p. 243.

Chapter 26: Diabetes

1. U.S. Bureau of Census, *Statistical Abstract of the United States: 1985*, 105th ed., Washington, D.C. (1984), p.74.
2. Krall, L. ed., *Joslin Diabetes Manual*, 11th ed. (Philadelphia: Lea & Febiger, 1978).
3. Freedland and Briggs, *A Biochemical Approach to Nutrition* (New York: John Wiley, 1977).
4. Pi-Sunyer, F. et. al., in *Present Knowledge in Nutrition*, 4th ed. (Washington, D.C.: Nutrition Foundation, 1984), chapter 40.
5. Mayer, J., in *Modern Nutrition in Health and Disease*, ed. Goodhart, R. et. al. (Philadelphia: Lea & Febiger, 1976), chapter 22.
6. Anderson, R.A. et. al., *American Journal of Clinical Nutrition*, vol. 41 (June 1985), p. 1177.
7. Elias, A.N. et. al., *General Pharmacology*, vol. 15, no. 6 (1984), p. 535.
8. Baldwin, C., *Prevention*, Dec. 1979, p. 146.
9. Mertz, W., in *Present Knowledge in Nutrition*, 4th ed. (1976), chapter 36.
10. McCarty, M., *Medical Hypotheses*, vol. 13 (1984), p. 139.
11. McCann, V.J. et. al., *Australian and New Zealand Journal of Medicine*, vol. 8 (1978), p. 259.
12. Harris, I. et. al., *Lancet*, vol. 2 (1971), p. 735.
13. Horrobin, D., article submitted to *Lipids*.

Chapter 27: Osteoporosis

1. *Journal of the American Medical Association*, vol. 252 (Aug. 10, 1984), p. 799.
2. Boyce, W. et. al., *Lancet* (Jan. 19, 1985), p. 150.
3. Sandler, R. et. al., *American Journal of Clinical Nutrition*, vol. 42 (Aug. 1985), p. 270.
4. See note 1 above.
5. *Lancet*, June 15, 1985, p. 1370.
6. Raisz, L., *Journal of the American Geriatrics Society*, vol. 30 (Feb. 1982), p. 127.
7. Boyce, B. et. al., *Lancet*, Nov. 6, 1982, p. 1009.
8. See note 3 above.
9. Korcok, M., *Journal of the American Medical Association*, vol. 247 (Feb. 26, 1982), p. 1106.
10. *Lancet*, Aug. 21, 1982, p. 423.
11. See note 6 above.
12. Schnitzler, C. et. al., *South African Medical Journal*, vol. 66, no. 19 (Nov. 10, 1984), p. 730.
13. Robinson, C., *Fundamentals of Normal Nutrition*, 3rd ed. (New York: Macmillan, 1978), p. 105.

Chapter 28: Arthritis

1. Jayson, M. et. al., *Understanding Arthritis and Rheumatism* (New York: Pantheon, 1974).

2. Kelly, W. et. al., eds., *Textbook of Rheumatology*, vol. 1, 2nd ed. (Philadelphia: W.B. Saunders, 1985).
3. Holvey, D., ed., *The Merck Manual*, 12th ed. (Rahway, N.J.: Merck & Co., 1972), p. 1206.
4. Williams, R., *Nutrition Against Disease* (New York: Bantam Books, 1973).
5. Regtop, H., in *Yearbook of Nutritional Medicine*, ed. J. Bland (New Canaan: Keats, 1985), pp. 55-70.
6. Kremer, J. et. al., *Lancet*, Jan. 26, 1985, p. 184.
7. Lee, T., et. al., *New England Journal of Medicine*, vol. 312 (May 9, 1985), p. 1217.
8. Simpkin, P., *Lancet*, 1976, p. 539.
9. Bauman, J. et. al., *Prostaglandins*, vol. 20 (1980), p. 627.

Chapter 29: Food Allergies and Sensitivities

1. Buckley, R. et. al., *Journal of the American Medical Association*, vol. 248 (Nov. 26, 1982), p. 2627.
2. Monro, J., *Lancet*, Sept. 29, 1984, p. 719.
3. Fontana, V., in *Modern Nutrition in Health and Disease*, ed. Goodhart, R. et. al. (Philadelphia: Lea & Febiger, 1976), p. 924, passim.
4. Cant, A., *Human Nutrition: Applied Nutrition*, vol. 38A (Dec. 1984), p. 455.
5. Vietmeyer, N., *Smithsonian*, Dec. 1985, p. 34.
6. Whitney, E. et. al., in *Understanding Normal and Clinical Nutrition* (St. Paul: West Publishing, 1983), p. 814.
7. Halsted, C., *American Journal of Clinical Nutrition*, vol. 33 (1980), p. 2736.
8. Koepke, J. et. al., *Annals of Allergy*, vol. 54, no.3 (Mar. 1985), p. 213.
9. Winner, H. et. al., *Symposium on Candida Infections* (Edinburgh: E & S Livingstone, 1966).

Chapter 30: Smokers

1. *Los Angeles Times*, part 7, Nov. 4, 1984, p. 18.
2. Pelletier, O., *Annals of the New York Academy of Sciences*, vol. 258 (1975), p. 156.
3. Remington, P. et. al., *Journal of the American Medical Association*, vol. 253 (May 24, 1985), p. 2975.
4. Sprince, H. et. al., *Agents and Actions*, vol. 4, no. 2 (1974), p. 125.
5. Sandler, D. et. al., *Lancet*, Feb. 9, 1985, p. 312.
6. Ibid.
7. Sexton, M. et. al., *Journal of the American Medical Association*, vol. 251 (Feb. 17, 1984), p. 911.
8. Stich, H., *International Journal of Cancer*, vol. 34 (1984), p. 745.
9. Carney, R.M. et. al., *New England Journal of Medicine*, vol. 310 (Mar. 1984), p. 614.

Chapter 31: Mental Functions

1. Seaker, M., *East West Journal*, vol. 12, no. 7 (July 1982), p. 26.
2. Barnes, B., *Hope: Hypoglycemia* (Los Angeles: Cancer Book House, 1977).
3. Groves, P. et. al., *Biological Psychology* (Dubuque: Wm. C. Brown, 1979).
4. Leiberman, H. et. al., *American Journal of Clinical Nutrition*, vol. 42 (Aug. 1985), p. 366.
5. Gelenberg, A. et. al., *American Journal of Psychiatry*, vol. 136, no. 6 (June 1979), p. 772.
6. Signoret, J. et. al., *Lancet*, Oct. 14, 1978, p. 837.
7. Lehnert, H. et. al., *Brain Research*, vol. 303 (1984), p. 215.

8. Lieberman, H.R. et. al., *Food Technology*, vol. 40 (Jan. 1986), p. 139.
9. Zamenhof, S. et. al., *Journal of Nutrition*, vol. 101 (1971), p. 1265.

Chapter 32: Sex

1. Willett, W. et. al., *New England Journal of Medicine*, vol. 310 (Mar. 8, 1984), p. 633.
2. Church, C., *Food Values of Portions Commonly Used* (Philadelphia: J.B. Lippincott, 1975).
3. Sudesh, K. et. al., *Annals of Internal Medicine*, vol. 97, no. 3 (Sept. 1982), p. 357.
4. Pfeiffer, C., *Zinc and Other Micro-nutrients* (New Canaan: Keats, 1978), p. 45.
5. Verma, K. et. al., *Acta Dermato-Vereneologica*, vol. 60 (1980), p. 337.
6. Hendler, S., *The Complete Guide to Anti-aging Nutrients* (New York: Simon & Schuster, 1985), p. 192.
7. Gonzalez, E., *Journal of the American Medical Association*, vol. 249, no. 20 (May 27, 1983), p. 2747.
8. Schachter, A. et. al., *Journal of Urology*, vol. 110 (Sept. 1973), p. 311.
9. Fahim, M. et. al., *Federation Proceedings*, vol. 35, no. 3 (Mar. 1, 1976), p. 361.
10. Abraham, G. et. al., *American Journal of Clinical Nutrition*, vol. 34 (Nov. 1981), p. 2364.
11. Goei, G. et. al., *Journal of Reproductive Medicine*, vol. 28, no. 8 (Aug. 1983), p. 527.
12. Williams, M. et. al., *Journal of International Medical Research*, vol. 13 (1985), p. 174.
13. Abraham, G., *Journal of Reproductive Medicine*, vol. 28, no. 7 (July 1983), p. 446.
14. Horrobin, D., *Journal of Reproductive Medicine*, vol. 28 (1983), p. 465.
15. Minton, J. et. al., *American Journal of Obstetrics and Gynecology*, vol. 135, no. 1 (Sept. 1, 1979), p. 157.
16. Howard, L. et. al., *American Journal of Clinical Nutrition*, vol. 36 (Dec. 1982), p. 1243.
17. Watrach, A. et. al., *Cancer Letters*, vol. 25 (1984), p. 632.
18. Orr, J. et. al., *American Journal of Obstetrics and Gynecology*, vol. 151 (Mar. 1, 1985), p. 632
19. Koop, C.E., *The Surgeon General's Report on AIDS*, Los Angeles Times supplement, Dec. 7, 1986.
20. Moseson, M., *Nutrition Research*, vol. 6 (1986), p. 729.
21. Weiner, R.G., *Journal of the American Medical Association*, vol. 252 (Sept. 1984), p. 1409.
22. Jain, J.K. et. al., *Nutrition Research*, vol. 6 (1986), p. 729.
23. Cathcart, R.F., *Medical Hypotheses*, vol. 14 (1984), p. 423.
24. Locke, S. et. al., *Foundations of Psychoneuroimmunology* (New York: Aldine Publishers, 1985).
25. Nonavinakere, V., *Nutrition Reports International*, vol. 23 (Apr. 1981), p. 297.
26. Adams, P. et. al., *Lancet*, Apr. 28, 1973, p. 7809.

Chapter 33: The Athlete

1. Bergstrom, J. et. al., *Journal of the American Medical Association*, vol. 221 (Aug. 28, 1972), p. 1000.
2. Robinson, C., *Fundamentals of Normal Nutrition* (New York: Macmillan, 1978), p. 63.
3. Williams, M., *Nutritional Aspects of Human Physical and Athletic Performance* (Springfield, Ill.: C.C. Thomas, 1976).
4. Howald, H., *Annals of the New York Academy of Sciences*, vol. 258 (1975), p. 458.
5. Leibovitz, B., *Carnitine* (New York: Dell, 1984), p. 169.
6. McCarty, M., *Medical Hypotheses*, vol. 7 (1981), p. 515.
7. Richardson, J., *Journal of Sports Medicine*, vol. 19 (1979), p. 133.
8. Bicknell, F. et. al., *The Vitamins in Medicine* (London: Heinneman, 1945).
9. Ivy, J. et. al., *Medicine and Science in Sports*, vol. 11, no. 1 (1979), p. 6.
10. Dorling, E., *Notabene Medici*, vol. 10, no. 5 (1980), p. 241.

11. Forgo, I., et. al., *Aerztliche Praxis*, vol. 33, no. 44 (1981), p. 1784.
12. Costill, D. et. al., in *Biochemistry of Exercise*, ed. Howard, H. (Baltimore: University Park Press, 1975).
13. Olsson, K. et. al., *Scandinavian Journal of Rehabilitative Medicine*, vol. 3 (1971), p. 31.
14. Peterson, D. et. al., *American Journal of Epidemiology*, vol. 92 (1970), p. 90.
15. Schrauzer, G. et. al., *Annals of the New York Academy of Sciences*, vol. 258 (1975), p. 377.
16. Kotze, H. et. al., *Journal of Applied Physiology*, vol. 42 (1977), p. 711.
17. Dillard, C. et. al., *Journal of Applied Physiology*, vol. 45 (1978), p. 927.
18. Brady, P. et. al., *Journal of Nutrition*, vol. 109 (1979), p. 1103.
19. Consolazio, C. et. al., *American Journal of Clinical Nutrition*, vol. 28 (Jan. 1975), p. 28.
20. Ashworth, A. et. al., *British Journal of Nutrition*, vol. 21 (1967), p. 833.
21. Williams, M., *Drugs and Athletic Performance* (Springfield, Ill.: C.C. Thomas, 1974).
22. Isidori, A. et. al., *Current Medical Research and Opinion*, vol. 7, no. 7 (1981), p. 475.
23. American College of Sports Medicine Position Statement, *Medicine and Science in Sports and Exercise*, vol. 9 (1977), p. 79.
24. Bonen, A. et. al., *Journal of Applied Physiology: Respiratory, Environmental and Exercise Physiology*, vol. 50, no. 4 (1981), p. 766.
25. *Lancet*, June 29, 1985, p. 1490.

Chapter 34: United States Recommended Daily Allowance

1. Kenney, K., *Glendale Daily News*, Nov. 4, 1985, p. 4.

Chapter 35: Senate Dietary Goals

1. U.S. Department of Agriculture, *Nutrition and Your Health, Dietary Guidelines for Americans*, Home and Garden Bulletin No. 232, Superintendent of Documents, Washington, D.C.

Chapter 36: Regulation of the Vitamin Industry

1. Kabir, H. et. al., *Journal of Nutrition*, vol. 113 (1983), p. 2412.
2. Yung, S. et. al., *Journal of Pharmaceutical Sciences*, vol. 71 (Mar. 1982), p. 282.
3. Whittington, R. et. al., *Lancet*, Jan. 22, 1983, p. 184.
4. Hendler, S., *The Complete Guide to Anti-aging Nutrients* (New York: Simon & Schuster, 1985), p. 101.

Chapter 37: Food Labeling

1. U.S. Department of Health, Education, and Welfare, *Current and Useful Information From the Food and Drug Administration*, DHEW Publication No. (FDA) 74-2022, (Washington, D.C., Mar. 1974).
2. Hamilton, E. et. al., *Nutrition: Concepts and Controversies* (St. Paul: West Publishing), p. 313.
3. Schroeder, H., *American Journal of Clinical Nutrition*, vol. 24 (May 1971).

Chapter 38: The Exchange System

1. Guthrie, H. et. al., *Journal of Nutrition Education*, vol. 13, no. 2 (1981), p. 46.

Chapter 40: Super Foods

1. Carroll, K., *Federation Proceedings*, vol. 41 (Sept. 1982), p. 2792.

2. Fleming, S. et. al., *American Journal of Clinical Nutrition*, vol. 41, no. 5 (May 1985), p. 909.
3. Jenkins, D. et. al., *American Journal of Clinical Nutrition*, vol. 34 (Mar. 1981), p. 362.
4. Saynor, R. *Lancet*, Sept. 22, 1984, p. 696.
5. Kromhout, D. et. al., *New England Journal of Medicine*, vol. 312 (May 9, 1985), p. 1205.
6. Bordia, A., *American Journal of Clinical Nutrition*, vol. 34 (Oct. 1981), p. 2100.
7. Sharma, V. et. al., *Indian Journal of Experimental Biology*, vol. 15 (1977), p. 466.
8. Amer, M. et. al., *International Journal of Dermatology*, vol. 19 (1980), p. 285.
9. Fujiwara, M. et. al., *Nature*, vol. 216 (1967), p. 83.
10. Bordia, A. et. al., *Atherosclerosis*, vol. 21 (1975), p. 15.
11. See note 6 above.
12. Miller, T., *Journal of the American Dietetic Association*, vol. 77 (Nov. 1980), p. 561.
13. *Indian Journal of Physiology and Pharmacology*, vol. 24 (1980), p. 233.
14. Amonkar, S. et. al., *Journal of Economic Entomology*, vol. 63 (1970), p. 1172.
15. Chang, M. et. al., *Journal of Nutrition*, vol. 110 (1980), p. 931.
16. Mowrey, D., *Lancet*, Mar. 20, 1982, p. 655.
17. Giri, J. et. al., *Indian Journal of Nutrition and Dietetics*, vol. 21 (Dec. 1984), p. 433.
18. Visudhiphan, S., *American Journal of Clinical Nutrition*, vol. 35 (June 1982), p. 1452.
19. Kumar, N. et. al., *British Medical Journal*, vol. 288 (June 16, 1984), p. 1803.
20. Cummings, M., *American Journal of Clinical Nutrition*, vol. 34 (Feb. 1981), p. 297.
21. Fordham, J. et. al., *Journal of Food Science*, vol. 40 (1975), p. 552.
22. Chen, L. et. al., *Journal of Food Science*, vol. 42 (1977), p. 1666.
23. Chen, L. et. al., *Journal of Food Science*, vol. 40 (1975), p. 1290.
24. Lai, J. et. al., *Nutrition and Cancer*, vol. 1 (1978), p. 27.
25. Anderson, J., *American Journal of Clinical Nutrition*, vol. 41 (May 1985), p. 1103.
26. *Food Engineering*, vol. 57 (Mar. 1985), p. 74.
27. Brown, W. et. al., *American Journal of Clinical Nutrition*, vol. 41 (May 1985), p. 1163.
28. Bierman, E., *American Journal of Clinical Nutrition*, vol. 41 (May 1985), p. 1113.
29. Shaw, J., *American Journal of Clinical Nutrition*, vol. 41 (May 1985), p. 1117.
30. Hendler, S., *The Complete Guide to Anti-aging Nutrients* (New York: Simon & Schuster, 1985), p. 259.
31. National Research Council, *Diet, Nutrition, and Cancer* (Washington, D.C.: National Academy Press, 1982).
32. Spector, H. et. al., *Proceedings of the Society for Experimental Biology and Medicine*, vol. 100 (1959), p. 405.
33. See note 30 above, p. 262.
34. Hesseltine, C., *Nutrition Reviews*, vol. 41, no. 10 (Oct. 1983), p. 293.
35. Hepner, G. et. al., *American Journal of Clinical Nutrition*, vol. 32 (Jan. 1979), p. 19.
36. *New England Journal of Medicine*, vol. 310 (1984), p. 1.
37. Reddy, N. et. al., *Journal of Food Science*, vol. 45 (1980), p. 1708.
38. Zamora, R. et.,al., *Journal of Nutrition*, vol. 109 (1979), p. 1333.
39. Steinkraus, K., *Antonie Van Leeuwenhoek*, vol. 49, no. 3 (Sep. 1983), p. 337.
40. *Nutrition and Cancer*, vol. 1 (1979), p. 19.
41. Held, S. et. al., *Forecast for Home Economics*, Apr. 1975, p. F-27.

Afterword

1. Ziporyn, T., *Journal of the American Medical Association*, vol. 253 (Apr. 5, 1985), p. 1846.
2. Sommer, A. et. al., *Lancet*, June 27, 1981, p. 1407.
3. Bhat, K.S., *Nutrition Reports International*, vol. 36, no. 3 (Sept. 1987), p. 685.
4. Hamilton, E. et. al., *Nutrition: Concepts and Controversies* (St. Paul: West Publishing, 1985), p. 149.
5. Smotherton, R., *Transforming* (San Francisco: Context, 1982), p. 124.

INDEX

Acetylcholine, 95, 100, 127
Acid-base (pH) balancers, 75, 163
Acne, 207-8, 268
Adenosine triphosphate (ATP), 106, 135
Adolescents
    acne in, 207-8
    alcohol/drug abuse by, 208-9
    anemia in, 210
    eating problems of, 209-10
    emotional changes in, 207
    physical changes in, 206-7
    pregnancy of, 188, 211
    recommended diet for, 211
    stress in, 210-11
Aflatoxins, 171
Aging
    eating problems of, 216
    mental powers in, 213
    nutritional problems of, 212
    physical changes of, 213-16
    recommended diet for, 216-17
AIDS (acquired immune deficiency syndrome), 271-73
Alcohol
    absorption of, 145-46
    calorie content of, 150
    contaminants in, 149
    hangover remedies for, 151-52
    -nutrient interaction, 14
    physiological effects of, 146-49
    and potency, 268
    in pregnancy, 147, 181, 187, 287
    production of, 145
    rational consumption of, 152
Alcoholism, 98, 115, 127, 128, 145, 249
    in adolescence, 208, 209
    nutrient treatment for, 150-51
Allergies. See Food allergies
Aluminum, 124, 163, 166, 248, 266
Alzheimer's disease, 124, 128, 163, 166, 213, 265, 266
Amino acids, 56, 57, 75, 95, 253
Amphetamines, 14
Anderson, James, 47
Anecdotal evidence, 21
Anemia, 56, 83, 90, 98, 100, 115, 185, 196, 203, 210, 288
    pernicious, 97, 99
Animal food
    carnitine in, 129

chicken dinner, easiest (recipe), 309
cholesterol in, 67
drug residues in, 174-75
fat in, 64, 68-70
See also Fish; Liver
Animal studies, 22
Anorexia nervosa, 226
Antacids, 14, 115
Antibiotics, 14, 174
Anticonvulsants, 14
Antihistamines, 14
Antihyperlipidemics, 14
Antihypertensives, 14
Appetite
    drugs and, 14-15
    poor, 201, 216
    See also Eating
Apples, 322
Apricot pits, 140
Arsenic, 102, 124
Arteriosclerosis, 234
Arthritis, 24, 72, 132, 133
    causes of, 249-50
    treatment of, 250-51
Asbestos poisoning, 149, 176, 238
Ascorbic acid. See Vitamin C
Aspartame, 164
Aspirin, 24, 115
Atherosclerosis, 233-34
Athletic performance
    and blood supply, 279
    bodybuilding, 278
    energy metabolism in, 274-76
    fluid/electrolyte balance in, 276-77
    pre-event meal in, 158, 278-79
    recommended nutrients for, 279-80
    and stress adaption, 277
    See also Exercise
Attitude
    and health, 8-9
    and weight control, 230-31
Avidin, 170

Bacteria
    in food poisoning, 176-77
    preservatives against, 160
    useful, 39, 139, 165, 320
Bananas, 321
Basophil histamine release, 255
Behavior modification, and weight control,

229-30
Beldekas, John, 273
Beri-beri, 92
Beta-carotene, 83, 84, 208, 239, 321
Beta cell burnout, 44
Biguanides, 14
Bile salts, 53, 67, 90
Bilirubin, 135
Bioflavonoids, 133-34
Biotin, 99-100
Birth control, 193
birth defects, 23-24, 98, 156, 181, 184, 187
Blindness, 23, 84, 87
Blind studies, 22-23
Blood
        clotting, 72, 317
        glucose, 40-42, 44, 48, 151, 155, 209,
            241-42, 263, 273
        ion levels in, 264
        and nutrient status, 27
        platelet aggregation, 234
        supply, 201, 279
        water in, 74
Bodybuilding, 278
Body fat, 221-23
Body maintenance, 8
Body temperature, 75, 117, 157, 277
Botulism, 160, 176-77
Brain
        cell loss in, 213, 214
        chemicals of, 56, 57, 94, 95, 127, 265
        development of, 108, 127, 184, 193,
            200, 266, 316
        function, 44, 56, 94, 95, 100, 127, 147
        interfering agents to, 265-66
        nutrient demands of, 94, 262-65
Breads/cereals
        additives to, 166
        in exchange system, 300
        See also Grains
Breast disease, 156, 270-71
Breast-feeding, 131, 137
        advantages of, 191-94, 253, 316
        duration of, 198
        lactation process in, 190-91
        nutrient needs of mother in, 89, 191,
            195, 284
        nutrient supplements for, 195-96
        obstacles to, 194-95
Brewer's yeast, 120, 136, 243, 244
Bulimia, 225-26
Butylated hydroxyanisole (BHA), 160, 240
Butylated hydroxytoluene (BHT), 160, 240

Cadmium, 124-25, 239, 269
Caffeine, 115

benefits of, 158, 276
and blood glucose levels, 41-42
effects on body, 154-57, 238, 271
sources of, 153-54
substitutes for, 157-58
See also Coffee
Calcium, 11, 13, 14, 15, 17, 20, 27, 42, 61,
        85, 90, 103-5, 116, 119, 148, 201, 234,
        236, 246-47, 264, 277, 285
Calories
        in alcohol, 150
        estimating needs for, 34, 287
        in old age, 214
Cancer
        causes of, 237-38
        and nutrition, 12, 53, 59, 72, 83, 84, 87,
            90, 98, 114, 118, 122, 123, 132, 133,
            140, 238-40, 271, 315, 320
        prevention program for, 240
        risk factors in, 63, 67, 77-78, 146, 156,
            171, 172, 258, 259
Candida albicans, 177
Carbohydrates
        in alcohol, 150
        basic unit of, 38
        daily intake of, 46, 286
        dietary functions of, 39, 265, 279
        food sources of, 38, 46
        and glucose tolerance, 40-42
        and lactose intolerance, 42
        loading, 274-75
        metabolism of, 39-40
        modified starch, 165
        types of, 37-38
        See also Fiber; Sugar
Cardiovascular system
        in aging, 213-14
        See also Heart disease
Carnitine, 25, 59, 71-72, 90, 128-29, 217,
        228, 275, 278
Carob, 157
Cassava, 169
Cell division, 83
Cellulose, 49
Chelation therapy, 234
Chicory, 157
Children
        and caffeine, 154, 155
        food preferences of, 199, 201-3
        nutritional problems of, 199, 203-4
        overfeeding of, 199, 203
        physical development of, 108, 137, 199,
            200-201
        recommended diet for, 205
        See also Hyperactivity; Infants
Chloramphenicol, 174

Chloride, 109
Chocolate, 154, 208
Cholesterol, 12, 48, 53, 90, 95, 135
    daily intake of, 66, 286
    and disease, 67-68
    food sources of, 67
    functions in body, 67
Choline, 68, 127, 217, 265, 316
Chondroiton sulfate, 141
Chromium, 12, 17, 28, 43, 44, 53, 102, 119-20, 136, 186, 217, 235, 243-44
Ciguatera, 170
Circulatory system, effects of alcohol on, 148
Cirrhosis of liver, 146
Clinical observations, 21-22
Clostridium botulinum, 176-77
Cobalt, 124
Coenzyme Q (CoQ), 134
Coffee
    caffeine content of, 154
    decaffeinated, 157
    See also Caffeine
Colchicine, 14
Collagen, 90, 114, 116
Colon cancer, 53, 72, 77
Comfrey tea, 170
Congeners, 149
Constipation, 53
Controlled scientific studies, 22-24
Copper, 116-17
Corticosteroids, 14
Cycasin, 169
Cyclamates, 164, 165
Cystic mastitis, 271
Cytotoxic testing, 255

DBCP, 173
Cehydration, 48, 75, 76-77, 148, 276
Delerium tremens, 147
Dental caries, 43, 121, 122, 124, 203, 260
Department of Health, Education and Welfare, 7, 11
Diabetes
    artificial insulin in, 245
    blood glucose and, 40-41, 44, 241-42
    causes of, 242-43
    incidence of, 241
    juvenile, 241, 242
    and nutrition, 47, 53, 59, 72, 75, 83, 84, 119, 120, 128, 132, 133, 135, 186, 243-44
    testing for, 242
Diethyl stilbestrol (DES), 175
Digestion/absorption
    and aging, 215

and alcohol consumption, 146
and caffeine, 156
enzymes in, 70, 140, 200, 215, 263-64
of fats, 48, 70-71, 90
of protein, 253
and stress, 210-11, 216
Digitalis, 14
Dioxin, 173, 238
Diuretics, 14, 226
Djenkolic acid, 170
DNA, 55, 87, 97, 98, 106, 112, 114, 118, 122, 124, 135, 238
Docosahexanoic acid (DHA), 65, 130, 131, 194, 316
Dopamine, 56, 265
Drug abuse, 208-9
Drugs
    caffeine content of, 154
    -nutrient interactions, 13-15, 226
    in pregnancy, 187-88
    residues in food supply, 174-75
    for weight loss, 227
Dyes, food, 161-62

Eating
    and behavior modification, 229-30
    disorders of, 183, 225-26
    and food preference, 201-2
    psychosocial aspects of, 202, 209, 210, 211, 216, 225
    See also Appetite; Obesity/overweight; Weight control
Eicosapentaenoic acid (EPA), 59, 65, 130-31, 194, 251, 316
Electrolytes, 264, 276-77
Elimination diet, 256
Emulsifiers/stabilizers, food, 161
Energy, 94, 100, 112, 273
    and carbohydrates, 37, 39, 42, 44
    and fats, 62, 71
    and fiber, 53
    maximum metabolism for, 274-76
    and vitamin E, 134
Environment, and health, 7
    See also Pollution
Enzymes, 55-56, 103, 134
    digestive, 70, 140, 200, 215, 263-64
    food additives, 165
Epilepsy, 45, 137
Ergot, 168, 171
Estrogen, 246, 248
Ethyl alcohol (ethanol), 145
Ethylene diamine tetracetic acid (EDTA), 162
Ethylene dibromide (EDB), 172
Evolutionary heritage, deviation from, 16-17

Exchange system, 297-303
Excretory system
    analysis of nutrient status, 28
    effects of alcohol on, 148
    and fiber diet, 47, 48
Exercise, 39, 42, 120, 260
    accelerated oxidation in, 277-78
    and caffeine, 158
    health benefits of, 6-7, 234, 247-48
    in pregnancy, 188
    and weight control, 228-29
    See also Athletic performance
Eyes, eyesight, 93, 147, 215
    See also Blindness

Fad diets, 227
Fat, 13, 14, 104, 120
    blockage of, 233-34
    body, 221-23
    burning of, 71-72, 129, 228, 274-75
    and cholesterol, 66-68
    deficiency of, 71
    digestion/absorption of, 48, 70-71, 90
    and disease, 72, 240, 248
    energy value of, 62, 71
    in exchange system, 299, 300
    food sources of, 68-70, 73, 314
    functions of, 62
    hydrogenated, 13, 66, 132
    and lecithin, 68, 127-28
    polyunsaturated, 63, 88, 239, 314
    recommended intake of, 73, 286
Fatty acids, essential, 13, 64-65, 71, 129-32
Fava beans, 170
Fertility, 268-69
Fetal alcohol syndrome (FAS), 112, 147, 181, 187
Fetal development
    risk factors in, 156, 259, 269
    stages of, 183-84
    See also Pregnancy
Fiber, 37, 39
    daily intake of, 215, 287
    excess, 48-49, 104
    and flatulence, 48, 51-52
    food sources of, 49-51, 315
    functions of, 47-48
    health benefits of, 52-54, 240
    types of, 49
Fish, 235
    fat in, 65, 69, 70
    nutrients in, 130, 315-16
    recipe for, 309-10
    toxins in, 170-71, 177
Fish oil, 131, 315-16
Flatulence, 48, 51-52, 136

Flavoring agents, 162
Fluoride, 121, 196, 201, 204, 248
Fluorine, 121
Folacin (folic acid), 13, 14, 15, 23-24, 90, 97, 98-99, 134, 186, 187, 209, 215, 217, 271, 288, 321
Food
    baby food, 196-98, 253-54
    caffeine in, 153-54
    canned, 17, 177
    carbohydrates in, 38, 46
    cholesterol in, 67
    fat in, 64-65, 68-70, 73
    fermented, 42, 52, 139, 320-21
    fiber in, 49-51
    fresh produce, 17-18, 172-73
    hypoallergenic, 256
    and nutrient loss, 17-18
    preferences, 201-3
    refined, 17, 33-34, 37-38, 92, 165, 319
    smoked, 171-72
    super foods, 314-23
    See also Animal foods; Fruits; Grains;
        Legumes; Milk/dairy; Nutrients;
        Vegetables
Food additives, 124, 127, 159-60
    acid-base balancers, 163
    anti-caking, 163
    coloring, 161-62
    emulsifiers/stabilizers, 161
    enzymes, 165
    firming and crisping, 163-64
    flavoring, 162
    flour and bread, 166
    humectants, 163
    nutritive, 165-66
    preservatives, 160
    safety of, 166-67
    sensitivities to, 257
    sequestrants, 162
    sweeteners, 164-65
Food allergies, 34, 192, 196, 204, 208, 250, 265-66
    allergic response in, 253
    causes of, 253-54
    nutritional treatment for, 256
    and sensitivities, 257
    symptoms of, 254-55
    testing for, 254-55
Food and Drug Administration (FDA), 281, 283, 290, 291, 292
Food industry, 23, 167
    health food, 288-90
    labeling by, 45, 291-93
Food preparation
    cookbooks for, 313

exchange system in, 297-303
substitutions in, 305
toxins produced in, 171-72
Food toxins
bacterial, 176-77
in food preparation, 171-72
from microorganisms, 171
natural, 168-71
precautions against, 178
residual, 172-76
Free radicals, 86, 87, 122, 239
Fructose, 38-39, 44, 45
Fruits
apples, 322
bananas, 321
carbohydrates in, 38
citrus, 91, 321
in exchange system, 299
fiber in, 50, 51
Fusarium mold, 171

Galactose, 38-39, 42
Gallstones, 53
Gamma amino butyric acid (GABA), 265
Gamma linolenic acid (GLA), 65, 130, 132,
194, 244, 270
Garlic, 235, 316-17
Genetics, and health, 5-6, 233
Ginger, 317
Ginseng, 137-39, 217, 276
Glucose, 38-39, 42, 119, 120, 128, 136, 186
See also Blood, glucose
Glucose tolerance factor (GTF), 119, 120,
136, 223, 241, 243-44
Glucose tolerance test, 41, 242
Goiter, 13, 117, 159, 165, 169
Grains
carbohydrates in, 38, 46
fiber in, 49-51
grasses of, 319-20
natural toxins in, 169
nutrients in, 319
refined, 33, 165, 319
See also Breads/cereals; Rice

Hair analysis, 28
Hardening of arteries, 234
Headache, caffeine and, 156
Health
crucial factors in, 5-9
status of labor force, 1-2
Health care
costs of, 1
and medical science, 2-3
preventative, 3
Hearing loss, 215

Heart disease
basic problems in, 233-34
and nutrition, 59, 63, 71, 72, 86, 90,
114, 124, 129, 130, 141, 316, 317
and potency, 268
prevention and control of, 234-35
risk factors for, 43, 52, 68, 71, 72, 114,
148, 156, 232-33, 258
Hemorrhoids, 47, 53
High blood pressure. See Hypertension
High-density lipoproteins (HDL), 68, 148,
234, 244, 317
Hospitals, 1, 18
Humectants, 163
Hydrochloric acid, 140, 215
Hyperactivity, 44, 53, 114, 132, 147, 154,
166, 204, 263
Hypertension, 109-10, 131, 132, 134, 148,
182, 183, 234, 236
Hypertrophy, 186, 224
Hypoglycemia, 40, 41, 44, 147, 263

Immune system, 201, 237, 253, 254, 272-73
Infants
food introduction to, 196-98, 253-54
low birth weight, 181, 182
mortality, 1, 211
See also Birth defects; Breast-feeding;
Fetal alcohol syndrome
Insulin, 15, 41, 44, 112, 136, 186, 241, 242,
245, 265
Iodine, 13, 117-18, 165, 169
Iron, 11, 14, 15, 58, 90, 114-16, 191, 196,
203

Ketosis, 72, 244, 275
Kidneys, 39, 61, 107, 110, 148, 214, 268, 289

Labeling, food, 291-93
Lactose, 39, 193
intolerance, 42, 52, 139, 215
Lead, 7, 15, 125, 175-76, 266
Lecithin, 68, 127-28, 161, 217, 265, 314
Legumes, 108
carbohydrates in, 38, 46
soybeans, 314-15
See also Beans
Leukotrienes, 251
Lind, James, 24, 89
Linoleic acid, 65, 129-30, 131-32, 194, 217,
244
Linseed oil, 132
Lipoic acid, 135
Lipoproteins, 68, 74, 234
Liver, 61, 128, 135, 146
Liver, in diet, 83, 84, 91, 97, 322

Magnesium, 14, 15, 105, 111-12, 235, 244, 264, 269, 270, 277
Malnutrition
    deviation from evolutionary design in, 16-17
    factors in, 11
    nutrient-drug interaction in, 13-15
    See also Nutrients, deficiency
Manganese, 17, 118-19, 239
Mastectomy, 270-71
Meat. See Animal foods
Mercury, 125, 239
Metabisulfite, 257
Milk/dairy
    acidophilus, 139
    cholesterol in, 67
    in exchange system, 301
    fat in, 68-70
    nonfat, 93
    vitamin D-fortified, 58, 159, 165
    See also Breast-feeding; Lactose; Yogurt
Minerals, 102-5, 289
    See also Nutrients; specific minerals
Molybdenum, 123
Monosodium glutamate (MSG), 84, 162, 256
Muscular system, 148, 274-76, 278
Myoinositol, 128

Nervous system, 146-47, 214
    See also Brain
Neural tube defects, 23-24, 98, 181, 187
Neurochemical transmitters, 56, 264-65
Niacin. See Vitamin B₃
Nickel, 124
Nitrates/nitrites, 15, 78, 160, 238
Norepinephrine, 56, 95, 265
Nucleosides, 135-36
Nutrients
    assessing body's status of, 27-31
    bioavailability of, 289
    deficiency, 11-13, 17-19, 43-44, 200, 201, 284
    -drug interactions, 13-15, 226
    in exchange system, 298
    industry regulation for, 288-90
    for offsetting pollution, 15-16
    recommended daily allowance (RDA), 12, 13, 18-19, 89, 283-85
    Senate dietary goals, 12, 38, 286-87, 304
    supplements, 11, 15, 24, 34, 189, 191, 195, 196, 204, 217, 243-44, 270, 288-90
    See also Minerals; Vitamin(s); specific nutrients
Nutrition

    biochemical individuality and, 25
    certification in, 26, 290
    controversy over, 20-21, 25-26
    and disease. See specific disease
    as factor in health, 7, 24-25
    through life cycle. See Adolescents; Aging; Children; Infants; Pregnancy
    rules of, 33-35
    and medical community, 25
    research methods in, 21-24

Oats, 319
Obesity/overweight, 8, 34, 43, 44, 52, 148
    assessing, 221-23
    in childhood and adolescence, 199, 203, 209
    health effects of, 223
    types of, 224
    undernourishment in, 10-11
    in women, 209, 224-25
    See also Eating; Weight control
Okara, 314
Oral contraceptives, 15, 83, 91, 94, 96, 99, 207, 273
Organogenesis, fetal, 183-84
Orotic acid, 135
Osmosis, 56
Osteoporosis, 12-13, 20, 61, 85, 148, 214-15, 244, 246-48
Overweight. See Obesity/overweight
Oxalates, 104, 169
Oxygen, and brain function, 263
Oxytocin, 193

Pangamic acid, 140-41
Pantothenic acid, 13, 17, 20, 100-101, 134, 206
Paraquot, 173
PCB (polychlorinated biphenyl), 78, 130, 175
Pectin, 49, 53
Pellagra, 24, 94
Peppers, 317-18
Pesticides, 15, 172-73
Phosphorus, 14, 15, 105-106, 248
Photosynthesis, 37, 82, 133
Physical examination, of nutrients status, 27
Phytates, 104, 169
Pica, 183
Placebo effect, 22
Plantains, 170
Platelet aggregation, 234
Poisons. See Food toxins
Pollution
    health effects of, 7, 233, 266
    industrial, 175-76

offsetting effects of, 15-16
radioactive, 174
water, 7, 77-78, 80, 149, 176, 177
Polycyclic hydrocarbons, 171-72, 174, 176
Polyunsaturated fat, 63, 88, 239, 314
Potassium, 14, 15, 27, 106-8
Potassium chloride, 15
Potency, male, 268-69
Pregnancy
adolescent, 188, 211
caffeine in, 156
nutrition and, 57, 96, 98, 120, 181-82, 185-87, 189, 266, 269
problems of, 182-83
risk factors for, 147, 154, 156, 187-89, 259, 287
See also Fetal development
Prematurity, 23, 84, 87, 211
Premenstrual syndrome (PMS), 206, 270
Preservatives, food, 160
Pritikin program, 236, 295
Prostaglandins, 65, 66, 130, 244
Prostate gland, 269
Protein, 11, 14
allergies, 265-66
amino acids of, 56, 57, 95
daily intake of, 61, 286
deficiency of, 56-57, 83
enhancement of, 59-60
excess of, 248, 278
in exchange system, 300
functions of, 55-56
quality of, 57-58
requirements for, 60-61, 207
in vegetarian diet, 58-59, 61
Provocative sublingual testing, 255
Psoralens, 171
Psychogenic disease, 8
Psychotropic drugs, 15
Pyridoxine. See Vitamin B6
Pyrimethamine, 15

Radiation exposure, 122, 174, 238, 320
Radioallergosorbent test (RAST), 255
Radon gas, 174, 238
Random chance, 23
Recipes, 305-313
Recommended daily allowance (RDA), 12, 13, 18-19, 89, 283-85
Reproducible results, 23-24
Reproductive system. See Sexual system
Respiratory system, 149
Riboflavin. See Vitamin B2
Rice, 319
Rickets, 58, 85, 86, 159, 165, 196
RNA, 55, 87, 92, 106, 114, 118, 124, 135

Rotation diet, 256
Rutin, 133, 251, 321

Saccharine, 164, 165
Salicylates, 15
Salmonella, 177
Salt, 109, 110, 162
Sassafras, 157, 169
Saxitoxin, 171
Scurvy, 24, 89, 90, 91, 321
Sedatives, 15
Selenium, 12, 15, 63, 102, 122-23, 125, 170, 239, 271
Senate dietary goals, 12, 38, 286-87, 304
Sequestrants, 162
Serotonin, 56, 57, 94, 95, 265
Set point theory, of weight loss, 229
Sexual system
and AIDS, 271-73
alcohol effects on, 147
development of, 207
energy/attitude/appearance and, 273
and fertility, 268-69
and potency, 267-68
and premenstrual syndrome, 270
and protein deficiency, 56
purposes of intercourse, 267
surgical procedures of, 270-71
Silicon, 124
Skeletal system, 148, 200-201, 214-15, 247
See also Osteoporosis
Skin
and acne, 207-8
aging of, 215
cancer, 238
Smoking. See Tobacco
Sodium, 78, 107, 109-11, 286
Sodium nitrite, 160
Soft drinks
caffeine in, 153-54
sugar in, 45
Soil, and nutrient depletion, 18
Solanine, 170
Soybeans, 68, 314-15
Soy sauce, 315, 320
Sperm production, 269
Sprouts, 318-19
Staphylococcus aureus, 176
Starch, modified, 165
Statistical significance, 23
Steroids, anabolic, 278
Stress
and allergic response, 254
and cancer, 237
and heart disease, 233
and nutrient needs, 210-11

Sucrose, 39, 44
Sugar, in diet, 20, 43-45, 164, 165
Sulfur, 108-9, 122
Sulfur dioxide, 160
Sun exposure, 85, 86, 217, 238
Superoxide dismutase (SOD), 141
Sweat/perspiration, 75, 105, 110, 111, 115, 120, 276
Sweeteners, 44, 45, 164, 65

Taste buds, 200, 215-16
Taurine, 108, 136-37, 193
Tea, 157
Tempeh, 320
Test tube studies, 22
Tetradotoxin, 170
Thaumatin, 164
Thiamin. *See* Vitamin B₁
Thiaminase, 171
Thirst, mechanism of, 75-76
Thrombus, 72
Thyroxin, 117, 185
Tin, 124
Tobacco, 15, 187, 235
 chewing, 260
 health risks of, 91, 258-59, 269
 quitting smoking, 260-61
 second hand smoking, 259
Tofu, 315
Toxemia, 96, 182, 211
Toxins in food. *See* Food toxins
Trichinosis, 177
Triglycerides, 63
Trypsin, 170
Tryptophan, 56, 57, 94, 95, 265, 316
Tyrosine, 56, 57, 265

Ulcers, 146
Uterus, surgical removal of, 271

Vaginal infections, 139
Vanadium, 33, 124
Vegetable fat, 64, 66
Vegetables
 carbohydrates in, 38, 46
 cruciferous, 320
 dark-green leafy, 321-22
 in exchange system, 299
 fiber in, 50, 51
 home-grown, 322-23
 peppers, 317-18
 sprouts, 318-19
Vegetarian diet, 58, 61, 97, 273
Vision. *See* Blindness; Eyes, eyesight
Vitamin(s), 81-82
 essential, 81, 126

fat-soluble, 82-89
in fortified foods, 165-66
industry regulation, 288-90
quasi-vitamins, 126-41
water-soluble, 89-101
See also Nutrients; *specific vitamins*
Vitamin A, 13, 14, 15, 18, 82-84, 147, 165, 208, 239, 284, 289, 319, 321
Vitamin B₁ (thiamin), 13, 14, 15, 92-93, 146, 240, 276
Vitamin B₂ (riboflavin), 11, 93-94
Vitamin B₃ (niacin), 15, 24, 94-95, 134, 217
Vitamin B₆ (pyridoxine), 14, 15, 17, 58-59, 95-96, 134, 206, 239, 244, 269, 270, 278, 285, 290, 315, 316
Vitamin B₁₂ (cyanocobalamin), 14, 15, 25, 58, 96-98, 124, 134, 217, 288
Vitamin B₁₅. *See* Pangamic acid
Vitamin C (ascorbic acid), 13, 14, 15, 17, 25, 89-91, 116, 159-60, 217, 239, 275, 277, 284, 289-90, 317, 318
Vitamin D (cholecalciferol), 13, 14, 15, 58, 85-86, 104, 165, 196, 217, 240
Vitamin E (tocopherol), 15, 17, 23, 63, 83, 86-88, 115, 122, 134, 159-60, 196, 239
Vitamin H. *See* Biotin.
Vitamin K (menadione), 88-89, 196
Vitro (test tube) studies, 22

Water
 chlorinated, 77-78
 deficiency, 75, 76-77, 276
 and electrolyte balance, 276-77
 and fiber, 48
 fluoridated, 121, 196
 functions in body, 74-75
 pollution, 7, 77-78, 80, 149, 176, 177
 purifying, 79, 80, 118
 and thirst mechanism, 75-76
 types of, 78-79
 and weight loss, 39
Weight. *See* Obesity/overweight
Weight control
 in adolescence, 209-10
 and eating disorders, 225-26
 gimmicks, 226-27
 high-fiber diet in, 52
 lifetime program for, 227-31
 Pritikin diet in, 236, 295
Wheat, 319

Yogurt, 42, 52, 139, 320

Zinc, 14, 15-16, 17, 28, 58, 61, 83, 112-13, 116, 147, 200, 201, 207, 208, 217, 239, 251, 266, 268, 269, 272, 275